REHABILITATION
ETHICS FOR INTERPROFESSIONAL PRACTICE

LAURA LEE SWISHER, PT, MDIV, PHD, FNAP, FAPTA

Professor and Director
School of Physical Therapy & Rehabilitation Sciences
Associate Dean, USF Health Morsani College of Medicine
University of South Florida
Tampa, Florida

CHARLOTTE BRASIC ROYEEN, PHD, OTR/L, FAOTA, FASAHP, FNAP

Dean, College of Health Sciences
A. Watson Armour III Presidential Professor
College of Health Sciences
Rush University
Chicago, Illinois

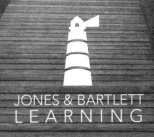

JONES & BARTLETT
LEARNING

World Headquarters
Jones & Bartlett Learning
5 Wall Street
Burlington, MA 01803
978-443-5000
info@jblearning.com
www.jblearning.com

Jones & Bartlett Learning books and products are available through most bookstores and online booksellers. To contact Jones & Bartlett Learning directly, call 800-832-0034, fax 978-443-8000, or visit our website, www.jblearning.com.

Production Credits

VP, Product Management: Amanda Martin
Director of Product Management: Cathy L. Esperti
Product Manager: Sean Fabery
Product Assistant: Andrew LaBelle
Senior Project Specialist: Vanessa Richards
Project Specialist, Navigate: Rachel DiMaggio
Digital Project Specialist: Rachel Reyes
Marketing Manager: Michael Sullivan
VP, Manufacturing and Inventory Control: Therese Connell
Composition: Exela Technologies
Project Management: Exela Technologies
Cover Design: Kristin E. Parker
Rights Specialist: John Rusk
Media Development Editor: Troy Liston
Cover Image (Title Page, Part Opener, Chapter Opener): © PPAMPicture/Getty Images
Printing and Binding: McNaughton & Gunn
Cover Printing: McNaughton & Gunn

Library of Congress Cataloging-in-Publication Data

Names: Swisher, Laura Lee, author. | Royeen, Charlotte Brasic, author.
Title: Rehabilitation ethics for interprofessional practice / Laura Lee Swisher and Charlotte Brasic Royeen.
Description: Burlington, MA : Jones & Bartlett Learning, 2020. | Includes bibliographical references and index.
Identifiers: LCCN 2018046756 | ISBN 9781449673376 (paperback)
Subjects: | MESH: Rehabilitation–ethics | Ethics, Professional
Classification: LCC RM735.4 | NLM WB 320 | DDC 174.2/958515–dc23
LC record available at https://lccn.loc.gov/2018046756

6048

Printed in the United States of America
23 22 21 20 19   10 9 8 7 6 5 4 3 2 1

Brief Contents

Contents

Chapter 10   Neuroethics: A Guide for the Perplexed Rehabilitation Professional 213

Chapter 11   The Future of Interprofessional Rehabilitation Ethics 235

Foreword

Rehabilitation professionals have long worked on interprofessional teams, so a renewed focused on interprofessional education and collaborative practice is familiar territory for us. The clarion call for interprofessional education and collaborative practice continues to be grounded in the health professionals' obligation to meet the needs of society and population health. Based upon this call, we are challenged to change or transform how we practice, and even how we educate.

To this end, in 2003, a small like-minded group of ethics educators came together through a federally funded working conference on leadership in ethics education for physical therapy and occupational therapy (Educating for Moral Action, 2005). This working conference, Dreamcatchers and the Common Good: Allied Health Leadership in Generational Health and Ethics, or "the Dreamcatchers," was orchestrated by a leader and mentor to many of us, Dr. Ruth Purtilo. We all continue to be inspired by the work of Dr. Purtilo, and to carry the torch for ethics education encapsulated by the moniker "the Dreamcatchers." Thus, the work of the Dreamcatchers has continued over the last 15 years with periodic working conferences at universities, publications, as well as national and international presentations (Jensen, Royeen & Purtilo, 2010).

In 2009, the Interprofessional Education Health Core Competencies (IPEC) were developed across four domains (values and ethics for collaborative practice, roles and responsibilities, interprofessional communication, and teams and teamwork). As we argued in the work of the Dreamcatchers, and the text that was an outcome of the conference, Educating for Moral Action: A Sourcebook for Rehabilitation (2005), there is no substitute for a moral foundation for all health professionals. Health professionals cannot be truly successful with sufficient technical education alone. Rather, a true grounding in moral foundations is now essential. If one can fully understand what it means to engage in moral foundations such as mutual respect, then the work of the team is more likely to be successful. Like understanding the deeper meaning of respect, the challenge of translating how that moral foundation is put into the action is the centerpiece of this text edited by Swisher and Royeen. Only with moral foundations as explored, communicated about, deliberated upon, and discussed in this text regarding the moral commons, can an authentic platform for success regarding patient engagement and services be made possible.

To date, there is no common language or theory for interprofessional ethics education and practice. This text by Swisher and Royeen provides us with a powerful structure, **the moral commons**, that provides a common ground for the important foundational work of moral dialogue that is essential in the work of interprofessional teams. The proposed tool to achieve such deliberation is the moral commons *within* the moral commons, the **Dialogic Engagement Model (DEM),** centered on the need for consideration and dialogue between individual and team. Only through such "talking" and conversation can humans really achieve understanding of the other and the team. Related to this, individual ethical judgments are necessary; however, they are not sufficient for the judgments that are part of team-based care. The DEM is simple yet powerful in its application. Human understanding through the process of language is as old as man himself huddled around a fire collaborating to socialize and survive. The DEM is the modern equivalent of a virtual bonfire, allowing humans the needed space to create learning and understanding. Preparation for such includes ethical analysis and consideration of the moral commons which then leads one to the individual and team dialogic process and finally the summative reflection.

This text, *Rehabilitation Ethics for Interprofessional Practice*, led by editors Dr. Laura Swisher and Dr. Charlotte Royeen, both of whom were original Dreamcatchers, builds on past work and most importantly, gives all of the health professions (not just those involved in rehabilitation) a substantive text that is grounded in both theory and practice and aligned with the present and future of clinical practice. The current book can be applied to many fields including the wide variety of allied health sciences, speech language pathology, audiology, physician assistant education, and anyone interested in moving beyond the traditional paradigm of the medical model of education and/or practice.

While many traditional ethics texts address well-known ethical principles and theories, the current text takes ethical principles and theories and translates them into easily understood units (Rule-Based, Ends-Based, Virtue-Based, and Narrative-Based). One can then make the application of ethical traditions in the dialogic engagement process with the DEM tool. A common structure is used in all chapters (topical outline, objectives, key terms, and integration of cases and reflection materials) and delivers a consistent message of practical application to education and clinical practice. For, ultimately, practical application is what each of us is trying to do, to change our little bit of the world.

Rehabilitation Ethics for Interprofessional Practice is a text that is timely, provocative, yet extremely practical and will help all of us enhance the quality of learning for our students and the quality of care for our patients and communities.

Gail M. Jensen, PT, PhD, FAPTA
Professor
Dean, Graduate School and
College of Professional Studies
School of Pharmacy and
Health Professions
Creighton University
Omaha, Nebraska

Charlotte Brasic Royeen, PhD, OTR/L,
FAOTA, FASAHP, FNAP
Dean, College of Health Sciences
A. Watson Armour III Presidential Professor
College of Health Sciences
Rush University
Chicago, Illinois

References

1.   Purtilo, R., Jensen, G., & Royeen, C. (Eds). (2005). *Educating for moral action: A sourcebook in health and rehabilitation ethics.* FA Davis Company.
2.   Jensen, G.M., Royeen, C.B.,& Purtilo, R.B. (2010). Interprofessional Ethics in Rehabilitation : The Dreamcatcher Journey. *Journal of Allied Health, 39*(3): 246–250.

Preface

This text reflects not just the six years it took to conceptualize, refine, and grow it, but also a journey across our lifetimes to mature into reflective practitioners of the scholarship of integration and application. While the current world of "science" continues to work on the scholarship of discovery, we have taken a path of equal import, responding to the human needs we have witnessed in practice across individual, group, and organizational systems. We believe that regardless of "evidence" from science, which is greatly needed, the guidance of how to apply "facts" from science always requires commitment to work across professions, cultures, and—often—geography. Included in this book are our companions who have walked this path with us. We thank them for embarking on this journey together.

We have aspired to exude an elusive commodity, i.e., *wisdom*, in this book since commitment as previously described requires wisdom in order to apply and integrate facts into practice. It has been said that wisdom, in part, is tolerance for ambiguity. Thus, you are wandering into a world of application where shades of gray color the application of facts. What from one perspective looks appropriate may look entirely different when viewed from another vantage point, and what appears as black and white can turn into shades of gray. Even a simple shadow can change the image you see in the light of the sun.

This book also reflects our commitment to helping readers learn. Thus, the publisher has worked with us to include a glossary, key terms, learning points, closing reflections, and take away messages. All of these reflect the experience and knowledge we have garnered from serving in the academy and teaching for many years. We have, therefore, tried to make readable that which by its very nature is very hard to read.

Finally, this book also reflects our commitment to doctoral-level educational learning in physical therapy and occupational therapy. Whenever we would discuss what our vision was for this text, it always ended up as this: "We want a text that reflects learning at the level of clinical doctoral education." The book, therefore, is accessible and readable, while being very dense and heavy with theoretical reference. We suggest that you first read the key terms for each chapter and glance through the Learning Points before reading the chapter. That will orient you to the nature and scope of the chapter and application opportunities. Additionally, at the end of each chapter, there are reflection materials designed to enhance integration and application of the knowledge presented.

We wish you well on your journey through the content of the text!

Laura Lee (Dolly) Swisher
Charlotte Brasic Royeen

Features of This Text

In order to enhance the reader's experience, each chapter of *Rehabilitation Ethics for Interprofessional Practice* includes an array of pedagogical features, including the following:

The **Chapter Outline** previews what topics are to be covered in that chapter.

CHAPTER OUTLINE

- Chapter Overview
- Why Interprofessional Rehabilitation Ethics?
- Clarification of Terms
- Professional and Interprofessional Ethics
- Rehabilitation (and Habilitation) Ethics as the Focus of this Book
- Major Theme of the Text
- Summary and Conclusion

CHAPTER OBJECTIVES

At the conclusion of this chapter, the reader will be able to:

1. Define basic ethical terms used to discuss ethical issues in health care.
2. Determine the limitations and barriers to using traditional medical ethical models in rehabilitation settings.
3. Delineate the qualities of individuals and teams necessary for interprofessional ethics.
4. Evaluate the idea of individual and team moral agency as central to interprofessional ethics.
5. Discuss the term "moral commons" and its implications for resolving ethical situations in interprofessional practice.
6. Analyze how moral agency relates to team conflict.

Chapter Objectives focus the reader on key concepts and the material they will learn.

KEY TERMS

Reading these key terms before reading the chapter will introduce you to key concepts which will then be somewhat familiar to you as you read this chapter. This is an important learning technique that will enhance your learning as a multi-step process. You may even wish to make a flash card set of key terms and quiz yourself on them once or twice before reading the chapter. This will better prepare you to immerse in the language of ethics and better prepare you to integrate the content.

Community of Practice: In health care, this refers to a group of people who work alongside each other and share common professional interests and goals. In pediatric rehabilitation practice, there are a range of practitioners bringing different practice paradigms, but sharing a common interest in order to provide a benefit to a child both within and separate to the family unit.

Interprofessional Collaborative Practice: Refers to health professionals from different disciplinary backgrounds working together with patients, families, carers [sic], and communities to deliver the highest quality of care" (WHO, 2010).

Moral Authority: Refers to the scope of authority a person has to make moral decisions on behalf of and in the interests of themselves or another. In the pediatric context, parents have moral authority to make decisions on behalf of their child. However, this authority does not extend to causing harm to their child.

Moral Commons: A safe zone for ethical deliberation characterized by mutual respect for personal and professional identity, common language, inclusion of relevant stakeholders, and the dialogic process. The three key elements of the moral commons are identity (personal and professional)), ethical tradition, and context.

Moral Deliberation: This refers to the process of conversation, reflection, and dialogue focused on weighing ethically relevant considerations. In the pediatric rehabilitation context, it includes consideration of the interests of the child, the child's family, and the interprofessional team.

Reading the **Key Terms**, along with their definitions, before engaging with the chapter material will help ensure they are somewhat familiar to the reader as they dive into the content. These have also been collected in an end-of-text Glossary.

Learning Point 10.1   Why might interfield theory be especially relevant to interprofessional education and practice?

Learning Points scattered throughout each chapter encourage the reader to consider how key concepts can be applied.

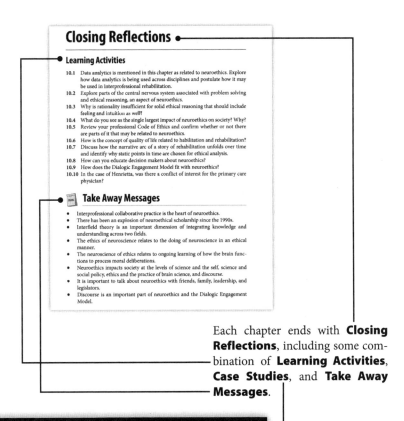

Closing Reflections

Learning Activities

10.1 Data analytics is mentioned in this chapter as related to neuroethics. Explore how data analytics is being used across disciplines and postulate how it may be used in interprofessional rehabilitation.

10.2 Explore parts of the central nervous system associated with problem solving and ethical reasoning, an aspect of neuroethics.

10.3 Why is rationality insufficient for solid ethical reasoning that should include feeling and intuition as well?

10.4 What do you see as the single largest impact of neuroethics on society? Why?

10.5 Review your professional Code of Ethics and confirm whether or not there are parts of it that may be related to neuroethics.

10.6 How is the concept of quality of life related to habilitation and rehabilitation?

10.7 Discuss how the narrative arc of a story of rehabilitation unfolds over time and identify why static points in time are chosen for ethical analysis.

10.8 How can you educate decision makers about neuroethics?

10.9 How does the Dialogic Engagement Model fit with neuroethics?

10.10 In the case of Henrietta, was there a conflict of interest for the primary care physician?

Take Away Messages

- Interprofessional collaborative practice is the heart of neuroethics.
- There has been an explosion of neuroethical scholarship since the 1990s.
- Interfield theory is an important dimension of integrating knowledge and understanding across two fields.
- The ethics of neuroscience relates to the doing of neuroscience in an ethical manner.
- The neuroscience of ethics relates to ongoing learning of how the brain functions to process moral deliberations.
- Neuroethics impacts society at the levels of science and the self, science and social policy, ethics and the practice of brain science, and discourse.
- It is important to talk about neuroethics with friends, family, leadership, and legislators.
- Discourse is an important part of neuroethics and the Dialogic Engagement Model.

Each chapter ends with **Closing Reflections**, including some combination of **Learning Activities**, **Case Studies**, and **Take Away Messages**.

🔍 CASE STUDY

Case of Joan

Joan had been an avid hiker and bicycler, and passionate swimmer for most of her life. At the age of 40, she was involved in a major bike accident that changed her whole life. The accident resulted in a severe polytrauma including various fractures (ribs, breastbone, skull, bone spurs), internal bleeding, traumatic injury to the skull and brain, and complete paraplegia. After three months of rehabilitation, Joan begins to experience the neuropathic pain of constant burning and shooting. Over the subsequent months, Joan was treated for pain with medication and acupuncture. However, the pain management interventions offered little to no improvement, and the pain significantly lowered her quality of life. Pain prevented her from participating socially and negatively impacted her ability to complete her daily routine. She also experienced difficulties with sleeping and eating.

Joan was admitted to the hospital for pain management. An interprofessional team that consisted of a physician, nurse, social worker, occupational therapist, physical therapist, pharmacist, and psychologist collaborated to implement pain management. On the VAS scale, Jane rated the intensity of her pain as 8. The team classified the pain as neuropathic. Joan experienced poor sleep quality, i.e., she would sometimes wake up, due to pain. She presented with low motivation, emotional instability, and was afraid that the pain would get worse. This led to a diagnosis of minor clinical depression. Joan reported significant limitations in carrying out her daily routine. Her mobility-related issues included problems in transferring to and from the wheelchair and driving due to constant pain and the pain medications. This was supported by the team's assessment. These mobility problems severely limited her ability to meet friends and hindered her from working. As a result, Joan felt isolated.

Since previous efforts to manage Joan's chronic pain focused on pharmacological interventions and proved unsuccessful, a more comprehensive approach is needed. Under the fee-for-service system, Medicare would pay each provider along with the hospital for her care.

▶ Navigate 2 Companion Website

Each new print copy of this text is accompanied by an access code for the Navigate 2 Companion Website, including the following learning and study tools:

- Chapter Quizzes
- Glossary
- Flashcards
- Crossword Puzzles

Instructor Resources

Instructors can also request access to the following resources available for use in conjunction with the text:

- Test Bank
- Slides in PowerPoint format
- Instructor's Manual

Acknowledgments

We thank our respective spouses Marsha and Matin. We also wish to acknowledge those who have engaged in conversations who learn with us, and those whose work continues to inspire us.

We thank the staff of Jones & Bartlett Learning, who has worked with us through a complex process to complete this text.

Dr. Royeen wishes to acknowledge support from the A. Watson Armour III Presidential Professor endowment from Rush University Medical Center.

We acknowledge those of you who will be reading this work with a view to application in practice. You are the future!

Contributors

Jeffrey Lee Crabtree, MS, OTD, FAOTA
Associate Professor
Department of Occupational Therapy
School of Health & Rehabilitation
 Sciences
Indiana University—Purdue University
 Indianapolis
Indianapolis, Indiana

Clare M. Delany, PhD
Professor
Department of Medical Education
The University of Melbourne
Melbourne, Australia

Bruce H. Greenfield, PT, MA, PhD, FNAP
Professor
Division of Physical Therapy
Department of Rehabilitation Science
School of Medicine
Senior Fellow
Center for Ethics
Emory University
Atlanta, Georgia

Gail M. Jensen, PT, PhD, FAPTA
Professor
Dean, Graduate School and College of
 Professional Studies
School of Pharmacy and Health
 Professions
Creighton University
Omaha, Nebraska

Shirley A. Wells, DrPH, OTR, FAOTA
Associate Professor
Department of Occupational Therapy
College of Health Professions
University of Texas Rio Grande Valley
Brownsville, Texas

Mary Ann Wharton, PT, MS
Physical Therapy Consultant
Adjunct Faculty
PTA Program
CCAC Boyce Campus
Monroeville, Pennsylvania
Adjunct Faculty
UPMC Geriatric PT Residency
Pittsburgh, Pennsylvania

Reviewers

Leesa DiBartola, PT, EdD, DPT, MCHES
Assistant Department Chair and
    Assistant Director of Clinical
    Education
Department of Physical Therapy
Rangos School of Health Sciences
Duquesne University
Pittsburgh, Pennsylvania

Diane Ferrero-Paluzzi, PhD
Associate Professor
Department of Speech
    Communication Studies
School of Arts and Science
Iona College
New Rochelle, New York

Diane Habash, PhD, MS, RDN, LD
Associate Clinical Professor
Division of Health Sciences and
    Medical Dietetics
Associate Director of Education,
    Center for Integrative Medicine
College of Medicine
Ohio State University
Columbus, Ohio

Yvette Hachtel, JD, MEd, OTR/L, FAOTA
Professor
School of Occupational Therapy
Gordon E. Inman College of Health
    Sciences and Nursing
Belmont University
Nashville, Tennessee

Chip Hahn, MS, AuD, CCC-A/SLP
Clinical Professor
Department of Speech Pathology and
    Audiology
College of Arts and Science
Miami University
Miami, Florida

Mary J. Hickey, PT, DPT, MHP, OCS
Associate Professor
Department of Physical Therapy,
    Movement and Rehabilitation
    Science
Bouvé College of Health Sciences
Northeastern University
Boston, Massachusetts

Carol Kruger-Brophy, PT, JD
Adjunct Professor
School of Physical Therapy
Gordon E. Inman College of Health
    Sciences and Nursing
Belmont University
Nashville, Tennessee

Tonya Miller, DPT, PhD
Assistant Professor
Graduate School of Physical Therapy
Health Professions Program
Lebanon Valley College
Annville, Pennsylvania

Senora D. Simpson, PT, PhD, MPH
Assistant Professor
Department of Physical Therapy
College of Nursing and Allied Health
    Sciences
Howard University
Washington, DC

Annette R. Tommerdahl, PhD
Adjunct Professor
Health Studies Program
College of Health Sciences
University of Louisiana Monroe
Monroe, Louisiana

Sheila Thomas Watts, PT, DPT, MBA, MS, GCS
Program Director, Clinical Physical
  Therapist
Physical Therapy Program
College of Health Professions
Sacred Heart University
Fairfield, Connecticut

Mary Ann Wharton, PT, MS
Physical Therapy Consultant
Adjunct Faculty
PTA Program
CCAC Boyce Campus
Monroeville, Pennsylvania
Adjunct Faculty
UPMC Geriatric PT Residency
Pittsburgh, Pennsylvania

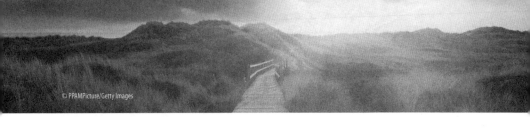

CHAPTER 1

Prologue, History, and Introduction: Why a Book about Interprofessional Rehabilitation Ethics?

Laura Lee Swisher and **Charlotte Brasic Royeen**

CHAPTER OUTLINE

- Chapter Overview
- Why Interprofessional Rehabilitation Ethics?
- Clarification of Terms
- Professional and Interprofessional Ethics
- Rehabilitation (and Habilitation) Ethics as the Focus of This Book
- Major Theme of the Text
- Summary and Conclusion

CHAPTER OBJECTIVES

At the conclusion of this chapter, the reader will be able to:

1. Define basic ethical terms used to discuss ethical issues in health care.
2. Determine the limitations and barriers to using traditional medical ethical models in rehabilitation settings.
3. Delineate the qualities of individuals and teams necessary for interprofessional ethics.
4. Evaluate the idea of individual and team moral agency as central to interprofessional ethics.
5. Discuss the term "moral commons" and its implications for resolving ethical situations in interprofessional practice.
6. Analyze how moral agency relates to team conflict.

KEY TERMS

Reading these key terms before reading the chapter will introduce you to key concepts which will then be somewhat familiar to you as you read this chapter. This is an important learning technique that will enhance your learning as a multi-step process. You may even wish to make a flash card set of key terms and quiz yourself on them once or twice before reading the chapter. This will better prepare you to immerse in the language of ethics and better prepare you to integrate the content.

Autonomy: The ethical principle obligating healthcare professionals to respect a patient's right to self-determination in health care.

Beneficence: The ethical principle obligating healthcare professionals to promote the good for the patient.

Ethics: Rational and systematic reflection on matters of morality, right, wrong, and the good. Some refer to ethics as second order ethics because it requires reflection on the first order beliefs about right and wrong involved in morality. The academic or philosophical field of study that examines the definition of, and analysis of, morality, right and wrong.

First Order Ethics: Ethical decisions based on the ethical values and principles learned through the primary cultural and social experiences of one's origin. (See morality)

Habilitation: The process of seeking maximal functional attainment.

Interprofessional Collaborative Practice: "Collaborative practice occurs when multiple health workers from different professional backgrounds provide comprehensive services by working with patients, their families, carers, and communities to deliver the highest quality of care across settings" (WHO, 2010, p. 13).

Interprofessional Education: "When students from two or more professions learn about, from and with each other to enable effective collaboration and improve health outcomes" (WHO, 2010, p. 13).

Interprofessional Ethics: Rational and systematic reflection on matters of morality, right, wrong, and the good encountered by healthcare professionals deliberatively working together in order to meet the goals of interprofessional collaborative practice. Interprofessional ethics should be patient/family centered, relationship focused, relevant across professions, and framed in language that is common to, and meaningful, across professions (Interprofessional Education Collaboratve Expert Panel, 2011). Interprofessional ethics may refer to the process of ethical collaboration or to the emerging field of study that focuses on ethical issues in interprofessional collaborative practice.

Interprofessional Rehabilitation Ethics: Rational and systematic reflection on matters of morality, right, wrong, and the good encountered by the rehabilitation team with emphasis on interprofessional collaboration and the work of the interprofessional team.

Justice: The ethical principle obligating healthcare professionals to fairness in fulfilling their professional roles.

Moral Agency: The capacity to act in an ethical manner. Individuals, teams, and organizations can exercise moral agency.

Moral Commons: A safe zone for ethical deliberation characterized by mutual respect for personal and professional identity, common language, inclusion of relevant stakeholders, and the dialogic process. Three key elements of the moral commons are identity (individual, personal, and interprofessional), ethical traditions, and context.

Morality: Personal and social beliefs, customs, values, and behavioral conventions regarding right, wrong, and the good that are learned through enculturation and social institutions that are often taken for granted and not subjected to reflection or analysis. Some refer to morality as first order ethics because the beliefs about right and wrong are taken for granted and not subjected to critical analysis.

Nonmaleficence: The ethical principle obligating healthcare professionals to prevent harm to the patient.

Principle: Ethical principles are general normative standards or guidelines for ethical behavior. Beauchamp and Childress (2009) identified four major categories of ethical principles: respect for autonomy, beneficence, nonmaleficence, and justice. Principles are less comprehensive than ethical theories and more specific than rules. Principles may conflict, requiring ethical analysis to resolve which principle may be more important in a particular situation.

Professional Ethics: Analysis of the ethical duties, obligations, virtues, and values for a specific profession.

Rehabilitation: The process of restoring function or seeking maximal functional ability (see habilitation) traditionally promoted by occupational therapy, physical therapy, and speech and language pathologists. The contemporary rehabilitation team embraces members of any profession or discipline pursuing the goals of attaining functional ability.

Rehabilitation Ethics: Rational and systematic reflection on matters of morality, right, wrong, and the good encountered by the rehabilitation team or in the process of restoring function.

Value: Values represent those commitments, qualities, and behaviors that are viewed as morally good and take priority over other commitments, qualities, or behaviors. Many professions have identified core values of professionalism.

Virtue: A trait, characteristic, or quality that is desirable or good. Virtue ethics emphasizes the cultivation of virtues (for example, honesty, compassion, fairness).

▶ Chapter Overview

This chapter focuses on defining basic terms, establishing a foundation for the text within interprofessional rehabilitation practice, and providing a rationale for a text dedicated to interprofessional rehabilitation ethics. Definitions and considerations for ethics and morality and for interprofessional ethics are put forth. Rehabilitation as a central focus of this text is discussed along with definitions of basic concepts such as rehabilitation. The multiple perspectives on rehabilitation are presented. All of this leads to a discussion of traditional medical ethics and bioethics and their lack in really addressing the need of interprofessional rehabilitation ethics. Finally, the themes of this book such as moral agency and the moral commons as precursors to development of a Dialogic Engagement Model presented later in this text are discussed.

▶ Why Interprofessional Rehabilitation Ethics?

With so many texts about ethics in health care, one might wonder whether there is a need for a book about interprofessional rehabilitation ethics. There is increasing momentum within health care for interprofessional collaborative practice (IPCP) and interprofessional education (IPE) (Goldberg, 2015, p. 32; Reeves, Perrier, Goldman, Freeth, & Zwarenstein, 2013; Schmitt, Gilbert, Brandt, & Weinstein, 2013; Sheldon et al., 2012). The push for interprofessional collaboration is based on the increasing recognition that collaborative teams may increase the quality, efficiency, and value of health care. There is a widespread consensus that interprofessional care depends on shared foundational ethical values and principles (Interprofessional Education Collaborative Expert Panel, 2011). In spite of the widespread agreement on the need for interprofessional collaboration, there has been little attention given to how interprofessional teams should address ethical issues (Clark, Cott, & Drinka, 2007; Engel & Prentice, 2013). Additionally, many existing ethics texts or resources do not address the role and perspective of rehabilitation professionals. The purpose of this text is to provide an interprofessional perspective on ethics relevant to all members of the healthcare team, with a particular focus on ethical issues encountered in rehabilitation.

Learning Point 1.1   How should interprofessional teams address ethical issues?

▶ Clarification of Terms

The question of what we mean by "interprofessional rehabilitation ethics" rests in part on the question as to what the term "ethics" means. Debate about the meaning of the term "ethics" extends to the ancient origins of philosophy. Definitions of the terms "ethics" and "morality" range from relatively straight-forward to very technical and philosophically complex. In this book ethics refers to systematic and rational analysis (Purtilo & Doherty, 2011, p. 16) of matters of morality, right, and wrong. As this definition suggests, ethics and morality are related terms. In everyday conversation we frequently use the terms ethics and morality interchangeably. In more academic discussion, ethics and morality may be contrasted by noting that ethics involves conscious rational reflection on morality (Hinman, 2013; Horner, 2003; Purtilo & Doherty, 2011), whereas morality refers more to the personal and social conventions about right and wrong that we learn through social enculturation. Moral conventions of this type may not be easily subjected to rational analysis. Bernheim and Childress (2015) capture the distinctions in our inconsistent and at times contradictory use of the terms:

> Drawing a rough but useful distinction, we can say that morality refers more to a social institution or practice—what people believe, value, and do—while ethics refers more to the reflective task of interpreting, understanding, and criticizing morality. By contrast, the terms ethical and moral are often used interchangeably. (p. 4)

Learning Point 1.2   Distinguish the concept of ethics from the concept of morality.

As this quote suggests, the collective beliefs, customs, duties, obligations, conventions of etiquette, and values that constitute morality are often "taken for granted." While all of these are imparted to us through communities (family, culture, religion, or other social institutions) as matters of "right or wrong behavior," we may not actually rationally examine tenets of morality without the stimulus of apparently conflicting moral values or obligations. Indeed, the taken for granted nature of morality may present serious barriers to ethical reflection and significant personal or social values as discomfort may be needed for individuals to place taken for granted moral values under the scrutiny of ethical analysis and reflection. One example of this kind of ethical analysis resulting in changed moral convictions is the Civil Rights movement whereby people in the United States recognized that the morality of segregation was not consistent with ethical standards of human rights and justice (Purtilo & Doherty, 2011, p. 16).

Learning Point 1.3   Can you think of a "taken for granted" ethical value or principle that you came to disavow based on later reflection and analysis?

Learning Point 1.4   What might be another example of society's ethical analysis changing moral convictions?

Hinman refers to this distinction between ethics and morality as first order and second order beliefs about right, wrong, good and evil to guide behavior, indicating that ethics requires conscious reflection on morality (Hinman, 2013, pp. 440, 442). First order ethics (or morality) refers to learned values and beliefs into which one is enculturated. Second order ethics represents "on-second thought" ideas about right and wrong that have been subjected to rational evaluation. This distinction captures the idea that we may accept moral norms and conventions without the rational examination expected in true ethical analysis. Consequently, this distinction implies that appealing to one's upbringing and values of origin falls short of true ethical analysis because simply living out personal or family values does not include rigorous rational evaluation associated with ethics. The distinction between morality and ethics is important because history demonstrates that moral beliefs may be flawed or ultimately found to ethically flawed. The term ethics also refers to the field of study focusing on ethical matters as a discipline within the field of philosophy.

Learning Point 1.5   Explain first order and second order ethics.

▶ Professional and Interprofessional Ethics

Professional ethics involves analyzing the ethical duties, obligations, virtues, and values for a specific profession. Each profession articulates the expectations for members of the profession through its Code of Ethics. Professional codes of ethics contain some general obligations for all healthcare professionals (respect for autonomy, beneficence, non-maleficence, justice, fidelity, informed consent, confidentiality), and some ethical obligations that are specific to the practice of the profession. For example, the medical code of ethics includes ethical obligations regarding termination of life support but rehabilitation professionals play a more collaborative than decision-making role with patients and families and the ethical issues they encounter at end of life may be quite different than those of the physician (Swisher & Hiller, 2010). Although many professional codes of ethics contain obligations to practice in a collegial manner, the obligations to team members, or process for collaborating as an interprofessional team, are not comprehensively addressed in most codes of ethics.

Despite the current emphasis on interprofessional education and clinical practice (see key terms), there has been limited attention to the ethical realm of interprofessional education and practice. The interprofessional education competencies (IPEC, 2011) were developed by an expert panel from six professions (dentistry, medicine, nursing, osteopathic medicine, pharmacy, and public health). The IPEC competencies report indicates that the primary goal of interprofessional education is to "prepare all health professions students for deliberatively working together with the common goal of building a safer and better patient-centered and community/population oriented U.S. healthcare system" (IPEC Panel, 2011, p. 3). These core competencies provide foundational expectations for interprofessional knowledge and practice of all healthcare professionals, and are excellent resources for educational programs, accrediting agencies, practitioners, and students. The IPEC authors identified ten principles for interprofessional practice, which are especially relevant to ethics:

1. Patient/family centered (hereafter termed "patient centered")
2. Community/population oriented
3. Relationship focused
4. Process oriented
5. Linked to learning activities, educational strategies, and behavioral assessments that are developmentally appropriate for the learner
6. Able to be integrated across the learning continuum
7. Sensitive to the systems context/applicable across practice settings
8. Applicable across professions
9. Stated in language common and meaningful across the professions
10. Outcome driven (p. 3)

Learning Point 1.6   What do you think should be in the realm of ethics and interprofessional education and interprofessional practice and why?

The IPEC Panel (2011) believed that ethics and values are at the heart of interprofessional collaboration and they assigned a prominent role to ethics by making Values/Ethics for Interprofessional Practice one of the four domains of competency for interprofessional practice. The four domains are presented in the subsequent quote from the IPEC Panel report:

> Interprofessional values and related ethics are an important, new part of crafting a professional identity, one that is both professional and interprofessional in nature. These values and ethics are patient centered with a community/population orientation, grounded in a sense of shared purpose to support the common good in health care, and reflect a shared commitment to creating safer, more efficient, and more effective systems of care. (p. 17)

Learning Point 1.7 What are the four domains of competency for interprofessional practice? Do you agree that ethics/values is a separate domain, or should it be seen as part of each of the other domains?

The Centre for the Advancement of Interprofessional Education (CAIPE) delineated principles of interprofessional education that link values, attitudes behaviors, and outcomes. For example, the CAIPE principles indicate that promoting professional parity requires the participants to abide by common "ground rules." Similarly, "sustaining" professional identity requires that individuals put aside power and status. **TABLE 1.1** links values and behavioral processes identified by CAIPE.

Learning Point 1.8 What are examples of power and status that you may see exhibited in teams?

The IPEC and CAIPE interprofessional principles point to the importance and limitations of values. Committing to values is important, but unembodied values without action or enabling processes may be meaningless. Interprofessional ethics requires "values in action" by individual professionals and interprofessional teams.

TABLE 1.1 Principles of Interprofessional Education: Values

Values in Interprofessional Education	Achieved
• Focuses on the needs of individuals, families and communities to improve their quality of care, health outcomes and well-being	• By keeping best practice central throughout all teaching and learning
• Applies equal opportunities within and between the professions and all with whom they learn and work	• By acknowledging but setting aside differences in power and status between professions
• Respects individuality, difference and diversity within and between the professions and all with whom they learn and work	• By utilizing distinctive contributions to learning and practice
• Sustains the identity and expertise of each profession	• By presenting each profession positively and distinctively
• Promotes parity between professions in the learning environment	• By agreeing 'ground rules'
• Instils interprofessional values and perspectives throughout uniprofessional and multiprofessional learning	• By permeating means and ends for the professional learning in which it is embedded

Reproduced from Barr, Helme, & D'Avary (2011).

Learning Point 1.9   Can you think of an example of a behavior that is not consistent with values in action by professionals?

According to Banks (2010), the term interprofessional ethics refers to the ethical principles, norms, guidelines, and a code of ethics that guides collaborative interprofessional practice.

> [Interprofessional ethics] includes the ethical issues, conflicts and dilemmas relating to rights, responsibilities, roles, and relationships that arise as a result of different professionals working together (e.g. dilemmas about information sharing, use of power, value conflicts, and interchangeability of roles). It also includes the study and development of ethical theories, frameworks and guidelines designed to take account of these issues and dilemmas. In this sense the term "interprofessional ethics" is singular—it is an area of study. (p. 282)

A true interprofessional ethic would therefore address issues of right and wrong encountered in "deliberatively working together" with the goal of patient-centered, relationship-focused, systems-sensitive health care directed toward quality care. Moreover, a true interprofessional ethic would respect the need for individual and team processes and behaviors necessary to translate values into action.

Learning Point 1.10   What does ethics in interprofessional education and practice mean to you?

▶ Rehabilitation (and Habilitation) Ethics as the Focus of This Book

Rehabilitation has historically been defined and practiced as an interprofessional endeavor (Stucki, Reinhardt, Grimby, & Melvin, 2007). A basic dictionary definition states that rehabilitation is "the restoration of a person to former privileges, status, or possessions by official decree, declaration, etc." or "Restoration of a person to health or normal activity after injury, illness, disablement, or addiction by means of medical or surgical treatment, physical and occupational therapy, psychological counselling, etc." (Oxford English Dictionary, 2014). Some sources (World Health Organization, 2011) include habilitation as a part of rehabilitation. We ascribe to that viewpoint (Siegert, Taylor, & Dean, 2012). Siegert, Taylor, and Dean (2012) indicate that the term rehabilitation has become a "buzzword" during the 21st century and that the meaning may vary considerably based on the writer, speaker, or context. Wade provides a preliminary definition of rehabilitation focusing on process.

Learning Point 1.11   Contrast rehabilitation to habilitation.

> Rehabilitation is an educational, problem-solving process that focuses on activity limitations and aims to optimize patient social participation and well-being, and so reduce stress on career/family. (Wade 2005, p. 814)

Definitions of rehabilitation have changed and evolved over the last century, fueled in part by our evolving ideas about illness, health, and disability. A number of sources (Siegert, Taylor, & Dean, 2012; Stucki, Cieza, & Melvin, 2007) trace the history of the term from its medical origins and focus during the 19th century to a "dramatic shift" toward the broader notion of health supported by the biopsychosocial model of health within the World Health Organization's definition of rehabilitation in 1992. The development of the ICF (WHO, 2001) has been one of the important drivers of the on-going dialogue about persons with disability and rehabilitation. While earlier models of disability (and rehabilitation) located disability as within the person, the ICF model defines disability as a product of interaction with environmental barriers. Stucki, Cieza, and Melvin (2007) propose the need for consensus on a conceptual definition of rehabilitation in support of implementing the ICF model of rehabilitation:

> Rehabilitation is the health strategy that, based on the WHO's integrative model of human functioning and disability, aims to enable people with health conditions experiencing or likely to experience disability to achieve and maintain optimal functioning in interaction with the environment....
>
> Rehabilitation is the core strategy for the medical specialty PRM, a major strategy for the rehabilitation professions and a relevant strategy for other medical specialties and health professions, service providers and payors in the health sector. (p. 282)

Learning Point 1.12　Contrast locating disability within a person compared with locating it within a society.

Dean et al. (2012) express reservations about any single definition of rehabilitation and also about exclusive identification of specific professions (such as the traditional designation of occupational therapy, physical therapy, and speech-language pathology) with rehabilitation. Instead, they identify five themes of rehabilitation:

1. The ICF as a conceptual framework and language
2. Interprofessional teamwork
3. Processes of rehabilitation: goal setting and mediators or factors influencing goal setting and goal attainment
4. Outcomes
5. The individual person in context (pp. 6–7)

This discussion of terminology related to interprofessional rehabilitation ethics has broadened the scope of interest for interprofessional rehabilitation ethics considerably. Our initial thoughts may have been that interprofessional rehabilitation ethics focuses primarily on the moral concerns of therapists, engineers, nurses, and physical medicine physicians as they address a person's recovery from injury and disease. In light of newer definitions of both the experience of disability and of rehabilitation, it becomes clear that interprofessional rehabilitation ethics is relevant to a much broader group of healthcare providers, family members, caregivers, philosophers, and others, even broadening its application to society and populations.

> **Learning Point 1.13**   Why is ethics related to interprofessional education and practice relevant to a larger group of stakeholders?

We believe that the long-term interprofessional teamwork experiences of rehabilitation professionals, recent experience in collaborating to implementing the ICF model in rehabilitation settings, and commitment to the biopsychosocial model position those involved in rehabilitation to play an important role in developing interprofessional ethics. We suggest that interprofessional rehabilitation ethics may even serve as the starting point for pedagogy and practice that is truly interprofessional in nature. A fresh look at interprofessional rehabilitation ethics should allow for, or accommodate, seven main limitations of more traditional medical ethics (bioethics), see **TABLE 1.2**.

TABLE 1.2   Limitations of Traditional Medical Ethics for Interprofessional Rehabilitation Ethics

1. Focus of traditional medical ethics or bioethics on disease, diagnosis, cure, and end-of-life issues.
   - Focus of rehabilitation is not to cure or diagnose per se, but to improve function and ability to live a better quality of life.

2. Traditional medical ethics and bioethics have not consistently included rehabilitation stakeholders, and at times have had contentious relationships with people with disabilities.
   - Rehabilitation ethics must include the views and voices of those who have a disability or those who live with people with disability.

3. Western-centric bias of medical ethics and bioethics.
   - Given that we in the rehabilitation fields work with a culturally diverse population, the western centric notion of ethics can no longer well serve the clients whom we serve.

4. Focus on current popular trends or issues in bioethics.
   - Rehabilitation ethics should rather focus upon the real and everyday issues that people needing habilitation or rehabilitation experience.

5. Geared towards a single provider profession (such as bioethics that is medicine centric).
   - Rehabilitation ethics must allow for a collaborative and team orientated view across all stakeholders.

6. Individualistic focus of medical ethics.
   - Rehabilitation professionals work in interprofessional teams within complex organizations. Resolution of ethical situations requires an appreciation of organizational and societal complexities.

7. Reactive focus—responding to ethical situations.
   - Need to be proactive in rehabilitation. Rehabilitation ethics must allow for a collaborative and team orientated view across all stakeholders.

Addressing the limitations of traditional medical ethics requires an inclusive process that embraces diversity, includes relevant stakeholders; addresses different professional, clinical and ethical perspectives and frameworks; and addresses collective entities (not merely individuals).

Learning Point 1.14   What are the limitations of traditional ethics focused upon medicine?

▶ Major Theme of the Text

The major theme of this text is that interprofessional rehabilitation ethics requires individual and team moral agency enacted within the moral commons (**FIGURE 1.1**). As described later in this text, individuals and the team must be actively engaged in developing moral agency and in creating the moral commons. In light of the limitations of traditional ethics (described previously), this process will be challenging and there are few existing models for this process. Development of team moral agency and collaborating in creating the moral commons requires new interprofessional skills for individual professionals, teams, and organizations.

Figure 1.1 provides a visual representation of elements of moral agency enacted within the "moral commons" for interprofessional rehabilitation ethics that are consistent with the purpose of this text to create a conceptual "moral commons" for interprofessional dialogue and ethical analysis. The idea of a moral commons builds upon the historical idea of land shared by the community for farming, recreation, and discussion; the commons created space for community interaction, play, and dialogue. Extending the metaphor of the ancient commons, the moral commons is a "safe zone" for discussion, interaction, and consensus building. Later in this text, we will elaborate on three key elements of the moral commons:

1. Identity (personal and professional)
2. Ethical traditions
3. Context and realms

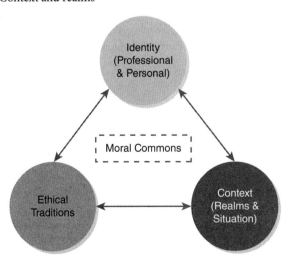

FIGURE 1.1 Individual and team moral agency enacted within the moral commons.

The current fragmented structure of the healthcare system does not provide a consistent forum or setting for the interprofessional team to discuss ethical situations. Additionally, short time constraints for team meetings often result in focusing only on clinical issues without consideration of ethical issues. Communication between team members and the family may be indirect or via telephone or virtual interaction. A forum or safe zone for ethical dialogue (moral commons) may not be readily available. Individual rehabilitation practitioners must be willing and able to create space for ethical discussion and to ensure that ethical issues do not drop out of interprofessional collaboration. Without shared space for dialogue to reach agreement, it is difficult for interprofessional teams to exercise team moral agency. It is the process of building the moral commons that is critical for the formulation of consensus to occur, and we believe this is essential for interprofessional rehabilitation ethics. In the following paragraphs, we say a few words about how this text will address common barriers to engaging in interprofessional ethics.

Learning Point 1.15   What do you think would be the BEST way to develop a moral commons?

Learning Point 1.16   What is consensus and why is it important?

Some authors describe the aggregate multiple capabilities needed to be ethical as "moral agency." For example, Gray and Wegner (2009) define moral agency simply as the "capacity to do right or wrong" (p. 505). Fry, Veatch, and Taylor (2006) add that moral agency involves cultivating the ability to do this consistently by defining moral agency as "the capacity to habitually act in an ethical manner" (p. 62). Although we often limit our thinking about ethics to individuals, they note that individuals, groups, teams, and organizations are moral agents.

Learning Point 1.17   Define and relate moral agency and moral commons.

Rehabilitation professionals (and the organizations in which practice) should have the following ethical competencies or elements of moral agency (Fry, Veatch, & Taylor, 2006, p. 62):

1. Moral Sensitivity
2. Moral Responsiveness
3. Moral Reasoning
4. Moral Discernment
5. Moral Accountability
6. Moral Character
7. Moral Valuing
8. Transformative Moral Leadership

Learning Point 1.18   Summarize the key concept of moral agency and what it means to you.

These observations about the components of moral agency indicate that ethics is far more than ethical decision making. Additionally, ethics is not only about what one does but about the character or virtues of the person who will act.

Learning Point 1.19   How are virtue and character similar?

▶ Summary and Conclusion

There are increasing calls for interprofessional education and collaborative practice. Although it is intuitively apparent that ethics and values are critical foundations for interprofessional practice, the area of interprofessional ethics has received scant attention within medical ethics and within rehabilitation. To borrow a colonial metaphor, there is no moral commons for interprofessional rehabilitation ethics. Providing a foundation for interprofessional rehabilitation ethics is therefore forging new ground, requiring rehabilitation practitioners to examine uniprofessional perspectives on ethics and clinical practice. The difficulty of this undertaking is further compounded by the fact that each profession has different clinical language and models.

Learning Point 1.20   Why does each profession have a unique language and set of conceptual models?

In this chapter we have attempted to provide a shared foundation for engaging in interprofessional rehabilitation ethics by defining keys terms, outlining the history of healthcare ethics with reference to rehabilitation, and discussing barriers to interprofessional rehabilitation ethics. To address these barriers, we have discussed key elements for creating the missing moral commons.

Learning Point 1.21   What are the three key elements for creating a moral commons?

The theme of rehabilitation ethics as individual and team moral agency enacted on the moral commons has been elaborated in the following ways:

- An interprofessional moral commons requires creative action in order to develop a safe zone for dialogue between team members, including the patient and family.
- Creation of the moral commons provides a foundation for ethical dialogue regarding personal and professional identity, the perspective offered by different ethical traditions, and contextual factors.
- Dialogue within the moral commons is necessary for individual and team moral agency enabling both to bring about the "good."

Learning Point 1.22   Can you identify a situation where you developed a forum to resolve differences? How did you create a "commons"?

In attempting to build the moral commons, we have also suggested that the ICF could be helpful in its explicitly moral foundation and in providing common language.

In chapter 2, we further develop the case process by delineating the steps involved in this process, outlining the ethical issues commonly encountered during rehabilitation, and using the Dialogic Engagement Model to analyze ethical cases. Subsequent text explores a specific ethical case or issue using the framework discussed in Chapter 2.

Several important themes have emerged in providing a foundation for the moral commons. One important theme is that of diversity and inclusion versus dogmatism and exclusion. Divergent ethical theories, professional hierarchy, different clinical models, and competing values all have the potential to create barriers to interprofessional rehabilitation ethics. People with disabilities have historically perceived themselves as marginalized from ethicists, academic studies, healthcare providers, and policy makers. There has been extensive discussion of silos between professions that inhibit interprofessional practice, and it may be that including patients and clients in interprofessional ethics may prove to be yet another silo to overcome. We believe that healthcare practitioners may play a crucial role in the emerging area of interprofessional ethics and we hope that this text may contribute to this effort.

Learning Point 1.23   Contrast diversity to dogmatism as concerns ethics.

Closing Reflections

Learning Activities

1.1   **Analysis of Beliefs**
Consider a time when you changed your beliefs about right or wrong. What prompted you to change and why?

1.2   **Reflection upon Beliefs**
Regarding learning activity 1.1, how long did the change last and why?

1.3   **Word Cloud**
Using an application from the internet, create a word cloud to capture the source of your ethical and moral beliefs. Compare your word cloud with those of others taking this class. How is the content similar and different?

1.4   **Moral Conflict**
Consider a time when you disagreed with a friend or colleague on an ethical matter. How did you resolve the issue?

1.5   **Codes of Ethics**
Pair with two others and investigate your own profession's Code of Ethics and that of two other professions. In what ways are the Codes of Ethics similar? In what ways are the Codes of Ethics not similar?

1.6   **Debate and Controversy**
There is some debate as to whether interprofessional ethics is a new field of study (Clark, Drinka, & Cott, 2007) or whether interprofessional ethics is merely an extension of professional ethics (Banks, 2010; IPEC, 2011;

Schmitt & Stewart, 2011, p. 76). Schmitt and Stewart (2011, p. 76) see interprofessional ethics as a "revitalizing" of professional ethics to address the needs of interprofessional practice. What do you think and why?

1.7   Understanding of Rehabilitation
Does your experience or understanding of rehabilitation reflect the five themes of the rehabilitation; interprofessional teamwork; processes of rehabilitation: goal setting and mediators or factors influencing goal setting and goal attainment; outcomes and the individual person in context rehabilitation? If so, how?

1.8   International Classification of Functioning, Disability and Health (ICF)
Look up the ICF on the internet. What are the implicit and explicit ethical and moral values of the ICF?

1.9   Moral Agency
Define and explain and provide an example in context from your own experience.

1.10   Teams and Moral Agency
How can teams organize and exercise moral agency?

1.11   Medical Ethics and Rehabilitation Ethics
In what ways do rehabilitation ethics differ from traditional medical ethics?

1.12   Moral Commons
What is meant by the term moral commons and why is it important?

1.13   Building Moral Commons
Consider a specific practice setting. How would you design a moral commons for that setting?

 # Take Away Messages

- The terms ethics and morality refer to issues of right, wrong, duty, values, and the "good."
- In everyday conversation, the terms ethical and moral are often used interchangeably.
- Personal and moral convictions are learned through a variety of sources (family, religion, school, media, professions, and others).
- Many of our most deeply held moral convictions are simply taken for granted and we do not examine their validity.
- Difficult ethical dilemmas invariably involve conflicting principles, values, virtues, or moral goods.
- In contrast to the unexamined nature of morality, ethics requires conscious, systematic thought and reflection.
- Ethical discussion requires the willingness of all participants to rationally examine moral convictions, analyze conflicting values, and provide a sound rationale for action.
- Unexamined moral values and reasoned ethical analysis are sometimes referred to as first and second order ethics.
- The implicit agreement of all participants to engage in ethical reasoning about moral conflict is part of a creating a "moral commons" rather than devolving into polarized argument.

References

Banks, S. (2010). Interprofessional ethics: A developing field? Notes from the Ethics & Social WelfareConference, Sheffield, UK, May 2010. *Ethics and Social Welfare, 4*(3), 280–294. doi:10.1 080/17496535.2010.516116

Barr, H., Helme, M., & D'Avray, L. (2011). *Developing interprofessional education in health and social care courses in the United Kingdom. A progress report. Paper 12.* The Higher Education Academy: Health Sciences and Practice. Retrieved from www.health.heacademy.ac.uk

Beauchamp, T. L., & Childress, J. F. (2009). *Principles of Biomedical Ethics* (6th ed.). New York: Oxford University Press.

Bernheim, J. F., & Childress, R. G. (2015). Introduction: A framework for public health Ethics. In Bernheim, J. F., Childress, R. G., Melnick, A., & Bonnie, R. J. (Eds.), *Essentials of Public Health Ethics* (pp. 3–19). Burlington, MA: Jones & Bartlett Learning.

Clark, P. G., Cott, C., & Drinka, T. J. (2007). Theory and practice in interprofessional ethics: A framework for understanding ethical issues in health care teams. *Journal of Interprofessional Care, 21*(6), 591–603. doi:10.1080/13561820701653227

Dean, S. G., Siegert, R. J., & Taylor, W. J. (2012). *Interprofessional rehabilitation a person-centred approach.* Chichester, West Sussex, U.K: Wiley-Blackwell.

Engel, J., & Prentice, D. (2013). The Ethics of Interprofessional Collaboration. *Nursing Ethics, 20*(4), 426–435. doi:10.1177/0969733012468466

Fry, S. T., Veatch, R. M., & Taylor, C. R. (2006). *Case studies in nursing ethics* (3rd ed.). Sudbury, Mass: Jones and Bartlett Publishers.

Goldberg, L. R. (2015). The importance of Interprofessional Education for students in Communication Sciences and Disorders. *Communication Disorders Quarterly, 36*(2), 121–125. doi:10.1177/1525740114544701

Gray, K., & Wegner, D. M. (2009). Moral typecasting: Divergent perceptions of moral agents and moral patients. *Journal of Personality and Social Psychology, 96*(3), 505–520. doi:10.1037 /a0013748

Hinman, L. M. (2013). *Ethics: A pluralistic approach to moral theory* (5th ed.). Boston, MA: Wadsworth, Cengage Learning.

Horner, J. (2003). Morality, ethics, and law: Introductory concepts. *Seminars in Speech and Language, 24*(4), 263–274. doi:10.1055/s-2004-815580

Interprofessional Education Collaborative Expert Panel (IPEC). (2011). Core competencies for interprofessional collaborative practice: Report of an expert panel. Washington, D.C.

Purtilo, R. B., & Doherty, R. F. (2011). *Ethical dimensions in the health professions* (5th ed.). St. Louis: Elsevier/Saunders.

Reeves, S., Perrier, L., Goldman, J., Freeth, D., & Zwarenstein, M. (2013). Interprofessional education: effects on professional practice and healthcare outcomes (update). *Cochrane Database of Systematic Reviews 3*, Cd002213. doi:10.1002/14651858.CD002213.pub3

Schmitt, M. H., Gilbert, J. H., Brandt, B. F., & Weinstein, R. S. (2013). The coming of age for interprofessional education and practice. *American Journal of Medicine, 126*(4), 284–288. http:// dx.doi.org/10.1016/j.amjmed.2012.10.015

Sheldon, M., Cavanaugh, J. T., Croninger, W., Osgood, W., Robnett, R., Seigle, J., & Simonsen, L. (2012). Preparing rehabilitation healthcare providers in the 21st century: Implementation of interprofessional education through an academic-clinical site partnership. *Work, 41*(3), 269–275. doi:10.3233/wor-2012-1299

Siegert, R. J., Taylor, W. J., & Dean, S. G. (2012). Introduction. In *Interprofessional rehabilitation* (pp. 1–8). West Sussex, UK: John Wiley & Sons, Ltd.

Stucki, G., Cieza, A., & Melvin, J. (2007). The International Classification of Functioning, Disability and Health (ICF): A unifying model for the conceptual description of the rehabilitation strategy. *Journal of Rehabilitative Medicine, 39*(4), 279–285. doi:10.2340/16501977-0041

Stucki, G., Reinhardt, J. D., Grimby, G., & Melvin, J. (2007). Developing "Human Functioning and Rehabilitation Research" from the comprehensive perspective. *Journal of Rehabilitative Medicine, 39*(9), 665–671. doi:10.2340/16501977-0136

Swisher, L. L., & Hiller, P. for the APTA Task Force to Revise the Core Ethics Documents. (2010). The revised APTA code of ethics for the physical therapist and standards of ethical conduct for the physical therapist assistant: Theory, purpose, process, and significance. *Physical Therapy, 90*(5), 803–824. doi:10.2522/ptj.20090373

Wade, D. T. (2005). Describing rehabilitation interventions. *Clinical Rehabilitation, 19*(8), 811–818.

WHO (World Health Organization). (2010). Framework for action on interprofessional education & collaborative practice. Geneva: World Health Organization. Retrieved November 13, 2018 from http://whqlibdoc.who.int/ hq/2010/WHO_HRH_HPN_10.3_eng.pdf

WHO (World Health Organization), & World Bank. (2011). World Report on Disability. Geneva: WHO. Retrieved from http://www.who.int/disabilities/world_report/2011/en/

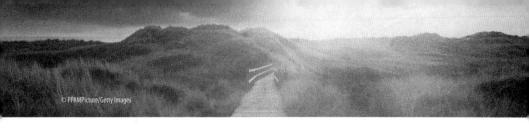

CHAPTER 2

Historical and Clinical Context for the Interprofessional Rehabilitation Moral Commons

Laura Lee Swisher and **Charlotte Brasic Royeen**

CHAPTER OUTLINE

CHAPTER OBJECTIVES

At the conclusion of this chapter, the reader will be able to:

1. Delineate historical, social, and healthcare factors that have shaped the development of the rehabilitation professions.

(continues)

CHAPTER OBJECTIVES (continued)

2. Identify the ethical implications of the biomedical, medical, biopsychosocial, and International Classification of Functioning, Disability and Health (ICF) models of health and disability.
3. Discuss the interrelationship between clinical and ethical spheres.
4. Discuss important themes and commonly encountered ethical issues in interprofessional rehabilitation practice.
5. Evaluate the role played by effect of team or organizational culture on moral agency.
6. Analyze key elements of the situational, social, and organizational context of rehabilitation practice and their implications for individual and team moral agency.

KEY TERMS

Reading these key terms before reading the chapter will introduce you to key concepts which will then be somewhat familiar to you as you read this chapter. This is an important learning technique that will enhance your learning as a multi-step process. You may even wish to make a flash card set of key terms and quiz yourself on them once or twice before reading the chapter. This will better prepare you to immerse in the language of ethics and better prepare you to integrate the content.

Disability: An impairment, functional limitation, activity limitation, or participation restriction resulting from a negative interaction between the individual and context (environment and personal factors) (Based on the ICF). Note that older ideas about disability define disability in terms of effects of disease on social role or task.

Ethical or Moral Distress: An ethical situation in which one knows the right thing to do but is unable to do it.

Ethical or Moral Reasoning or Judgment: The dimension of moral agency that refers to making a decision about the "right" action. Moral judgment may depend in part on ethical traditions as the ethical traditions present different aspects of the ethical action.

Ethical or Moral Sensitivity: The dimension of moral agency that involves recognition and interpretation of the situation.

Ethical or Moral Silence: Situation characterized by silence and lack of moral discourse when confronting an obvious ethical problem or issue.

Ethical or Moral Temptation: Situation in which one is faced with a right versus wrong situation and is tempted to choose to do the wrong thing based on self-interest.

Ethical Situation: A classification of different ethical contexts that may suggest a specific response. Situation types include ethical ambiguity/uncertainty, ethical issue or problem, ethical dilemma, moral distress, moral temptation, and ethical silence. Classifying an ethical issue into known types, may provide insight into a correct response. For example, moral temptation should typically be resisted.

Groupthink: Dysfunctional group dynamic identified by Janis (1972) in which group members may ignore rational strategies in order to promote group harmony or avoid conflict.

International Classification of Health, Disability, and Functioning (ICF): A conceptual model developed by the World Health Organization (WHO) that delineates how health, disability, environment, personal factors, and function are interrelated. The ICF also provides a taxonomy for standard evaluation and outcomes measures through the development of shared language, terminology, and classification systems.

Models of Disability: Conceptual model of the relationship between the individual person; illness, pathology, disease; impairment, functional limitation, activity limitation, or participation restriction and the environment.

Organizational Culture: The implicit and explicit values, culture, rituals, customs, or ways of behaving within an organization that are often "taken for granted."

Professional Identity: An internal sense of the professional self that evolves and matures over time and provides a basis for clinical and moral action. Building on the work of Kegan (1982), Bebeau and others describe professional identity formation as developing from independent operator to team-oriented idealist to self-defining professional (Bebeau & Lewis, 2003; Bebeau & Monson, 2012).

Realms of Ethical Action: Distinguishes different ethical concerns based on whether the ethical situation is interpersonal (individual realm), within an organization or institution (organizational/institutional realm), or at the level of society as a whole (societal realm) (Glaser, 1994).

Team Identity: The collective attitudes and beliefs held by a team regarding ethics, values, teamwork, relationships, power, hierarchy, and clinical roles.

▶ Chapter Overview

An understanding of interprofessional rehabilitation ethics requires an appreciation of the historical development, clinical context, and scope of practice of rehabilitation professionals. This perspective must also be informed by the voices of patients, clients, and families served by rehabilitation professionals. This chapter discusses each of the three elements of the moral commons within the historical, clinical, and organizational context of rehabilitation. We provide a historical sketch of the development of rehabilitation, discuss the unique clinical environment of rehabilitation, provide an overview of ethical issues encountered in rehabilitation practice, and discuss the interrelationship between clinical and ethical issues. The chapter concludes by addressing the influence of organizational and team culture in shaping ethical environments and related implications for individual and team moral agency enacted within the moral commons.

Learning Point 2.1 Why should rehabilitation ethics consider the input of patients, clients, families, and rehabilitation professionals?

▶ Rehabilitation's Historical Roots

A previous discussion in chapter one indicated the challenges of defining the term "rehabilitation." Rehabilitation refers to a process focused on function or enablement, but it also refers to the collective professions and disciplines that participate in rehabilitation. It is, therefore, not surprising that there is no singular or linear perspective on the history of rehabilitation. The history of rehabilitation embraces individual professions involved in rehabilitation, but also the collective efforts of those involved in what we have called the process of rehabilitation. Rehabilitation historians trace its origins to several thousand years ago among the Greeks and Romans who used physical modalities to treat pain. Wars and treating the resulting war injuries have also been associated with the advancement of rehabilitation (Cruess, Cruess, Boudreau, Snell, & Steinert, 2014; Lei-Rivera, Sutera, Galatioto, Hujsak, & Gurley, 2013). According to Eldar and Jelić (2013, p. 1019), the origins of the "spirit of rehabilitation" can be traced to Europe in the 18th century and to the field of orthopedics following World War I. Occupational therapy and physical therapy both attribute early professional roots at least in part to the reconstruction aides used during and after World War I, although there were undoubtedly other factors influencing the new professions as well (Wikström-Grotell, Broberg, Ahonen, & Eriksson, 2013). These earliest years of rehabilitation following WWI were far from harmonious from an interprofessional standpoint as medicine, nursing, occupational therapy, physical therapy, and speech-language pathology conflicted regarding autonomy, scope of practice, and professional status (Gurley, Hujsak, & Kelly, 2013; Schiff, Salazar, Vetter, Andre, & Pinzur, 2014).

Learning Point 2.2 What is your definition of rehabilitation?

Another world war and the polio epidemic highlighted additional needs for rehabilitation. Howard Rusk attributed the birth of the modern concept of rehabilitation to the adversity and necessity of World War II (Lei-Rivera et al., 2013; Yu et al., 2011). As indicated in **TABLE 2.1**, the years after World War II witnessed the growth of the rehabilitation professions working in collaborative teams. Human rights efforts also played a significant role in the development of rehabilitation, especially regarding the rights of persons with disabilities. The widespread focus on human rights that swept the globe in the decades after WWII would also extend to the rights of persons with disabilities, fundamentally changing our views on the definition, language, and models used to describe disabilities. WHO was active in promoting the rights of persons with disabilities and ultimately created the foundation for the ICF framework (WHO, 2001). The move away from the biomedical model of health in favor of the biopsychosocial model of health and the development of the ICF model have established rehabilitation professionals as primary contributors to health around the world.

Learning Point 2.3 How do human rights relate to disabilities and rehabilitation?

Learning Point 2.4 How does the biomedical model of health compare to the biopsychosocial model of health?

TABLE 2.1   Timeline for Rehabilitation Ethics

Time	Events
Greek and Roman times	Use of electricity, heat, and cold for pain
Civil War	Treatment of war injuries and disabilities
1914–1918	• World War I calls attention to the needs of soldiers wounded in the war • Reconstruction aides created to assist recovery (early physical and occupational therapists)
1930s and 40s	Franklin Delano Roosevelt World War II • Continued need for rehabilitation • Nazi medical experimentation human rights violations • Rehabilitation teams care for wounded soldiers and civilians
1950s	Peak of U.S. polio epidemics Willowbrook and Tuskegee experiments
1951	Rusk Institute founded for rehabilitation
1960s and 70s	Civil Rights movement addresses human rights
1970s	Birth of medical ethics
Late 1970s	Emergence of Biopsychosocial Model of Disability
1979	Belmont Report delineates principles for ethical research
1970–1990	Dominant Period of Principlism in Medical Ethics
1990	Americans with Disabilities Act (ADA) enacted
1992	WHO defines rehabilitation
2001	International Classification of Functioning, Disability and Health
2006	United Nations Convention on the Rights of Persons with Disabilities
2011	Interprofessional Education Competencies published

Based on Eldar & Jelić (2003); Linker (2005); Opitz, Folz, Gelfman, & Peters (1997); Rusk (1949).

This brief history indicates the complex interplay between the competing forces of the development of individual professions and the shared goals of rehabilitation. As we will discuss later in the chapter, this tension between professional identity and interprofessional collaboration continues to influence rehabilitation team dynamics.

In the following paragraphs, we examine the unique context of rehabilitation ethics in relation to the three critical elements of the moral commons introduced in chapter 1.

▶ Elements of the Moral Commons: Ethical Traditions

During the 1970s the unprecedented focus on human rights and enhanced technology fueled development of the field of medical ethics. Paternalistic assumptions of the Hippocratic Oath seemed inadequate to respond to difficult questions and conflicts between conflicting societal standards and ethical standards. For example, the ability to save lives through dialysis raised the issue of fairness in allocation and rationing of healthcare resources such as dialysis and transplantation. Medical ethicists used a variety of philosophical ethical approaches (such as deontology, utilitarianism, virtue, and care) to address complex ethical issues. During the 1970s, Beauchamp and Childress (2009) developed an approach to ethics referred to as principlism or "the four-principles" approach.

> **Learning Point 2.5**   What are paternalistic assumptions?

1. Respect for persons and autonomy
2. Beneficence
3. Non-maleficence
4. Justice

These four primary principles also provided a foundation for other "intermediate" principles, such as informed consent, confidentiality, etc. (see **FIGURE 2.1**). Principles are common everyday ethical standards that function as general guidelines (Beauchamp, 1995; Beuachamp & Childress, 2009, p. 12) for making ethical decisions. Principles are neither full-blown abstract ethical theories nor specific rules for moral conduct. The "intermediate" position of ethical principles between theoretical and concrete considerations has made principles valuable tools for healthcare professionals in medical ethics. For example, the ethical principles of informed consent and confidentiality are often viewed as specific elaborations of the more general principle of autonomy. Intermediate principles provide "specification" of the guidance of the four basic principles by application to a more specific context.

> **Learning Point 2.6**   How does the intermediate principle of informed consent provide more specific guidance than the general principle of autonomy?

The period of principlism (extending roughly from the 1960s through the 1990s) (Pellegrino, 1993) gave way to a backlash against principlism during which

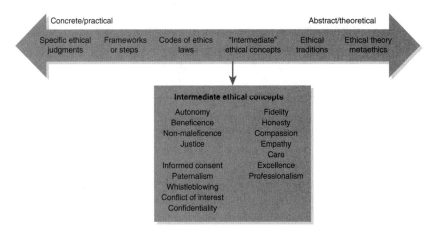

FIGURE 2.1 Ethical principles as intermediate concepts.

the approach was criticized for being reductionist, overly deductive, lacking adequate moral theory, sexist, focused on conflicting principles, subjective in interpretation, ignoring context, and providing too little guidance (Clouser & Gert, 1990; Davis, 1995). Nevertheless, principlism remains the dominant and most commonly used approach to medical ethics as evidenced by the number of editions for the seminal bioethics text *Principles of Biomedical Ethics* (Beauchamp & Childress, 2009).

Learning Point 2.7   What is meant by the period of principlism in ethics?

Learning Point 2.8   Why do you think that principlism remains a dominant approach in ethics in your profession?

Principle-based medical ethics has several limitations for rehabilitation ethics. Medical ethics has been criticized for its relative lack of interest in ethical issues in disability and rehabilitation. In a special edition of the *American Journal of Bioethics*, Kuczewski (2001) acknowledged this lack of attention:

> Bioethics has not devoted a good deal of attention to the study of issues related to disability or to rehabilitation care. What attention has been given to disability has largely focused on requests to terminate potentially life-sustaining treatment or requests for assistance in dying… (p. 36)

People with disabilities describe this lack of interest in more strident tones (Hurst, 2003), criticizing medical ethics as politically-focused and ignoring the voice and experience of people with disabilities. Newell addressed the "rejected knowledge" from the failure of medical ethics to listen to the voices, experiences, and perspectives of people with disabilities (2006). These comments point to the long-standing divide between the ethics community and people with disabilities. Although the principles approach has been medicine and physician-centric with little attention to rehabilitation or disability issues, the model has nevertheless been used extensively in professions associated with the rehabilitation process.

Learning Point 2.9   What is "rejected knowledge"?

Rule-Based Tradition	Ends-Based Tradition
Laws Codes of ethics Ethical Principles	Consequences Outcomes
Virtue-Based Tradition	**Narrative-Based Tradition**
Virtuous action Being a good person Character Traits	Listening for "voice" Sensitivity to others' experience Societal bias perspective

FIGURE 2.2 Four ethical traditions.

In this text (**FIGURE 2.2**), we identify four major ethical "traditions" (Rule-Based, Ends-Based, Virtue-Based, and Narrative-Based), and we suggest that principlism contributes significantly to the interprofessional moral commons as part of the Rule-Based ethical tradition. The common framework and shared language of the four principles support interprofessional ethical dialogue. At the same time, it is important to recognize the potential limitations of exclusive focus on principlism for interprofessional rehabilitation ethics.

Learning Point 2.10   Principlism best matches which of the four major ethics traditions discussed in this text?

We will explore each of the traditions in more detail in this chapter.

▶ Elements of the Moral Commons: Identity

The second critical element for creating the moral commons involves considering the personal and professional identity of others. Even though many health professions historically evolved from medicine and or nursing, each health profession or discipline has developed its own unique language and unique theoretical framework to support its role and scope of practice. As a result, members of the healthcare team may literally be speaking different languages without even knowing that they are doing so. There is a growing consensus that a shared conceptual framework for interprofessional collaboration would be helpful to healthcare providers (Allan, Campbell, Guptill, Stephenson, & Campbell, 2006; D'Amour, Ferrada-Videla, San Martin Rodriguez, & Beaulieu, 2005; Giacomini, Kenny, & DeJean, 2009). As Allan et al. (2006) note: "A shared language and conceptual framework is essential to successful interprofessional collaboration" (p. 235). Many rehabilitation professions use the WHO's ICF (2001) as a foundation for clinical reasoning. Major features of the ICF model include its intention to merge the medical and biopsychosocial models of disability, and incorporating environmental and contextual factors (WHO, 2001). Although the ICF was intended for use by all health professionals, it has gained more traction among rehabilitation professionals than in medicine. While most healthcare disciplines have endorsed some form of the biopsychosocial model of health, a literature review by Allan et al. (2006) suggests that the biomedical model continues to have influence and that biopsychosocial language has had less "diffusion" into the medical literature than the rehabilitation literature.

Learning Point 2.11   How can different health professionals speak from different perspectives?

Several authors have reported on the successful use of the ICF as a shared language and conceptual framework for interprofessional practice and its positive effects on interprofessional collaborative practice. Allan et al. (2006) suggest that the ICF may provide a way to "transcend" the boundaries of individual professions and can serve as a basis for full discussion of patients' needs and goals. Rentsch et al. (2003) used the ICF to organize the work of the neurorehabilitation team, reporting that its implementation provided a common foundation for goal planning, enhanced teamwork and communication, and resulted in improved quality of care. To illustrate, in a rehabilitation setting, Harty, Griesel, and van der Merwe (2011) used a visual tool (Talking MATS) representing the nine ICF activity and participation domains to reach consensus regarding rehabilitation goals between clients with communication disorders following stroke and their rehabilitation therapists.

Learning Point 2.12   Why is the ICF model appropriate to use in rehabilitation?

The need for a shared clinical framework presupposes an implicit shared moral obligation of the members of the interdisciplinary healthcare team which is committed to meet the needs of the patient/client within his/her environment (Engel & Prentice, 2013). Engel and Prentice (2013) describe interprofessional care as an inherently moral enterprise grounded in the ethical goal of beneficence (promoting good) for the patient. In spite of this shared patient-centered focus, they observe that practitioners from different perspectives will invariably construe the "good" differently, creating dissonance in acting collaboratively. In this case, "the good" refers to the various outcomes that may be possible from a particular scenario. Noting that there is little written about interprofessional ethics, Engel and Prentice (2013) conclude that there is an urgent need to attend to this important area of interprofessional care.

Learning Point 2.13   Why can there be multiple "good" outcomes from a particular ethical case?

Learning Point 2.14   Does the professional identity of each rehabilitation profession implicitly provide a different lens for what is perceived as "good?"

In addition to the implicit moral foundation of interprofessional practice, conceptual clinical frameworks are themselves grounded in explicit or implicit ethical values or principles. Although practitioners may view clinical and ethical as totally separate domains, further reflection would suggest that clinical frameworks are ethics and value-laden. They frame our thinking about the nature of the presenting problem, relationships between the patient and the healthcare team, interprofessional relationships, and resources needed by the patient. In this regard one might compare the implicit and explicit ethical values of the moral, medical (Engel, 1977; 1981), social (Llewellyn & Hogan, 2000; Masala & Petretto, 2008; Oliver, 2013; Scullion, 2010) and ICF clinical frameworks. Building on the work of Olkin (2002) and Roush and Sharby (2011), (see **TABLE 2.2**) compare the moral, medical, social, and ICF models of disability.

Learning Point 2.15   How can clinical frameworks be value laden?

As indicated in Table 2.2, disability models have different theoretical bases and assumptions regarding the nature of disability, and these contrasting ideas have implications for health, rehabilitation, and ethics. Rehabilitation professionals have endorsed the ICF and its underlying biopsychosocial model of disability largely based on its clinical framework. Although rehabilitation professionals support full participation, and of persons with disability within society, there has been less discussion of how truly revolutionary the ICF model has been in presenting a clinical model that is grounded in explicit ethical principles.

The ICF explicitly links its clinical framework to the United Nations Convention on Rights of Persons with Disabilities (UNCRPD) (United Nations, 2006), work that was simultaneously led by the WHO. Indeed, Bickenbach (2011) has fully delineated the close relationship between the United Nations Convention on Rights of Persons with Disabilities (UNCRPD) with the ICF (Bickenbach, 2011). The participation domains of the ICF are closely aligned with rights delineated within specific articles in the UNCRPD. For example, Article 20 of the UNCRPD delineates the right to mobility and Chapter 4 of the ICF addresses the domain of mobility (Bickenbach, 2011, p. 6).

Learning Point 2.16   Do you agree with using the United Nations work for a foundation for work in disabilities and rehabilitation?

A review of the work of the United Nations demonstrates on-going advocacy for persons with disabilities dating back to the 1940s, during which time the United Nations perspective evolved from a "welfare perspective" to one of human rights (United Nations, 2018). Bickenbach (2011) provides an excellent summary of how the ICF provides an effective bridge between clinical and ethical values:

> The ever-expanding literature on ICF implementation suggests that the ICF model of functioning and disability potentially offers more than merely a guide for structuring disability data.... At the same time, the ICF exemplifies in its model of functioning and disability the so-called 'biopsychosocial concept of disability', in which disability is a multi-dimensional concept that constitutes the outcome of interactions between intrinsic features of the person and the person's physical, built, attitudinal and social and political

TABLE 2.2 Comparison of Models of Disability

Models of Disability	Moral	Medical Model	Social Model	ICF
Historical origin	Ancient times	19th century	1970s	2001
Disability results from	Divine action or punishment/blessing for human shortcoming or actions	Physical abnormality or disease	Social structures or barriers "social oppression model" (Thomas)	Interaction between impairments and societal barriers
Individual or Social Emphasis	Individual	Individual	Social	Interaction between individual and social
Theoretical basis	Theological	Disease model Medical & basic sciences	Social Construction Minority Group Oppression	Biopsychosocial Model
Human rights and ethical foundations	Injustice of "blaming the victim"	Inequality of power relationships	Seeks equality and fairness in through social policy	Parallel and outgrowth of UN human rights declaration
Model for IP rehabilitation team	Rehabilitation may or may not be appropriate	Hierarchical with MD as head of team and focus on "cure"	Support patient and society in overcoming barriers; healthcare professionals may present barriers to overcoming disability	Interprofessional teamwork including stakeholders: patient-centered
Strengths or Limitations	May be seen as blaming the victim	Addresses medical aspects	Strong link to political action and social change Lack of attention to impairments and psychosocial aspects such as individual identity and relationships; less effective in dealing with mental impairments; problem of impairment-disability dichotomy	Does not include consideration of individual perceptions of personal factors and cuality of life (Huber, Sillick, & Skarakis-Doyle, 2010)

Based on Roush & Sharby (2011).

environment. This conception is fully aligned with the so-called 'rights approach to disability', in which the focus in disability policy is shifted from the 'personal misfortune' of a decrement in health to a fully contextualized lived experience of functioning as effected, positively or negatively, by the individual physical and social context. The ICF is at once both a scientific and a rights-based instrument. (Bickenbach, 2009, 2005)

Thus ICF is, in effect, a potential bridge, not merely between indicators and data sources—which is, in practical terms, an essential facilitator of a scientifically respectable monitoring process—but also a bridge between scientific values and the political and social values expressed in the rights in the CRPD. (p. 7)

Learning Point 2.17   How does the ICF bridge clinical and ethical values?

These observations provide an indication that the ICF might be used effectively for common discussion of interprofessional rehabilitation ethical issues, especially in light of on-going criticisms of the medical model and evidence suggesting lack of integration into medicine. In this text, use of the ICF framework is suggested as another way to create common ground for interprofessional education and interprofessional practice dialogue.

Learning Point 2.18   How can the ICF serve as a common ground for interprofessional education and ethics?

In spite of the apparent widespread acceptance of the ICF model, rehabilitation professionals should be aware of on-going debates by a variety of stakeholders regarding its underlying social model of disability (Anastasiou & Kauffman, 2013; Edwards, 2008; Llewellyn & Hogan, 2000; Masala & Petretto, 2008; Riddle, 2013; Shakespeare, 2006). Some academics have been critical of the social model interpreted as a social constructivist model, or structuralist model, that attributes disability only to social structures, and others have questioned the long-term consequences and continued resiliency of the social model (Gabel & Peters, 2004; Shakespeare, 2006). Although the ICF model appears to explicitly endorse an interactionist model that blends medical and social origins, these criticisms also reveal that the social model of disability may also have limitations. Thus, divisions between academics, healthcare providers, and people with disability continue to mark social action and disability scholarship. The slogan "Nothing About Us Without Us", first coined in 1993, captures the perception of disempowerment, exclusion, and loss of voice experienced by people with disabilities (Charlton, 1998, p. 3; Franits, 2005). This divide has moral and ethical significance, and speaks to the need for enhanced inclusion, partnerships, research, and careful attention to the experience of persons with disabilities. Based on the history of the rehabilitation professions, one could argue that our professional identity must include a moral commitment to those with disabilities to enhance function, the process of habilitation, access, and empowering the voice of persons with disability.

Learning Point 2.19   What are the limitations of the social model of disability?

Learning Point 2.20   What does the phrase, "Nothing About Us Without Us" encapsulate?

In addition to the differences in clinical perspective discussed earlier, each member of the team brings different individual values and perspectives. Ethics is not only about what one does but also about the character of the person who will

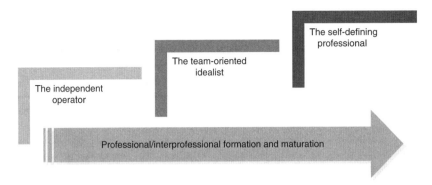

FIGURE 2.3 Professional/interprofessional identity formation and development.
Based on Kegan (1982); Bebeau & Lewis (2003); Bebeau & Monson (2012).

act. The virtue ethical tradition has focused extensively on character development and the development of habits of virtue. Development of virtues and becoming an effective moral agent are all part of the development of a personal, professional, and interprofessional identity grounded in ethical values. Many professions also have adopted core values that serve like core virtues when cultivated in daily practice. Ethical decisions and actions emanate from a continuously developing sense of self. Overlapping personal, professional, and interprofessional identities come together in self-identity. This sense of self changes and grows over your professional lifetime. In *The Evolving Self* Kegan (1982) examined the developmental process of identity formation. Bebeau and Lewis (2003) and Bebeau and Monson (2012) applied Kegan's developmental framework to professional identity formation, suggesting that professional identity matures from the independent operator to team-oriented idealist to self-defining professional (**FIGURE 2.3**).

Learning Point 2.21   If you are a student in a health professions educational program, please locate your relevant Code of Ethics and core values of professionalism for your field.

This framework has implications for professional education in that it suggests that professional students may not be ready for interprofessional team collaboration in the earliest phases of professional education. The task of attending to the dual identity as a professional and member of interprofessional team (Khalili, Orchard, Laschinger, & Farah, 2013) is an important dimension of interprofessional ethics as these ethical obligations may at times conflict.

Learning Point 2.22   Why do you think it may be hard for students to come to terms with interprofessional education early in their professional educational career?

▶ Elements of the Moral Commons: Context (Situation and Realms)

The third element of the moral commons involves consideration of context. The context of ethical situations may be complex and incorporates personal, interpersonal, family, organizational, political, social, professional, reimbursement, and cultural issues. Due to the complexity of ethical issues, it can be helpful to identify, classify, or "diagnose" the type of ethical situation to identify an appropriate response. Purtilo and Doherty (2011) and Kidder (1995) distinguish different types of ethical situations. **TABLE 2.3** is based, in part, on their descriptions and provides implications for moral agency for different ethical situations.

Ethical situation types may not be entirely distinct from each other. For example, moral silence may result in moral distress as one analyzes the source of silence. Prolonged moral distress may become "moral residue."

Moral distress may be especially relevant to interprofessional ethics (Jameton, 2017). Team conflict and hierarchical power differentials are frequent sources of moral distress to which nurses and rehabilitation providers may be especially vulnerable. These dynamics are amplified by reimbursement pressures and the ethical climate of the healthcare institution. Additionally, the close work of rehabilitation teamwork may actually discourage team members from voicing ethical

TABLE 2.3 Ethical Situation and Implications for Moral Agency

Type of Issue	Description	Implications for Moral Agency
Ambiguity or uncertainty	Circumstances or facts surrounding the situation are not clear enough to provide a definitive indication as to the nature of the ethical situation. Uncertainty may also arise with regard to your own values.	Clarify facts, deliberate with mentors to provide clarification and moral discernment.
Issue/problem	Important ethical or moral values present or challenged. Typically, broad concepts such as "technology at end of life: or "social media."	Requires further moral discussion and deliberation to specify or delineate future action.
Dilemma	Poses a choice between two important but competing duties, obligations or values. It is not possible to fulfill both duties or values. Kidder describes this as a "right versus right" situation, contrasting it to a "right versus wrong: situation." An example of ethical dilemma that has been extensively discussed in medical ethics is autonomy and beneficence.	Engage in extensive moral judgment. Consider how specific contextual factors, different ethical traditions, and personal factors may influence. Kidder recommends exploring alternatives that may honor both duties ("trilemma" options). Consult the ethics literature on the dilemma.

Distress	Ethical or moral distress occurs when a person is unable to address an ethical situation due to internal or external constraints (Jameton, 2017). Organizational and interprofessional hierarchy are important sources of moral distress. The inability to act in response to ethical situations may leave "moral residue" (Epstein & Hamric, 2009; Hardingham, 2004) and is a potential source of professional burnout. Some describe one source of moral distress as "constrained practice" (Carse, 2013; Nalette, 2010; Oh & Gastmans, 2015).	Weigh alternatives and consequences. Is it truly the case that you are unable to act? Confer with others who share your beliefs. Collective interprofessional action may be more effective and incur fewer consequences. Discuss potential actions with a trusted mentor. For very serious situations, may consider whistleblower options.
Temptation	A situation in which one of the alternative courses of action is unethical, inappropriate, or illegal. Kidder describes this as a "right versus wrong" situation. In many cases, choosing the "wrong" course of action will benefit self-interest.	Develop a plan to act with moral courage. Identify the barriers to acting ethically and the long-term consequences of unethical actions.
Silence	Important ethical values or principles are challenged, but nobody is speaking.	Develop a plan to act for moral courage and break the silence. Work with others to identify the most appropriate forum for speaking out.

Based on Kidder (1995); Purtilo & Doherty (2011).

disagreement due to a concern that this may result in team conflict or isolation from the team (Austin, 2016). Noting that healthcare organizations are "moral communities," Austin (2016) urges healthcare practitioners to attend to organizational ethics and the environment: "Empowerment for ethical practice can be supported by the encouragement of inter-professional contributions to ethical decision making and by ensuring opportunities for the processing of difficult care situations (eg, formal/informal ethics debriefing, ethics consultations, ethics committees) and for ethics education (e.g., ethics rounds to learn from cases, ethics training)" (Austin, p. 132). She encourages healthcare leaders and managers to discuss sources of moral distress with front-line practitioners.

Another contextual consideration is the "realm" of action. Glaser's description of three realms of human dignity and ethical action is helpful when thinking about the dimensions of moral agency necessary in different settings. He describes three realms (individual, organizational/institutional, and societal (1994; 2005), with the complexity of moral agency increasing from the individual realm through the organizational and societal levels. Each realm focuses on different aspects of moral agency (**FIGURE 2.4**). For example, the individual realm focuses on the duties and rights of individuals and in interpersonal relationships. Within the organizational realm, fair policies and processes are critical. The societal realm embraces social systems and policies. Each of the realms should be considered in an ethical matter, but in some cases one realm may be most important, and realms may not compensate for deficits in another realm. Glaser also referred to an emerging fourth realm of human dignity: the global realm. While the global realm may not be relevant to every ethical problem, global and international considerations have increasing importance. Glaser points out that ethical problems invariably have dimensions from each realm. Although some problems may have a critical or "cardinal" realm, it is important to recognize all three realms in each ethical problem. Professional ethics education has traditionally emphasized interpersonal ethics, and many professionals are less comfortable with organizational and social realm ethics.

Learning Point 2.23   Why does the complexity of moral agency increase when going from individual to societal levels?

Learning Point 2.24   What ethical issues are raised in each of the three realms for the issue of informed consent and health case access?

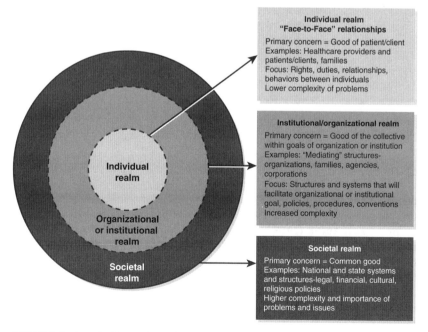

FIGURE 2.4 Realms of ethics and moral agency.
Based on Glaser (1991).

Effective moral agency by groups, or teams may involve different types of skills than skills for individual action. While direct communication is often the most effective skill for interpersonal issues, effective moral agency may require team collaboration (organizational realm) or policy-making (societal realm) in collective settings.

> **Learning Point 2.25**   Why is moral agency by a group different than that of an individual?

The Realm Individual Process Situation (RIPS) Model (Swisher, Arslanian, & Davis, 2005) is one example of an ethical decision-making model that incorporates ethical traditions, types of ethical situations and realm. The purpose of the RIPS framework is to expand the focus of decision-making steps beyond moral judgments, principles, ethical dilemmas, and the individual realm. The underlying premise of the framework is that many ethical decision-making models narrowly focus on ethical dilemmas requiring moral judgment in the individual realm. This focus is in contrast to the reality that rehabilitation professionals work on teams within complex organizations in which only a limited number of situations are true ethical dilemmas.

▶ Ethical Issues in Rehabilitation

Consistent with the emerging status of interprofessional ethics and the developing area of rehabilitation described in the last chapter, it is not surprising that there are few resources that explicitly address ethical issues in rehabilitation from an interprofessional perspective. That is, scant literature exists that is written by rehabilitation team members from an explicitly interprofessional perspective addressing ethical issues shared by the team. Many more resources, however, are written from a uniprofessional perspective and discuss the interprofessional implications of ethical issues encountered in rehabilitation practice.

Professionals are in constant dialogue relating professional, interprofessional, team-based, and personal aspects of their experience with practice. This section delineates some of the ethical issues experienced by rehabilitation professionals. The overall goal is to familiarize healthcare professionals with common ethical issues in rehabilitation in order to facilitate the ability to recognize issues (moral sensitivity) and to make decisions about common situations (moral judgments). In chapter 1, we addressed the fact that rehabilitation is a process and approach, thus broadening the possible members of the interprofessional team. It is not possible for us to include every discipline and professional perspective in this text. For the purposes of this text, we will focus on case examples drawn from medicine, nursing, occupational therapy, pharmacy, speech language pathology, physical therapy, psychology, rehabilitation counseling, and social work.

> **Learning Point 2.26**   What is the difference between moral sensitivity and moral agency?

One of the few studies of ethical issues in rehabilitation was performed by Kirschner, Stocking, Wagner, Foye, and Siegler (2002; 2001). The authors analyzed ethical issues encountered by clinicians and admitting staff in an urban inpatient rehabilitation setting. Practicing clinicians and admitting staff were asked to provide three ethical issues from practice. The authors' analysis of the survey responses generated 15 categories of ethical issues generated by the rehabilitation team. **FIGURE 2.5** summarizes the ethical issues found from this study, subthemes, and related ethical issues from other research literature.

ETHICAL ISSUES

1. Reimbursement Issues
    - Policy and regulatory constraints
    - Critique of care driven by reimbursement models
    - Length of stay determination

2. Goal Setting Conflicts (between team members, family members, and caregivers)
    - Goal Setting Process
    - Team Models and Process
    - Conflict and disagreement
    - Predicting Risk and Harm
    - Unclear prognosis a challenge for goal-setting

3. Decision-Making Capacity/Informed Consent
    - Autonomy – Interdependent, relational, and changing autonomy
    - Shared Decision Making
    - Adherence

4. Confidentiality (Team knowledge of criminal or dangerous patient behavior)
    - Reporting impaired driving

5. End-of-Life Issues (Advance Directives. Withholding intervention, do not resuscitate orders)
    - Unique perspectives of people with disabilities
    - Request to forego treatment perceived as devaluing life for people with disabilities
    - Utilitarian argument by Singer – some with disabilities may be declared "non-persons"

6. Discharge Planning (Unsafe, suboptimal, refused, or potentially abusive situation)
    - Balancing safety with patient values
    - Institutional constraints on continuing rehabilitation care

7. Quality of Life related to dysphagia
    - Refusal of treatment

8. Patient autonomy limits – requesting additional services
    - "Difficult Patient or Family"
    - Challenging Patients

9. Veracity regarding prognosis or treatment effectiveness
    - Evidence Based Practice
    - Deception for good ends

10. Personal/Professional Boundaries
    - Use of social media

FIGURE 2.5 Ethical issues in rehabilitation.
Based on Kirschner, Stocking, Wagner, Foye, & Siegler (2001).

The issues generated by the practitioners in this study provide valuable information about ethical issues in the inpatient rehabilitation clinical setting. As indicated by Figure 2.5, daily ethical issues in this setting include reimbursement, discharge planning, establishing goals, conflict between team members, truth-telling with patients, and maintaining appropriate boundaries. While the Kirschner et al. study provides a good indicator of some major categories of ethical issues in this rehabilitation setting, a number of ethical issues represented in the literature were not represented. For example, the ethical issues presented are not representative of those found in other settings, such as home health, outpatient, private practice, sub-acute, skilled nursing, sports, or settings that primarily serve children or adolescents.

> **Learning Point 2.27** Envision examples of ethical issues you may have seen similar to those delineated in Figure 2.5.

> **Learning Point 2.28** What other ethical issues would you add to those in Figure 2.5 to be more representative of all rehabilitation settings and across the lifespan?

Although this discussion of the literature falls short of a systematic and comprehensive literature review, it does provide some insight into the general nature of ethical issues in rehabilitation. Not surprisingly, many of the ethical issues focus on relationships with other team members, the patient, and family members. While some of the earliest literature focused on the unique nature of rehabilitation as contrasted to medical ethics, later literature appears to establish a more complete theoretical basis for rehabilitation ethics. It is clear that there is a need for further research to explore the many settings in which rehabilitation occurs. Much of the literature discusses conflicts within the team, with little research into the ethical dimensions of positive teamwork and the team as moral community. An apparent trend within the rehabilitation ethics literature has been a growing awareness of the need to involve the patient and family as full partners. This trend is reflected in the early process-oriented focus on informed consent to the more recent discussion of shared decision making (Elwyn et al., 2012; Kaizer, Spiridigliozzi, & Hunt, 2012), and is consistent with enhanced understanding of the ethical underpinnings of rehabilitation practice. This focus on patient and family centered care was paralleled by a focus on evidence-based practice (Rochette et al., 2014). At the same time, rehabilitation has been moving away from its focus on acute care, turning away from paternalism, and listening more carefully to patient voices (Kuczewski & Fiedler, 2001). In retrospect, one might see a young discipline attempting to establish its unique identity, develop theoretical underpinnings, and embrace strong core ethical values to support future development. Additional research is needed to assist rehabilitation professionals in order to identify and address the variety of ethical issues encountered in practice, education, and research. It is especially important to address the ethical dimensions of teamwork and interprofessional relationships.

> **Learning Point 2.29** Where should a discussion about informed consent with a patient take place?

> **Learning Point 2.30** How do rehabilitation teams engage in informed consent and shared decision making?

▶ The Organizational and Team Context for Interprofessional Rehabilitation Ethics

An understanding of the "gestalt" of the ethics environment in any setting or context is critical to approaching specific ethical issues in rehabilitation ethics because the organizational context inevitably shapes a professional's experience of ethical issues. **FIGURE 2.6** illustrates contributors to the environment and overlapping ethical spheres that contribute to the professional and interprofessional ethical perspectives and identities of healthcare professionals.

Figure 2.6 reveals a myriad of contributors to the gestalt of the ethics setting. Each of these contributors should be considered or analyzed in order to fully appreciate an ethical situation. Many sources contribute to the ethical environment for rehabilitation professionals' ethical thinking and action. The actual sphere of explicitly interprofessional rehabilitation ethics literature may be small at this stage in the evolution of interprofessional ethics, but many other sources are also relevant to interprofessional rehabilitation ethics. For example, ethical concepts such as informed consent, confidentiality, evidence-based practice, veracity, patient autonomy, moral reasoning, and decision making transcend professional boundaries even though these concepts may be applied or encountered differently by different professionals in different settings.

Organizational and team (or sub-unit) ethics are contributors to the ethical environment (see Figure 2.4). Organizational and team culture (Leape et al., 2012; Lind, Kaltiala-Heino, Suominen, Leino-Kilpi, & Valimaki, 2004; Nelson, Taylor, & Walsh, 2014; O'Donnell et al., 2008; Reiser, 1994; Walsh-Bowers, Rossiter, & Prilleltensky, 1996) play an important role in shaping healthcare professional's

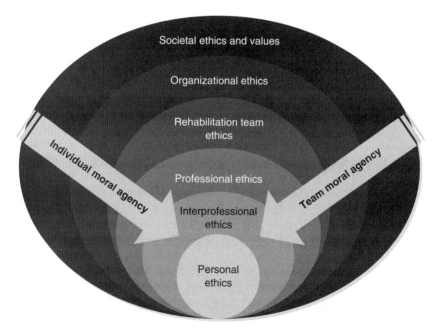

FIGURE 2.6 Environment of interprofessional rehabilitation ethics.

ethical values and behavior; indeed organizational and team values may at times "trump" professional and personal values in daily practice. The terms "organizational culture" and "team culture" refer to the implicit and explicit values, assumptions, and priorities that shape decision making, expectations, and behavior for the organization and team members. Most healthcare organizations have a mission statement that articulates the explicit values of the organization, and these are generally congruent with professional codes of ethics that focus on the patient's interest, professional behavior, and accountability to meet the needs of society.

Learning Point 2.31 How might organizational and/or team ethics be identical or different?

The implicit or hidden culture of the team or organization, however, may differ markedly from the publicly espoused values of that group. Current organizational concerns about the increasing cost of health care and declining reimbursement produce fiscal constraints that contribute to healthcare environments, which may subvert personal values, professional obligations, or mission statements. To illustrate, organizational and team cultures may also incorporate other positive or negative values (for example, excellence, research, power and hierarchy, gender or racial bias, and other biases). Organizational and team cultures may create barriers for interprofessional collaborative practice by reinforcing medical centric practice and perpetuating power differentials between professionals.

Learning Point 2.32 Can you give an example of a power differential between professionals?

Organizational culture and team culture are especially important contributors to interprofessional rehabilitation ethics for the following reasons:

1. **Emphasis on the need for teamwork:** Interprofessional rehabilitation ethics takes place in collective settings where team and organizational dynamics are critical to success of the team.
2. **Unresolved issues of power and hierarchy:** Issues of power and hierarchy constitute one the most difficult issues in interprofessional collaboration because of the longstanding power and status given to physicians. True interprofessional collaborative practice implies a team constituted by moral equals, with leadership assumed by different team members for different patient goals. Although most professional education currently requires interprofessional education, healthcare organizations and systems have not yet incorporated the collaborative values and commitments of interprofessional collaboration being implemented in academic education. For example, issues of power may become a moral issue when rehabilitation professions are "ordered" (by a clinical or administrative superior) to act in manner that is inconsistent with professional values and duties.
3. **Enhanced scope of practice for rehabilitation professionals:** Educational requirements for many rehabilitation professions now require or endorse doctoral education, and state practice acts have generally

broadened the scope of practice for many rehabilitation professions. Engel and Prentice (2013) describe the tension in interprofessional education that arises from encouraging students to work at the fullest limits of their education and legal scope of practice and competition between team members arising from overlapping areas of practice (p. 427). This tension is further exacerbated by political turf wars among professions regarding practice act legislation.

4.   **Changes in payment models within the U.S. healthcare system are facilitating integrated care systems and scrutiny of outcomes that require interprofessional teamwork and collaboration:** Changes in the healthcare system will emphasize reduction in cost and increased value in efficiency and collaboration.

5.   **Limited attention to the collective aspects of ethics:** Ethics literature in healthcare has emphasized individual ethical decision making and there is limited information about team and organizational decision making.

Learning Point 2.33   What are organizational dynamics?

Learning Point 2.34   How can power and hierarchy contribute to moral distress?

Learning Point 2.35   Refer to your state practice act if you are in professional education.

Due to the increasing emphasis on team and collaborative processes rehabilitation, professionals should be aware of team problems, dysfunctional processes, and malfunction that may occur in collective decision making. Janis (1972) was one of the first to discuss the effect of group dysfunction on collective decision making, attributing major political mistakes (such as the Bay of Pigs) to a faulty group decision-making process he called "groupthink." Groupthink involves an abnormal drive for group consensus that causes group members to ignore possible alternatives and express unanimity rather than engaging in critical problem-solving. Groupthink has been cited as the cause for other flawed decisions such as in the cases of Watergate, Challenger, and Enron (Hart, 1991), but there are other types of problems that groups may exhibit. For example, Whyte (1989) indicates that group polarization (a process where group discussion causes members to accept more extreme positions and greater risk) is a description for group processes leading to the Challenger event. The fatal launch of the Challenger has been extensively studied with various interpretations of the problems in decision making that resulted in the shuttle being launched against the recommendations of the engineers (McDonald, 2012; Vaughan, 1996; Werhane, 1991). Based upon these two examples, it is clear that collective decision making provides challenges to ethical decision making. For that reason, it is important that rehabilitation professions consider organizational and team culture, address organizational and team realms when responding to ethical issues, and collaborate with others in developing the moral agency of teams and organizations in which they work. Organizational and team environment are important in the work of professionals, having the potential to undermine professional and ethical goals of team members.

Moral distress is an individual response to organizational or other constraints on moral agency. While nursing was the first to examine moral distress, there are numerous studies of moral distress in many other disciplines demonstrating that the experience is not confined to nursing (Allen et al., 2013; Penny, Ewing, Hamid, Shutt, & Walter, 2014; Whitehead, Herbertson, Hamric, Epstein, & Fisher, 2015). Moral distress may occur when organizational or team culture create a situation where professionals feel unable to act in an ethical manner due to external or internal barriers (Brazil, Kassalainen, Ploeg, & Marshall, 2010; Carpenter, 2010; Hardingham, 2004; Kalvemark, Hoglund, Hansson, Westerholm, & Arnetz, 2004; Mukherjee, Brashler, Savage, & Kirschner, 2009). Moral distress has been associated with burnout, decreased employee retention, demoralization, frustration, anger, and other negative effects. These negative effects may persist over time, creating long-term problems (moral residue) (Shakespeare, 2006).

Learning Point 2.36 Why are there emotional outcomes from moral distress?

In spite of the widespread acceptance of moral distress, recent scholarship has been critical of the lack of clarity of the concept and of the quality of research about moral distress (Johnstone & Hutchinson, 2015). Thomas and McCullough (2015) attempted to clarify moral distress by developing a philosophical taxonomy. They note that the two primary components of moral distress are:

1. Professional and individual integrity
2. Impediments to acting on professional or individual integrity: challenges, threats, or violations (p. 113)

Others have urged greater consideration of the role of interprofessional organizations and teams in attending to relationships, as well as the implications for interprofessional teams. Pavlish, Brown-Saltzman, Fine, and Jakel's (2015) qualitative study of moral distress among oncology nurses found a "culture of avoidance" associated with remaining silent, and they encouraged proactive measures to address the system. Some commentators note that ethical disagreements between members of the team are inevitable, and urge attention to "preventative education" or proactive ethics in resolving and preventing ethical conflicts (Johnstone & Hutchinson, 2015). The same authors (2015) question whether the notion of moral distress serves to reinforce powerlessness and sanctions the lack of moral agency represented by silence, calling for a moratorium on the use of the term. Another perspective urges that we pay more attention to the socio-political roots of moral distress from a structural viewpoint (McCarthy & Gastmans, 2015; Varcoe, Pauly, Webster, & Storch, 2012) through examination of the effect of resource scarcity, power differentials, and systemic toxic effects. Austin (2012, p. 36) describes the problem of moral distress as the "ethical canary" in the mine, indicating the need for further analysis of the "habitability" (Vanderheide, Moss, & Lee, 2013) of the healthcare workplace.

Learning Point 2.37 Have you ever experienced moral distress? If so, where and why?

In summary, organizational and team culture shape the professional expectations for team members, professionals, and staff in both positive and negative ways. The fact that moral distress has been found to exist across disciplines indicates the need for further attention to organizational contexts for interprofessional care. Pavlish, Brown-Saltzman, Jakel, and Fine (2014) remind us that teams and organizations represent a kind of moral community, providing the following ideal characteristics of moral community:

1. Open, respectful team relationships
2. Processes for timely, honest, planned communication
3. Accessible, strong, ethics-minded leadership
4. Routine, readily available, system-wide ethics resources
5. Provider awareness and willingness to use ethics resources (pp. 134–135)

These five characteristics provide reference points for rehabilitation professionals in evaluating their organization and team. Rehabilitation professionals should be aware of the culture in which they work and have the ability to participate in and shape organizational and team cultures, and they should be aware of resources (for example, ethics consultation) available for individuals who experience moral distress. Moral distress should trigger further evaluation of the individual, the team, the organization, and the larger environment. It is especially important for rehabilitation professionals to appreciate the way in which the prevailing culture may systematically affect ethical decisions. Additionally, rehabilitation professionals should look beyond their own professional organizations to consider the effect of the socio-political environment on healthcare delivery.

> **Learning Point 2.38**   Is there any avenue for an ethics consultation in your institution if you are experiencing moral distress? If not, should there be?

These observations about organizational and team culture are excellent reminders of the discussion of moral agency in the last chapter. Recall that the concept of moral agency refers not only to individuals but also to collectivities such as the organization and the team. The problem of moral distress highlights that both the individual and team moral agency must be cultivated simultaneously. As the field of interprofessional ethics emerges, further research is needed to determine ways to foster the moral agency of rehabilitation teams and organizations.

▶ Summary and Conclusion

An understanding of the historical, social, clinical, and organizational context of rehabilitation is critical for interprofessional rehabilitation ethics. The views of patients, clients, and families who are served by rehabilitation providers should be heard and valued across the elements of the moral commons, and the clinical context of rehabilitation. This chapter provided a historical overview of the development of rehabilitation, a view of the unique clinical environment of rehabilitation, discussion of ethical issues encountered in rehabilitation practice, and the relationship between clinical and ethical issues. The chapter concluded by identifying the influence of organizational and team culture in shaping ethical environments and related implications for individual and team moral agency enacted within the moral commons.

Closing Reflections

Learning Activities

2.1 **Analysis of Historical Roots**: Explain the historical roots of rehabilitation.

2.2 **Tension Between Professional Identity and Interprofessional Collaboration**: Why is there a tension between professional identity and interprofessional collaboration?

2.3 **Ethical Traditions**: Contrast the four ethical traditions described in Chapter 2.

2.4 **International Classification of Disability, Health, and Functioning (ICF)**: How does the ICF lend itself to rehabilitation ethics?

2.5 **Models of disability**: Discuss various models of disability and identify the one that you like best and explain your rationale.

2.6 **Identity**: What is the role of identity (personal and professional) in the moral commons?

2.7 **Context and Realms**: What is the role of context and realms in the moral commons?

2.8 **Ethical Issues in Rehabilitation**: In addition to the ethical issues identified in this chapter from research by Kirschner et al. (2001), speculate as to other areas of rehabilitation in which ethical issues may, or are likely to, occur.

2.9 **Ethics as Discipline**: Is rehabilitation ethics an emerging new field or an expansion of ethics in general? Team with a classmate and debate these two points.

2.10 **Collective Decision Making**: What aspects of group behavior and interaction may negatively affect decision making of that group and why?

2.11 **Moral Distress**: How can moral distress be prevented or addressed?

2.12 **Moral Community**: How would you construct or design a moral community?

Take Away Messages

Reflecting on Organizational Ethics and Culture

- Consult on-line resources and your library to identify cases in organizational ethics about the Challenger disaster.
- How would you define the term organizational ethics?
- If you were a member of the engineering team, would you have recommended for or against the launch in light of your knowledge about the O-rings and the projected low temperatures?
- The Challenger disaster has been extensively studied as an example of organizational dysfunction and associated ethical concerns. A number of people have discussed the Challenger disaster as an example of Groupthink. Locate additional resources about the Challenger and Groupthink. Do you think that the organizations involved (NASA and Morton Thiokol) exhibited the eight symptoms identified by Janis (1972)
  1. Illusion of invulnerability
  2. Rationalizations

3. Inherent morality of the group
4. Stereotypes
5. Pressure to conform
6. Self-censorship
7. Unanimity
8. Mindguards

- During the teleconference between the engineers and the administrators, the managers asked the engineers to "take off their engineer's hat." Is this appropriate from an ethical standpoint?

- During congressional hearings after the Challenger exploded, the engineers realized that the astronauts had not been informed of the on-going problems with O-ring sealing and erosion. Should the astronauts have been informed of the risks? If so, who within the organization should have informed the astronauts?

- Were the conclusions of the Rogers Commission correct regarding the cause of the shuttle accident?

- Both Roger Boisjoly and Allan McDonald from Thiokol were whistleblowers although they did so in very different ways. How should one decide when it is right to be a whistleblower?

- The Healthsouth scandal involved a rehabilitation company. Use on-line resources to learn more about the Healthsouth scandal. What can we learn about organizational ethics in health care from the Challenger disaster and the Healthsouth scandal?

References

Allan, C. M., Campbell, W. N., Guptill, C. A., Stephenson, F. F., & Campbell, K. E. (2006). A conceptual model for interprofessional education: The international classification of functioning, disability and health (ICF). *Journal of Interprofessional Care, 20*(3), 235–245. doi:10.1080/13561820600718139

Allen, R., Judkins-Cohn, T., deVelasco, R., Forges, E., Lee, R., Clark, L., & Procunier, M. (2013). Moral distress among healthcare professionals at a health system. *JONA'S Healthcare Law Ethics and Regulation, 15*(3), 111–118. http://dx.doi.org/10.1097/NHL.0b013e3182a1bf33

Anastasiou, D., & Kauffman, J. M. (2013). The social model of disability: Dichotomy between impairment and disability. *Journal of Medicine and Philosophy, 38*(4), 441–459. doi:10.1093/jmp/jht026

Austin, W. (2012). Moral distress and the contemporary plight of health professionals. *HEC Forum, 24*(1), 27–38. doi:10.1007/s10730-012-9179-8

Austin, W. (2016). Contemporary healthcare practice and the risk of moral distress. *Healthcare Management Forum, 29*(3), 131–133. doi:10.1177/0840470416637835

Beauchamp, T. L. (1995). Principlism and its alleged competitors. *Kennedy Institute of Ethics Journal, 5*(3), 181–198.

Beauchamp, T. L., & Childress, J. F. (2009). *Principles of biomedical ethics* (6th ed.). New York, N.Y.: Oxford University Press.

Bebeau, M., & Lewis, P. (2003). *Manual for assessing and promoting identity formation.* Minneapolis, MN: Center for the Study of Ethical Development.

Bebeau, M. J., & Monson, V. E. (2012). Professional identity formation and transformation across the life span. In A. Mc Kee & M. Eraut (Eds.), *Learning trajectories, innovation and identity for professional development* (pp. 135–162). Dordrecht, Holland: Springer.

Bickenbach, J. E. (2011). Monitoring the United Nation's Convention on the Rights of Persons with Disabilities: Data and the International Classification of Functioning, Disability and Health. *BMC Public Health, 11 Suppl 4,* S8. doi:10.1186/1471-2458-11-S4-S8

Brazil, K., Kassalainen, S., Ploeg, J., & Marshall, D. (2010). Moral distress experienced by health care professionals who provide home-based palliative care. *Social Science & Medicine, 71*(9), 1687–1691. doi:10.1016/j.socscimed.2010.07.032

Carpenter, C. (2010). Moral distress in physical therapy practice. *Physiotherapy Theory and Practice, 26*(2), 69–78. doi:10.3109/09593980903387878

Carse, A. (2013). Moral distress and moral disempowerment. *Narrative Inquiry in Bioethics, 3*(2), 147–151.

Charlton, J. I. (1998). *Nothing about us without us: Disability oppression and empowerment*. Berkeley, CA: University of California Press.

Clouser, K. D., & Gert, B. (1990). A critique of principlism. *Journal of Medicine and Philosophy, 15*(2), 219–236.

Cruess, R. L., Cruess, S. R., Boudreau, J. D., Snell, L., & Steinert, Y. (2014). Reframing medical education to support professional identity formation. *Academic Medicine, 89*(11), 1446–1451. doi:10.1097/acm.0000000000000427

D'Amour, D., Ferrada-Videla, M., San Martin Rodriguez, L., & Beaulieu, M. D. (2005). The conceptual basis for interprofessional collaboration: core concepts and theoretical frameworks. *Journal of Interprofessional Care, 19*(Suppl 1), 116–131. doi:10.1080/13561820500082529

Davis, R. B. (1995). The principlism debate: A critical overview. *Journal of Medicine and Philosophy, 20*(1), 85–105.

Edwards, S. D. (2008). The impairment/disability distinction: A response to Shakespeare. *Journal of Medical Ethics, 34*(1), 26–27. doi:10.1136/jme.2006.019950

Eldar, R., & Jelić, M. (2003). The association of rehabilitation and war. *Disability & Rehabilitation, 25*(18), 1019–1023. doi:10.1080/0963828031000137739

Elwyn, G., Frosch, D., Thomson, R., Joseph-Williams, N., Lloyd, A., & Kinnersley, P. (2012). Shared decision making: A model for clinical practice. *Journal of General Internal Medicine, 27*. doi:10.1007/s11606-012-2077-6

Engel, G. L. (1977). The need for a new medical model: A challenge for biomedicine. *Science, 196*(4286), 129–136.

Engel, G. L. (1981). The clinical application of the biopsychosocial model. *Journal of Medicine and Philosophy, 6*(2), 101–124. doi:10.1093/jmp/6.2.101

Engel, J., & Prentice, D. (2013). The ethics of interprofessional collaboration. *Nursing Ethics, 20*(4), 426–435. doi:10.1177/0969733012468466

Epstein, E. G., & Hamric, A. B. (2009). Moral distress, moral residue, and the crescendo effect. *Journal of Clinical Ethics, 20*(4), 330–342.

Foye, S. J., Kirschner, K. L., Wagner, L. C. B., Stocking, C., & Siegler, M. (2002). Ethics in practice. Ethical issues in rehabilitation: A qualitative analysis of dilemmas identified by occupational therapists. *Topics in Stroke Rehabilitation, 9*(3), 89–101.

Franits, L. E. (2005). Nothing about us without us: Searching for the narrative of disability. *American Journal of Occupational Therapy, 59*(5), 577–579.

Gabel, S., & Peters, S. (2004). Presage of a paradigm shift? Beyond the social model of disability toward resistance theories of disability. *Disability & Society, 19*(6), 585–600. doi:10.1080/0968759042000252515

Giacomini, M., Kenny, N., & DeJean, D. (2009). Ethics frameworks in Canadian health policies: Foundation, scaffolding, or window dressing? *Health Policy, 89*(1), 58–71. doi:10.1016/j.healthpol.2008.04.010

Glaser, J. (1994). *Three realms of ethics*. Kansas City, MO: Rowan and Littlefield.

Glaser, J. (2005). Three realms of ethics: an integrating map of ethics for the future. In R. Purtilo (Ed), *Educating for moral action: A sourcebook in health and rehabilitation ethics* (pp. 169–184). Philadelphia, PA: FA Davis Co.

Gurley, J. M., Hujsak, B. D., & Kelly, J. L. (2013). Vestibular rehabilitation following mild traumatic brain injury. *Neuro Rehabilitation, 32*(3), 519–528. doi:10.3233/nre-130874

Hardingham, L. B. (2004). Integrity and moral residue: nurses as participants in a moral community. *Nursing Philosophy, 5*(2), 127–134. doi:10.1111/j.1466-769X.2004.00160.x

Hart, P. T. (1991). Irving L. Janis' Victims of Groupthink. *Political Psychology, 12*(2), 247–278. doi:10.2307/3791464

Harty, M., Griesel, M., & van der Merwe, A. (2011). The ICF as a common language for rehabilitation goal-setting: Comparing client and professional priorities. *Health and Quality of Life Outcomes, 9*, 87. doi:10.1186/1477-7525-9-87

Huber, J. G., Sillick, J., & Skarakis-Doyle, E. (2010). Personal perception and personal factors: Incorporating health-related quality of life into the International Classification of Functioning,

Disability and Health. *Disability and Rehabilitation, 32*(23), 1955–1965. http://dx.doi.org/10.3109/09638281003797414

Hurst, R. (2003). The International Disability Rights Movement and the ICF. *Disability and Rehabilitation, 25*(11–12), 572–576. doi:10.1080/0963828031000137072

Jameton, A. (2017). What moral distress in nursing history could suggest about the future of health care. *AMA Journal of Ethics, 19*(6), 617–628. doi:10.1001/journalofethics.2017.19.6.mhst1-1706

Janis, I. L. (1972). *Victims of groupthink: A psychological study of foreign-policy decisions and fiascoes.* Boston, MA: Houghton, Mifflin.

Johnstone, M.-J., & Hutchinson, A. (2015). 'Moral distress' – Time to abandon a flawed nursing construct? *Nursing Ethics, 22*(1), 5–14. doi:10.1177/0969733013505312

Kaizer, F., Spiridigliozzi, A.-M., & Hunt, M. (2012). Promoting shared decision-making in rehabilitation: Development of a framework for situations when patients with dysphagia refuse diet modification recommended by the treating team. *Dysphagia, 27*(1), 81–87. doi:10.1007/s00455-011-9341-5

Kalvemark, S., Hoglund, A. T., Hansson, M. G., Westerholm, P., & Arnetz, B. (2004). Living with conflicts-ethical dilemmas and moral distress in the health care system. *Social Science and Medicine, 58*(6), 1075–1084.

Kegan, R. (1982). *The evolving self.* Cambridge, MA: Harvard University Press.

Khalili, H., Orchard, C., Laschinger, H. K., & Farah, R. (2013). An interprofessional socialization framework for developing an interprofessional identity among health professions students. *Journal of Interprofessional Care, 27*(6), 448–453. doi:10.3109/13561820.2013.804042

Kidder, R. M. (1995). *How good people make tough choices: Resolving the dilemmas of ethical living.* New York, NY: Simon and Schuster.

Kirschner, K. L., Stocking, C., Wagner, L. B., Foye, S. J., & Siegler, M. (2001). Ethical issues identified by rehabilitation clinicians. *Archives of Physical Medicine & Rehabilitation, 82*(12), S2–8.

Kuczewski, M. G. (2001). Disability: An agenda for bioethics. *American Journal of Bioethics, 1*(3), 36–44. doi:10.1162/152651601750418026

Kuczewski, M. P., & Fiedler, I. P. (2001). Ethical issues in rehabilitation: Conceptualizing the next generation of challenges. *American Journal of Physical Medicine & Rehabilitation, 80*(11), 848–851.

Leape, L. L., Shore, M. F., Dienstag, J. L., Mayer, R. J., Edgman-Levitan, S., Meyer, G. S., & Healy, G. B. (2012). Perspective: A culture of respect. Part 2: Creating a culture of respect. *Academic Medicine, 87*(7), 853–858. doi:10.1097/ACM.0b013e3182583536

Lei-Rivera, L., Sutera, J., Galatioto, J. A., Hujsak, B. D., & Gurley, J. M. (2013). Special tools for the assessment of balance and dizziness in individuals with mild traumatic brain injury. *Neuro Rehabilitation, 32*(3), 463–472. doi:10.3233/nre-130869

Lind, M., Kaltiala-Heino, R., Suominen, T., Leino-Kilpi, H., & Valimaki, M. (2004). Nurses' ethical perceptions about coercion. *Journal of Psychiatric and Mental Health Nursing, 11*(4), 379–385. doi:10.1111/j.1365-2850.2004.00715.x

Linker, B. (2005). The business of ethics: Gender, medicine, and the professional codification of the American Physiotherapy Association, 1918–1935. *Journal of the History of Medicine and Allied Sciences, 60*(3), 320–354. doi:10.1093/jhmas/jri043

Llewellyn, A., & Hogan, K. (2000). The use and abuse of models of disability. *Disability & Society, 15*(1), 157–165. doi:10.1080/09687590025829

Masala, C., & Petretto, D. R. (2008). From disablement to enablement: Conceptual models of disability in the 20th century. *Disability & Rehabilitation, 30*(17), 1233–1244. doi:10.1080/09638280701602418

McCarthy, J., & Gastmans, C. (2015). Moral distress: A review of the argument-based nursing ethics literature. *Nursing Ethics, 22*(1), 131–152. doi:10.1177/0969733014557139

McDonald, A. J. (2012). *Truth, lies, and o-rings inside the space shuttle Challenger disaster.* Gainesville, FL: University Press of Florida.

Mukherjee, D., Brashler, R., Savage, T. A., & Kirschner, K. L. (2009). Moral distress in rehabilitation professionals: Results from a hospital ethics survey. *Physical Medicine and Rehabilitation, 1*(5), 450–458. doi:10.1016/j.pmrj.2009.03.004

Nalette, E. (2010). Constrained physical therapist practice: An ethical case analysis of recommending discharge placement from the acute care setting. *Physical Therapy, 90*(6), 939–952. doi:10.2522 /ptj.20050399

Nelson, W. A., Taylor, E., & Walsh, T. (2014). Building an ethical organizational culture. *Health Care Manager (Frederick), 33*(2), 158–164. http://dx.doi.org/10.1097/HCM.0000000000000008

Newell, C. (2006). Disability, bioethics, and rejected knowledge. *Journal of Medicine and Philosophy, 31*(3), 269–283. doi:10.1080/03605310600712901

O'Donnell, P., Farrar, A., Brintzenhofeszoc, K., Conrad, A. P., Danis, M., Grady, C., . . . Ulrich, C. M. (2008). Predictors of ethical stress, moral action and job satisfaction in health care social workers. *Social work in health care, 46*(3), 29–51. doi:10.1300/J010v46n03_02

Oh, Y., & Gastmans, C. (2015). Moral distress experienced by nurses: A quantitative literature review. *Nursing Ethics, 22*(1), 15–31. doi:10.1177/0969733013502803

Oliver, M. (2013). The social model of disability: Thirty years on. *Disability & Society, 28*(7), 1024–1026. doi:10.1080/09687599.2013.818773

Olkin, R. (2002). Could you hold the door for me? Including disability in diversity. *Cultural Diversity and Ethnic Minority Psychology, 8*(2), 130–137. doi:10.1037/1099-9809.8.2.130

Opitz, J. L., Folz, T. J., Gelfman, R., & Peters, D. J. (1997). The history of physical medicine and rehabilitation as recorded in the diary of Dr. Frank Krusen: Part 1. Gathering momentum (the years before 1942). *Archives of Physical Medicine and Rehabilitation, 78*(4), 442–445. http://dx .doi.org/10.1016/S0003-9993(97)90240-9

Pavlish, C., Brown-Saltzman, K., Fine, A., & Jakel, P. (2015). A culture of avoidance: Voices from inside ethically difficult clinical situations. *Clinical Journal of Oncology Nursing, 19*(2), 159–165. http://dx.doi.org/10.1188/15.CJON.19-02AP

Pavlish, C., Brown-Saltzman, K., Jakel, P., & Fine, A. (2014). The nature of ethical conflicts and the meaning of moral community in oncology practice. *Oncology Nursing Forum, 41*(2), 130–140. http://dx.doi.org/10.1188/14.ONF.130-140

Pellegrino, E. D. (1993). The metamorphosis of medical ethics. A 30-year retrospective. *Journal of the American Medical Association, 269*(9), 1158–1162.

Penny, N. H., Ewing, T. L., Hamid, R. C., Shutt, K. A., & Walter, A. S. (2014). An investigation of moral distress experienced by occupational therapists. *Occupational Therapy in Health Care, 28*(4), 382–393. doi:10.3109/07380577.2014.933380

Purtilo, R. B., & Doherty, R. F. (2011). *Ethical dimensions in the health professions* (5th ed.). St. Louis, Mo: Elsevier/Saunders.

Reiser, S. J. (1994). The ethical life of health care organizations. *Hastings Center Report, 24*(6), 28–35.

Rentsch, H. P., Bucher, P., Dommen Nyffeler, I., Wolf, C., Hefti, H., Fluri, E., . . . Boyer, I. (2003). The implementation of the 'International Classification of Functioning, Disability and Health' (ICF) in daily practice of neurorehabilitation: An interdisciplinary project at the Kantonsspital of Lucerne, Switzerland. *Disability and Rehabilitation, 25*(8), 411–421. doi:10.1080 /0963828031000069717

Riddle, C. A. (2013). Defining disability: Metaphysical not political. *Medicine Health Care and Philosophy, 16*(3), 377–384. doi:10.1007/s11019-012-9405-9

Rochette, A., Racine, E., Lefebvre, H., Lacombe, J., Bastien, J., & Tellier, M. (2014). Ethical issues relating to the inclusion of relatives as clients in the post-stroke rehabilitation process as perceived by patients, relatives and health professionals. *Patient Education and Counseling, 94*(3), 384–389. http://dx.doi.org/10.1016/j.pec.2013.10.028

Roush, S. E., & Sharby, N. (2011). Disability reconsidered: The paradox of physical therapy. *Physical Therapy, 91*(12), 1715–1727. doi:10.2522/ptj.20100389

Rusk, H. A. (1949). Rehabilitation: The third phase of medicine. *Canadian Medical Association Journal, 61*(6), 603–607.

Schiff, A., Salazar, D., Vetter, C., Andre, J., & Pinzur, M. (2014). Results of a near-peer musculoskeletal medicine curriculum for senior medical students interested in orthopedic surgery. *Journal of Surgical Education, 71*(5), 734–737. doi:10.1016/j.jsurg.2014.01.007

Scullion, P. A. (2010). Models of disability: their influence in nursing and potential role in challenging discrimination. *Journal of Advanced Nursing, 66*(3), 697–707. http://dx.doi.org/10.1111/j.1365-2648 .2009.05211.x

Shakespeare, T. (2006). *Disability rights and wrongs*. Retrieved from http://www.usf.eblib.com/patron/FullRecord.aspx?p=356014

Swisher, L. L., Arslanian, L. E., & Davis, C. M. (2005). The Realm-Individual-Process-Situation (RIPS) Model of Ethical Decision-Making. *HPA Resource, 5*(3), 1.

Thomas, T. A., & McCullough, L. B. (2015). A philosophical taxonomy of ethically significant moral distress. *Journal of Medicine and Philosophy, 40*(1), 102–120. http://dx.doi.org/10.1093/jmp/jhu048

United Nations. Convention on the Rights of Persons with Disabilities (CRPD). Retrieved from https://www.un.org/development/desa/disabilities/convention-on-the-rights-of-persons-with-disabilities.html

United Nations (2018). The United Nations and disability: 70 years of the work towards a more inclusive world. Retrieved from https://www.un.org/development/desa/disabilities/wp-content/uploads/sites/15/2018/01/History_Disability-in-the-UN_jan23.18-Clean.pdf

Vanderheide, R., Moss, C., & Lee, S. (2013). Understanding moral habitability: A framework to enhance the quality of the clinical environment as a workplace. *Contemporary Nurse, 45*(1), 101–113. doi:10.5172/conu.2013.45.1.101

Varcoe, C., Pauly, B., Webster, G., & Storch, J. (2012). Moral distress: Tensions as springboards for action. *HEC Forum, 24*(1), 51–62. doi:10.1007/s10730-012-9180-2

Vaughan, D. (1996). *The Challenger launch decision : Risky technology, culture, and deviance at NASA*. Chicago, IL: University of Chicago Press.

Walsh-Bowers, R., Rossiter, A., & Prilleltensky, I. (1996). The personal is the organizational in the ethics of hospital social workers. *Ethics & Behavior, 6*(4), 321.

Werhane, P. H. (1991). Engineers and management: The challenge of the Challenger incident. *Journal of Business Ethics, 10*(8), 605–616. doi:10.2307/25072192

Whitehead, P. B., Herbertson, R. K., Hamric, A. B., Epstein, E. G., & Fisher, J. M. (2015). Moral distress among healthcare professionals: Report of an institution-wide survey. *Journal of Nursing Scholarship, 47*(2), 117–125. doi:10.1111/jnu.12115

Whyte, G. (1989). Groupthink reconsidered. *The Academy of Management Review, 14*(1), 40–56. doi:10.2307/258190

Wikström-Grotell, C., Broberg, C., Ahonen, S., & Eriksson, K. (2013). From Ling to the academic era – An analysis of the history of ideas in PT from a Nordic perspective. *European Journal of Physiotherapy, 15*(4), 168–180. doi:10.3109/21679169.2013.833985

World Health Organization (WHO). (2001). International Classification of Functioning, Disability and Health (ICF). Retrieved from http://www.who.int/classifications/icf/icf_more/en/

Yu, T.-C., Wilson, N. C., Singh, P. P., Lemanu, D. P., Hawken, S. J., & Hill, A. G. (2011). Medical students-as-teachers: A systematic review of peer-assisted teaching during medical school. *Advances in Medical Education and Practice, 2*, 157–172. doi:10.2147/amep.s14383

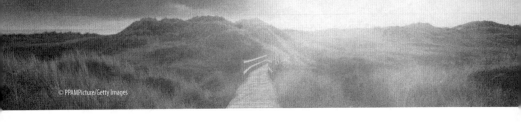

CHAPTER 3

Dialogic Engagement Model for Interprofessional Rehabilitation Ethics

Laura Lee Swisher and **Charlotte Brasic Royeen**

CHAPTER OUTLINE

- Chapter Overview
- Ethical Theories and Decision-Making Frameworks: The Challenge of Ethical Terminology
- Ethical Pluralism
- Practical Focus
- Ethical Traditions
- Models of Interprofessional Ethical Decision Making for Rehabilitation
- The Dialogic Engagement Model
- Application of the Dialogic Engagement Model
- Summary and Conclusion

CHAPTER OBJECTIVES

At the conclusion of this chapter, the reader will be able to:

1. Distinguish the purposes of ethical *theories* from ethical decision-making frameworks.
2. Provide a rationale for each of the elements of the Dialogic Engagement Model from an interprofessional perspective.
3. Describe the Dialogic Engagement Model as both ethical decision-making framework and process for interprofessional ethical deliberation.
4. Analyze each of the elements of the moral commons related to individual and team moral agency.

(continues)

KEY TERMS

Reading these key terms before reading the chapter will introduce you to key concepts which will then be somewhat familiar to you as you read this chapter. This is an important learning technique that will enhance your learning as a multi-step process. You may even wish to make a flash card set of key terms and quiz yourself on them once or twice before reading the chapter. This will better prepare you to immerse in the language of ethics and better prepare you to integrate the content.

Active Engagement Model: Model of applied ethics proposed by Delany, Edwards, Jensen, and Skinner (2010) that delineates three components or steps to active engagement: active listening, reflexive thinking, and critical reasoning. The active engagement model emphasizes connectedness and moral agency.

Dialogic Ethics: Dialogic ethics emphasizes that ethics requires interactive dialogue or "dialectical process" that resembles an interactive conversation (Abma, Molewijk, & Widdershoven, 2009). This dialogue takes place on multiple levels with regard to the self, other people, theory and practice, competing principles or values, and the perspectives of various stakeholders. Involves listening, reflexivity, and reciprocity.

Ends-Based Ethical Tradition: Ethical tradition that resolves ethical situations based on the ends, consequences, or outcomes. Utilitarianism is the classical historical example of Ends-Based thinking and it posits that we should seek the "greatest good for the greatest number of people."

Ethical Pluralism: The idea that ethical truth is not a single unitary proposition, and that there are multiple perspectives on moral truth, all of which capture part of the truth, and none of which embrace the entire truth (Hinman, 2013, pp. 45, 364). Ethical pluralism is not synonymous with normative ethical relativism.

Ethical Principle: A normative concept that provides guidance for ethical conduct that is more general than a rule. Examples of ethical principles include the four-principles (autonomy, beneficence, non-maleficence, and justice), as well as informed consent, confidentiality, conflict of interest, and many others. The principles approach was popularized by Beauchamp and Childress (2009).

Ethical Reciprocity: Ethical reciprocity is the process of putting oneself in someone else's shoes. It extends the idea of treating others as one would like to be treated. Ethical reciprocity is one part of dialogic ethics.

Ethical Relativism: In contrast to absolutism, ethical relativism proposes that ethical values may vary across different cultures (descriptive relativism) and that these values are "right" within those cultures (normative relativism) (Hinman, 2013, p. 32).

Ethical Theory: A comprehensive approach to ethics that provides a conceptual foundation delineating the fundamental nature of ethics and morality, how the component parts are interrelated, and how these relate to moral behavior. Examples of ethical theories include deontology, utilitarianism, virtue ethics, pragmatism, and cognitive moral development. While the majority of ethical theories are grounded in philosophy, the cognitive developmental theory is grounded in psychology. Most ethical decision making uses intermediate ethical concepts rather than fully developed ethical theory.

Ethical Tradition: An ethical perspective and related language that has developed over history with a specific focus on ethical analysis without consideration of its general theoretical adequacy. Kidder identified three major ethical traditions: Rule-Based, Ends-Based, and Care-based. In this text, we refer to four ethical traditions: Rule-Based, Ends-Based, Virtue-Based, and Narrative-Based. Referring to "ethical traditions" creates common moral ground by grouping ethical theories and perspectives based major emphases.

Moral Deliberation: This refers to the dialogic process outlined, in part, in this text. It refers to deliberating about decisions of a moral nature through meaningful conversation, deliberation, and dialogue. In contrast to traditional case discussion's focus on determining what to do, moral deliberation emphasizes facilitation of multiple perspectives. Moral deliberation views process and outcome as inseparably linked. Moral deliberation about patient care should include patient or family stakeholders (Abma et al., 2009, p. 223).

Moral Indeterminacy: Imprecise or uncertain outcome of moral discussion resulting from respect for diverse ethical, cultural, or personal values of perspectives of the participants. Given that there is no unitary or single ethical truth, analysis of ethical dilemmas or problems does not always produce a single best answer or course of action. Rather, moral indeterminacy refers to the multiple paths that may be a "right" course of action in response to an ethical situation. Moral indeterminacy may be a barrier for interprofessional ethics because the lack of one definitive "right" resolution may discourage professionals from persevering to determine the best course of action through moral dialogue.

Narrative-Based Ethical Tradition: Ethical tradition that resolves ethical situations by listening to the experiences, voices, and perspectives of the participants and stakeholders. Responds to the criticism that healthcare ethics has been inattentive to patients' experiences.

Normative: Refers to considerations as to what one ought to do, typically grounded in consideration of duties and obligations. Normative ethics are a significant part of professional ethics. Normative ethics is often contrasted to descriptive ethics.

Polarized Discussion: Discussion characterized by participants asserting conflicting positions without a willingness to listen or respond to the ideas or values of other participants and without the goal of reaching consensus.

Quadrant Approach: Ethical decision-making approach developed first by Jonsen, Siegler, and Winslade (2006) and widely used in medicine. This approach analyzes ethical issues with four primary concerns: medical indications, patient preferences, quality of life, and contextual fairness.

Reflexivity: A concept taken from qualitative research that involves self-reflection on one's beliefs, values, emotions, preconceptions, and social role assuming that cognitive reflection promotes the ability to "bracket" or set personal subjective experiences aside (Cutcliffe, 2003, p. 137). Reflexivity should examine hidden values and assumptions and aspects of everyday life that are so ingrained in life that they are "taken for granted."

Rights: An entitlement to possess something or behave in a particular manner. Duties are often viewed as corollaries of rights. If one has a fundamental human right to free speech, for example, society has an obligation to enable free speech.

Rule-Based Ethical Tradition: Ethical tradition that resolves ethical situations using duties, obligations, principles, and rules. Professional codes of ethics typically rely heavily on the Rule-Based tradition. Medical ethics has been criticized for its over-use of Rule-Based thinking grounded in ethical principles.

Virtue-Based Ethical Tradition: Ethical tradition that focuses on the cultivation of personal character, quality, or ethical virtues.

▶ Chapter Overview

This chapter provides a model (the Dialogic Engagement Model) for interprofessional rehabilitation ethics that serves as an ethical decision-making framework, but also as a process for interprofessional moral deliberation and action. An important premise of the Dialogic Engagement Model is that a disconnect frequently occurs between ethical decision making and ethical action, and the same disconnect may also occur between individual and team moral agency. Healthcare professionals typically make ethical decisions from a "siloed" professional perspective without consideration of the team or organizational context in which their decisions must be implemented. In practice, few teams routinely incorporate ethical deliberation into their work. Moreover, there is increasing evidence that teams and organizations may at times serve as barriers to moral deliberation and action. In response to increasing levels of moral distress in health care, Wall and Austin (2008) studied the impact of teams and organizations on practitioners' experiences in addressing ethical challenges. Results indicated that teams and organizations may actually exacerbate moral distress through the following mechanisms (See **TABLE 3.1**).

Learning Point 3.1 Can you think of an instance where team or organizational factors influenced our ethical action in a negative or positive way?

However, Wall and Austin's (2008) research also indicated that teams can serve a positive role in moral deliberation and action through encouragement, support, clarification, feedback, and contributing to solutions In this text, we have referred to the challenges found by Wall and Austin as the lack of a "moral commons." A limited number of participants were able to find or benefit from what we are calling the moral commons. The clear implication is that rehabilitation professionals must move beyond a focus on individual professional making ethical decisions to embrace team

TABLE 3.1 Team and Organizational Barriers to Ethical Action

Team Influences	Supervisory and Organizational Influences
1. Power imbalances and hierarchical behavior	1. Silencing based on fear of reprimand
2. Lack of support	2. Conflict with organizational goals
3. Isolation—nobody to talk with about ethical situations	3. Cross-disciplinary supervisory relationships mean that the supervisor may not understand standards and concerns of employees
	4. Avoiding formal ethics structures due to concerns about practicality or not understanding

Based on Wall & Austin (2008).

and organizational processes that support ethical action. Austin (2007) emphasizes that healthcare environments must view themselves as "moral communities" where dialogue is the primary work of ethics.

Learning Point 3.2 Do you agree with Austin that healthcare environments are moral communities? What qualities would a moral community exhibit?

[T]he dominant approaches to healthcare ethics that focus primarily . . . on moral reasoning are insufficient. They are neither relevant nor responsive enough to day-to-day experience . . . An interdisciplinary exploration of moral experience . . . would allow the questions, doubts, disagreements, and challenges that shape ethical practice to surface . . . It would move attention to . . . the institutional processes involved in making healthcare environments morally habitable places . . . An interdisciplinary approach would allow shared meanings to be created and . . . genuine dialogue to be acquired. (p. 86)

The Dialogic Engagement Model is both an ethical decision-making framework that incorporates interprofessional elements but also a process for creating a moral commons that will support moral deliberation and action. In that regard, individual ethical judgments are "necessary but not sufficient" to interprofessional moral ethical behavior because these frameworks must be implemented in team and organizational contexts. In this chapter, we discuss ethical decision-making frameworks and ethical theories, provide an overview of interprofessional ethical decision-making frameworks, and explore the Dialogic Engagement Model as an interprofessional decision-making framework and dialogic process that addresses some of the inherent limitations of other models.

▶ Ethical Theories and Decision-Making Frameworks: The Challenge of Ethical Terminology

Ethical decision-making models abound in professional ethics (Greenfield & Jensen, 2010; Hunt & Ells, 2013; Manson, 2012; Park, 2012; Purtilo & Doherty, 2011; Van Denend & Finlayson, 2007) and many ethics texts provide a step by step process for approaching ethical situations. Decision-making frameworks may be helpful in establishing a rational process for analyzing all of the factors needed to make a true ethical decision. Additionally, a step by step process may help to develop a comprehensive personal process for analyzing ethical situations.

Learning Point 3.3 What is one example of an ethical decision-making framework?

Decision-making frameworks applied to ethical situations should not be confused with ethical theories. Decision-making frameworks have different purposes than ethical theories. The purpose of a decision-making framework is to assist individuals in addressing all elements of an ethical situation with the goal of determining a course of action in response to that situation. In contrast to this practical purpose of decision-making frameworks, ethical theories provide a conceptual foundation grounded in philosophy or social science to delineate the fundamental nature of ethics and morality as it relates to human social and moral behavior. While decision-making frameworks provide a practical "how-to" guide, ethical theories address deeper and more general questions about the nature, meaning, and basis of all ethical thought and action. Many professions have ethical decision-making frameworks to help professionals negotiate ethical quandaries. The three most persistent classical philosophical ethical theories (See **TABLE 3.2**) include deontology, utilitarianism, and virtue ethics, each of which is associated with well-known philosophers from the past.

Learning Point 3.4 What is the difference between an ethical theory and an ethical framework?

While these well-developed ethical theories continue to have influence on healthcare ethics, there are many other ethical theories used in healthcare ethics. An almost dizzying array of ethical theories and frameworks for use is further complicated by the fact that what some would call a theory, others would call a framework. As discussed in Chapter 2, principlism (the four principles approach) has been the dominant approach to medical ethical issues since the 1970s in the United States. To further muddy the waters, some ethicists would say that principlism and many other ethical theories fall short of being a "true ethical theory" and others would distinguish major or lesser theories from approaches. No universal agreement exists regarding what constitutes a "major theory" in

TABLE 3.2 Classical Ethical Theories Used for Healthcare Ethics

Theory	Description	Comments
Deontology	Ethics as Duty or Obligation Ethics is based on universal duties known through reason. The categorical imperative stated that people should act in manner such that their behavior could be a universal law (that is ethical under any circumstances).	Associated with the philosopher Immanuel Kant. Strong suit: Useful when consensus exists on duties, obligations, and rights. Weak suit: • Cultural or contextual circumstances mitigate whether universal duties apply. • May not consider consequences. • Who decides duties that apply? • What to do with conflicting duties?
Utilitarianism	Ethics as Consequence or Outcome Ethics is based on promoting "utility" or "happiness" for the majority of people within the community. Utilitarianism is often characterized as the "greatest good for the greatest number."	Associated with the philosophers John Stuart Mill and Jeremy Bentham. Strong suit: Policy decisions to bring about good for the community or a large group of people. Weak suit: • May not protect universal human rights in promoting "greatest good." • How to balance competing goods? (Example: long-term environment versus jobs)
Virtue-Based	Ethics as virtue, character, or personal qualities Ethics is based on the cultivation of virtues, character, or personal qualities. Focus is on "who you are" versus "what to do." Most professions have adopted core values of professionalism that could be viewed as core virtues.	Associated with the philosopher Aristotle. Strong suit: Addressing issues of relation or adversity, "everyday ethics." Weak suit: • Policy decisions • Competing or conflicting virtues

ethics. Therefore, categorization of theories, approaches, and frameworks in ethics is problematic.

Additionally, ethical terminology describing similar ethical theories may vary (for example, teleology may or may not be related to consequentialism). A final complication is that there is no evidence that "better" ethical theories result in better moral action.

The numerous ethical theories and variations in ethical terminology create a rich tapestry of ethical resources, but also pose a serious challenge to creating a moral commons for interprofessional rehabilitation ethics. Different professions may also incorporate specific ethical theories or frameworks into practical decision-making tools. Because different frameworks use different major concepts and language, the plethora of ethical approaches may present challenges to interprofessional ethical discussions in that different groups may be using different frameworks or different terminology. And the constraints to moral dialogue resulting from this dissonance may be invisible: Participants may not even be aware that different ethical frameworks are confounding the conversation. Thus, a major intent of this text is to provide a platform for understanding different ethical viewpoints and the varied nature of who brings what to the conversation.

 The existence of so many theories and "truths" without apparent ways to resolve conflicts between them is a uniquely "postmodern problem" (Ess, 2006) in that the postmodern world endorses the validity of multiple perspectives. Ethical discussion may become frustrating when it devolves to some arguing for one perspective and others concluding that everyone is "right" from his or her own perspective, sometimes referred to as the problem of "moral indeterminacy." Moral indeterminacy refers to the fact that analyzing ethical dilemmas or problems may not produce a single best answer or course of action. When, in fact, action is still required at the end of the conversation.

Moral dialogue and moral agency require the possibility of common language, a shared framework, and dialogue to accommodate different perspectives. In this text, we have adopted the following three foundations to facilitate the interprofessional moral commons as regards ethical theory and language:

1.   Ethical Pluralism
2.   Practical Focus
3.   Ethical Traditions

▶ Ethical Pluralism

In support of interprofessional moral dialogue, we endorse ethical pluralism (Hinman, 2013) to accommodate the various ethical, theoretical, cultural, and global perspectives required in the postmodern global world. Ethical pluralism is the belief that ethical truth is not a single unitary proposition, and that there are multiple perspectives on moral truth, all of which capture part of the truth, and none of which embrace the entire truth (Hinman, 2013, pp. 45, 364). As Ess (2006, p. 216) suggests, embracing ethical pluralism provides a way to navigate the Scylla and Charybdis represented by ethical absolutism (or dogmatism) and ethical relativism. Ethical relativism asserts that ethical values vary across different cultures (descriptive relativism) and that these values are right within each culture (normative relativism) (Hinman, 2013, p. 32). It is critical to note that ethical pluralism is not synonymous with normative ethical relativism (Hinman, 2013, p. 32) which endorses any position as ethical as long as it is considered moral within a particular society or culture. Steering this middle course of ethical pluralism respects the following qualities necessary for effective ethical theories discussed by Hinman (2013, pp. 27–28): understanding of other cultures and beliefs, tolerance of others' ideas and culture, standing against evil and unethical actions, and willingness to recognize our fallibility and limitations. In a very practical way, ethical pluralism provides a way to negotiate the ethical extremes of "there is a single right way and it is my way" and "whatever or anything goes." Moral discourse requires dialogue, not simply engaging in polarized debate.

Learning Point 3.8   What are Scylla and Charybdis and how are they used as an analogy in this chapter?

Learning Point 3.9   Is it important to distinguish normative relativism from ethical pluralism?

Ethical pluralism is an especially appropriate foundation for interprofessional ethics because each profession has developed its own theoretical approach to ethics. For example, medicine has predominantly been grounded in principle-based ethics and nursing has developed care-based theories. Rehabilitation professions have used these frameworks and taken them in different directions. While each theory has merits and limitations, interprofessional dialogue requires that we respect each framework and appreciate the analysis within the cultural context of the involved professions.

▶ Practical Focus

As consistent with the pioneering work of Jane Addams (1902) this text takes a practical approach to ethics in placing a priority on ethics in practice over pure ethical theory. The primary role of theory within this text is to support moral dialogue, clarify ethical conflicts, and assist in reaching consensus about practical moral action. Our intention in emphasizing dialogue and action over theory is not to devalue ethical theory. There can be no doubt that ethical theory is important and helpful; however, there are many resources to address ethical theory. Although we may analyze the relative strengths and weaknesses of different ethical theories and their "fit" with a specific situation, we will not devote time to arguing for any one ethical framework. Ethical pluralism recognizes that moral conflicts and disagreement are inevitable. Resolution of ethical conflicts involves reflection, analysis, dialogue, and engagement. From that perspective, ethical pluralism requires that we become "multilingual" in ethical theories and appreciate the perspective that different ethical theories and frameworks may bring to moral dialogue.

Learning Point 3.10   What is a practical focus on ethics?

In keeping with the philosophy of the text, we do not provide a comprehensive overview of ethical theories and approaches. Most rehabilitation professionals have had a basic introduction to ethical theories and problem-solving. The emphasis of the text is on using aspects of ethical theories, engaging different ethical traditions in resolving practical ethical issues, and employing moral case deliberation in support of individual and team moral agency. Readers are encouraged to use resources from their own profession. The tools provided in the Dialogic Engagement Model are intended to complement professional tools rather than compete with or supplant them.

▶ Ethical Traditions

Consistent with ethical pluralism and creating a moral commons for dialogue, we propose the use of the term "ethical tradition" (Kidder, 1995) rather than ethical theories or approaches, and we suggest recognizing four major ethical traditions to encompass commonly used theories and approaches (**TABLE 3.3**).

In discussing ethical traditions, we are building on the work of Kidder (1995) who classified moral theories into three traditions (Rule-Based, Ends-Based, and Care-Based). We have replaced Kidder's Care-Based Ethics with the Narrative-Based Tradition that includes narrative, care, experience, and critical ethics and we have added the Virtue-Based Tradition. Table 3.3 illustrates the four major ethical traditions (Rule-Based, Ends-Based, Virtue-Based, and Narrative-Based Traditions) and specific ethical theories that would fall under each tradition. For example, deontology and the four principles approach fall within the Rule-Based Tradition. The term "ethical tradition" suggests a perspective and related language that have been developed over history with a specific ethical focus without drawing judgments as to its general theoretical adequacy. Each tradition represents similar ethical emphases and concerns, and we have suggested an important historical writer associated with that perspective. By grouping ethical theories and relating them to specific ethical thinkers, we are not arguing that all of the theories within that tradition evolved from the historical figure most associated with that tradition. For example, the Narrative Tradition brings together a number of ethical perspectives that focus on life experience and relationships (both personal and societal). This has been associated with Gilligan's (1993) ethics of care because Gilligan was one of the first to observe that men and women have different experiences in addressing ethical situations, and that women attend more to relationships in ethics.

Learning Point 3.11   Do you agree with Gilligan that men and women look at ethical issues through a different lens?

TABLE 3.3 Four Major Ethical Traditions

Rule-Based Tradition	**Ends-Based Tradition**
Historical Example: Immanuel Kant	**Historical Examples: Mill and Bentham**
Laws and Legal Standards	Consequentialism
Ethical Principles and Principlism	Utilitarianism
Deontology (Duty-based)	Outcomes (Includes fiscal, personal, interpersonal, organizational, fiscal, social, global)
Absolute Duties	
Absolutism	Communitarianism
Rules	Evidence Based Practice
Religious	Intentions (Implied consequences)
Codes of Ethics	
Entitlement to human rights	
Virtue-Based Tradition	**Narrative-Based Tradition**
Historical Example: Aristotle	**Historical Example: Gilligan**
Virtues	Narrative
Values-based	Ethics of care
Core Values	Voice
Professional Identity and Formation	Phenomenology
Moral Agency	Life Experience
	Critical theory
	Feminist ethics
	Individual liberalism
	Relationships
	Contextualism
	Situational Ethics
	Violation of human rights

Based on Kidder (1995).

A key focus of the Narrative Tradition is in appreciating different life experiences by "listening for voice" and considering relationships. Our intent is not to suggest that Gilligan was responsible for the phenomenological or critical theory perspectives.

Some would call these traditions "lenses" because each tradition represents a specific ethical focus, and because we recommend that a thorough ethical analysis should use all four of the traditions. The goal of identification of four primary ethical traditions presented in Table 3.3 is to minimize the paralysis of moral discourse that is focused exclusively on disagreements regarding theory. Participants in moral discussion may use this tool to locate their own perspective and that of others within a particular tradition. For example, a person might use the Ethical Tradition Tool to identify that he/she is using the language and analysis associated with the Rule-Based Tradition, whereas another person might be using the Narrative-Based Tradition. These four major traditions presented in Table 3.3 will also be integrated into subsequent case discussions in the chapters that follow, and the expectation for effective interprofessional dialogue is that all professionals should be able to consider what each tradition offers in analyzing an ethical situation.

Learning Point 3.12   Look at Table 3.3 and identify the major ethical tradition with which you are most familiar and comfortable.

Learning Point 3.13   What is meant by ethical tradition?

It should be noted that the purpose of considering the four ethical traditions is to create common moral ground for interprofessional ethics discussion. It is a tool for practical conceptualization, dialogue, and action and is not intended as a purely theoretical analysis. From a theoretical perspective, there are important distinctions between theories within the ethical traditions.

As illustrated in **TABLE 3.4**, each tradition provides a different focus or ethical lens for viewing an ethical situation. The traditions are not mutually exclusive; for example, the narrative perspective plays a role in considering each of the traditions.

TABLE 3.4 Fitting Ethical Situations to Ethical Tradition*	
If the Ethical Situation Concerns...	**The Most Useful Ethical Tradition May Be:**
Duties delineated in laws, rules, professional codes, or societal expectations	**Rule-Based**
Issues of Public Policy Common good Balancing multiple interests	**Ends-Based**
Relationships Narratives Personal experiences Lack of access Human rights Disempowered status	**Narrative-Based**
Personal qualities, moral courage, moral agency, or demonstrating core values	**Virtue-Based**

*We extend acknowledgement to Dr. Herman Triezenberg for contributing to this concept.

However, considering each of the traditions creates interprofessional moral ground for comprehensively discussing ethical considerations using common language.

Certain ethical traditions may also be a better "fit" for different ethical situations. For example, a Narrative-Based Ethic may be more appropriate than Ends-Based Ethics in dealing with complex personal or cultural issues. On the other hand, the Ends-Based Tradition (utilitarianism) has historically been used to address complex policy decisions focusing on the overall goods of policy.

Table 3.4 provides an indicator of how ethical traditions may provide a better "fit" to different types of ethical situations. You may be drawn to certain approaches presented in Table 3.2 more than others. The purpose of agreeing on a limited number of ethical traditions is to minimize debate about the plethora of theories and to provide four different major ways to view ethical situations shared by all participants. Baker's (2014) history of medical ethics describes how the authors of the principles-based approach intended to create a simple common language for all. Baker and others (O'Rourke & Crowley, 2013; Strike, 1995) refer to this simple principles-based language as a type of simplified *"lingua franca"* for medical ethics (Baker, 2014, p. 299). From the perspective of the ethical traditions, the expectation is to be multilingual in using each of the ethical traditions within which the principles approach provides ample solid ground. Moreover, working through the lens provided by each of the four traditions results in a comprehensive view of the ethical situation, is consistent with ethical pluralism, and supports dialogue from multiple perspectives.

Learning Point 3.14 Why do different ethical traditions have differing attraction for you?

Learning Point 3.15 What does the term *"lingua franca"* mean?

▶ Models of Interprofessional Ethical Decision Making for Rehabilitation

Very few ethical decision-making frameworks have been developed for interprofessional contexts, and even fewer address rehabilitation professionals. In this section, we explore several decision-making models developed for interprofessional ethical decision making. Manson's (2012) literature search for ethical decision-making "frameworks" appropriate for interprofessional education found few frameworks that were appropriate for interprofessional use, with some being too complex and others not being sufficiently comprehensive. Manson's search for interprofessional ethical frameworks revealed eleven different approaches that Manson thought might be appropriate. Of these eleven frameworks, two were variants of the well-known four quadrant approach (Jonsen, Siegler, & Winsdale, 2006), which proposes a four category grid of ethical concerns associated with ethical principles and pertinent information:

- Medical Indications [Beneficence and Non-Maleficence],
- Patient Preference [Autonomy],
- Quality of Life [Beneficence, Non-Maleficence], and
- Respect for Autonomy, and Contextual Factors [Loyalty and Fairness] (p. 11).

One drawback to using the four quadrant model in rehabilitation ethics is its focus on medicine.

Few of the decision-making frameworks in Manson's search had a foundation in evidence, nor had they been validated (Manson, 2012; Tsai & Harasym, 2010). Based on her review of the literature and the resulting eleven frameworks, Manson (2012) created the CoRE-Values Framework with four domains: codes of ethics, regulations, ethical principles, and values. Manson used this framework with medical and nursing students, receiving positive feedback from faculty and students.

Learning Point 3.16   Name one framework that may be used in ethical decision making.

Park (2012) reviewed and analyzed 20 ethical decision-making frameworks across a number of disciplines, finding similarities and integrating them into a common decision-making sequence with a detailed discussion of considerations for each step. The resulting six "generic" ethical decision-making steps are outlined here:

1. Identify the problem
2. Collect additional information
3. Develop alternatives
4. Select the best course of action with justification
5. Implement decisions
6. Evaluate effects and develop strategies to prevent future occurrences (p. 139)

While Park's review of ethical decision-making models included some representatives from rehabilitation, some models from rehabilitation disciplines were missing from this and other reviews (Betan, 1997; Burger, Kramlich, Malitas, Page-Cutrara, & Whitfield-Harris, 2014; Carrier, Levasseur, Bédard, & Desrosiers, 2010; Carter et al., 2011; Kenny, Lincoln, & Balandin, 2007).

Learning Point 3.17   What are the six steps common to most existing ethical decision-making frameworks?

Clark, Cott, and Drinka (2007) proposed an interprofessional framework to address principles, structures, and processes as they pertain to the individual, the team, and the organization. Noting the absence of decision-making models for rehabilitation and the importance of patient centered care, Hunt and Ells (2013) developed a six-step decision-making framework that integrates the ICF: 1) Identify ethical issues; 2) Collect information; 3) Review and analyze; 4) Identify and weigh options; 5) Make decision; and 6) Evaluate and follow-up. They provide extensive additional questions under each of the six steps that address the rehabilitation process from an ethical perspective.

In this section we have reviewed several ethical decision-making frameworks for interprofessional decision making. There are very few interprofessional models developed explicitly for rehabilitation, and many proposed models do not incorporate rehabilitation language or considerations into medically-focused models. Nevertheless, as Park (2012) demonstrates, there is remarkable congruency in the various discipline's frameworks that help one to navigate the process of analyzing an ethical situation, choosing an action, and implementing a plan.

We believe that ethical decision-making frameworks can be helpful for rehabilitation students and early career professionals as they are developing a rational, logical, and consistent approach to ethical situations. Nevertheless, ethical decision-making approaches have limitations in approaching complex ethical problems for teams. The virtue of delineating basic steps for ethical decision making is that it provides a simple linear process, reduces complexity, and facilitates reaching a decision. This is in contrast to the fact that most of the processes in our worlds are non-linear and steeped in complexity (Wheatly, 1998). These same virtues of ethical decision making frameworks do not capture the complexity and number of factors required for complex ethical decision making in interprofessional contexts. Indeed, group discussion may devolve into polarized opinions and indirectly suggest that there is one best answer that emerges for every ethical situation.

Learning Point 3.18　How do polarized group discussions negatively affect group ethical decision making?

One striking feature of professional ethical decision-making frameworks is that they do not often include explicit consideration of the interprofessional team. This suggests the need for a process for rehabilitation professionals to build on insights of decision-making frameworks learned in professional education in addressing interprofessional environments. We encourage readers to continue to use a variety of ethical decision-making frameworks for preliminary analysis. (For those who may not have a framework, you may consider the RIPs framework presented in the last chapter). However, as discussed later, we believe that interprofessional ethics deliberation requires a dialogic process to extend beyond simple frameworks for analysis.

Irvine, Kerridge, and McPhee (2004) discuss the inherent complexity of interprofessional teams and relationships, suggesting that traditional approaches to ethics may reinforce competition and hierarchy, thereby undermining teamwork. They suggest a "dialogic ethic" that focuses on relationships and moral deliberation: "Ethical deliberation is conceived as a historically situated, two-sided practice characterized by participants doing their utmost to achieve mutual understanding". Irvine et al. (2004) describe dialogic ethics as follows:

> Dialogic ethics is organized around an extended notion of collegiality. . . . [A]ll credentialed health care professionals are indispensable co-participants in a relationship of exchange. . . . We maintain that professionals of all stripes . . . gain from engaging the perspectives . . . of rival conceptions rather than being driven by the logic of their own particular . . . professional moral knowledge. It may produce new, possibly hybrid, systems of ethical thought and moral standards that are appropriate to today's multidisciplinary health care environments. (p 249)

A dialogic ethic grounded in moral deliberation is an appropriate forum for interprofessional rehabilitation ethics. Similar to clinical reasoning, as professionals mature, they should rely less on algorithmic or strict decision-making models and move toward more complex, layered, and deliberative dialogic models of ethical reasoning. The next section describes the theoretical basis for the Dialogic Engagement Model presented in this text.

Learning Point 3.19　How is clinical reasoning similar to ethical reasoning?

▶ The Dialogic Engagement Model

This section of the chapter describes the Dialogic Engagement Model that is used in the remainder of the text. We provide a theoretical background, describe the process, discuss the implications for interprofessional rehabilitation ethics, and provide beginning level case applications for using the model. This process brings together the critical elements of interprofessional rehabilitation ethics discussed in the first chapter, the moral case deliberation model, and active engagement facilitation (Delany et al., 2010). Moral deliberation has been used extensively in the Netherlands and Europe to facilitate moral dialogue and decision making in clinical and educational settings (Molewijk, Abma, Stolper, & Widdershoven, 2008; van der Dam, Abma, Kardol, & Widdershoven, 2012; van der Dam et al., 2013; Weidema, Molewijk, Widdershoven, & Abma, 2012; Widdershoven, Abma, & Molewijk, 2009).

Learning Point 3.20 What is moral deliberation?

Dialogic ethics provides the philosophical foundation for the Dialogic Engagement Model. Consistent with the hermeneutic tradition, dialogic ethics values narrative accounts, listening and engaging with others, dialogue between participants, and the mutual learning that emerges through the process of dialogue. Hermeneutic philosophy and dialogic ethics both emphasize the important role of dialogue in understanding. Dialogic ethics requires openness to the perspective of others and a willingness to learn from reflection and deliberation (Molewijk, Abma, Stolper, & Widdershoven, 2008). The process also includes active listening, paraphrasing for accuracy checking, responding with meaningful and relevant thoughts, and exploring through ethical traditions. The process of moral deliberation should facilitate not only ethical knowledge but ethical competence and expertise (Molewijk et al., 2008). Moral deliberation is practice-based experiential learning in which participants learn though dialogue and reflection. In order to foster positive relationships, personal experience, and dialogue, moral case deliberation embraces the following collegial processes:

- on-going dialogue
- practical rationality focused on patient-centered care
- experiential knowledge
- moral equality of caregivers, multiple perspectives
- open processes, and facilitation by someone knowledgeable in ethics (Abma, Molewijk, & Widdershoven, 2009).

The active engagement model was designed by Delany et al. (2010) as an integrative model for applied ethics emphasizing connectedness, moral agency, integrating ethical principles, narrative ethics approaches, and sociology. The model proposes three components or steps: active listening, reflexive thinking, and critical reasoning. Each step is associated with questions to facilitate the process involved in that step. A stated goal of the authors was to provide a bridge between polarized considerations of theory versus practice and relationships versus normative analysis.

Our proposed Dialogic Engagement Model incorporates aspects of both the moral deliberation model and the active engagement model (Delany et al., 2010). In contrast to the three steps of the active engagement model (active listening, reflexive thinking, and critical thinking), we propose the following three interdependent dimensions illustrated in **FIGURE 3.1**. We refer to these as "dimensions" rather than

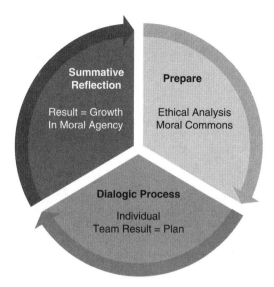

FIGURE 3.1 Dimensions of dialogic engagement model.

steps because these are iterative processes that occur for both the individual and the team in a manner that is not always a linear sequence of steps. For example, team dialogue and self-reflection may well cause one to return to preparation through analysis. Likewise, one may recognize the need to further develop the interprofessional moral commons to support team dialogue.

The primary emphasis of the Dialogic Engagement Model is the rehabilitation professional as moral agent in ethical dialogue with patients, families, team members, organizations, social entities, and the self. Emphasis on moral dialogue is consistent with supporting an interprofessional ethical process and the moral agency of the team. Our hope is that this process might become mainstream in rehabilitation and other interprofessional teams. In the following paragraphs, we briefly comment on each dimension of the process.

Learning Point 3.21   Why is the Dialogic Engagement Model unique?

The first dimension of moral deliberation is to prepare for moral dialogue and reflection. Preparation requires analyzing the ethical situation from your own professional/personal perspective and establishing the moral commons. During preparation, ethical analysis uses your own preferred tradition and decision-making tools from your professional perspective. The goal of preparatory ethical analysis is to be able to provide a brief summary of the issue and course of action. Sorting out your own ethical perspective provides a foundation for dialogue and reflection.

Preparation for group discussion requires that each group member engage in a process of personal discernment regarding each of the elements of the moral commons (identity, ethical tradition, and context) in relation to individual and team moral agency. In other words, there is conceptual homework to be done before any group meeting or conversation. For, without being thought about first individually, it is a challenge to come together and think collectively. In considering each element, group members should consider his/her own deeply held values and perspectives,

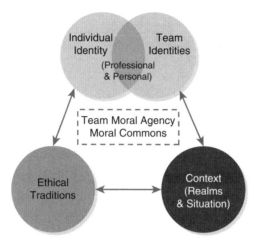

FIGURE 3.2 From individual moral agency to team moral agency.

as well as attempting to step outside the self to consider how others might consider each element. Preparation also involves locating appropriate resources (scholarly literature, codes of ethics, pertinent clinical information, situation-specific evidence, legal considerations, interprofessional role clarification, or clinical mentorship). Finally, preparation requires that each team member consider the ethical situation using a shared language and framework. As illustrated in **FIGURE 3.2** each individual should consider questions of identity, traditions, and context:

> **Learning Point 3.22** Describe the preparation process for the Dialogic Engagement Model.

    a.   Identity

Consider how personal, professional, and interprofessional identity influence your view of the moral issue to be discussed. What are the relevant ethical values and duties related to each aspect of identity? With regard to professional and interprofessional identity, how does the scope of practice and team expectations for role influence how you frame the issue? How might others on the team view you? Are there conflicting values and duties? In this portion of preparation, participants may also consider clinical scope of practice, role delineation, and overlapping practice considerations. Reflect on the clinical language and frameworks that are operative. Are different languages and perspectives being used? Are any of the clinical languages or frameworks conflicting or an impediment to other stakeholders (including patients)?

> **Learning Point 3.23** How does identity affect the Dialogic Engagement Model?

    b.   Ethical Traditions (including legal issues)

Consider the case from each of the ethical traditions. What are the legal issues to be considered under the Rule-Based tradition? What relevant information does each ethical tradition provide for the case? Identify critical duties, virtues, consequences/outcomes, and narrative considerations (voice, perspective). Do you have a preference for a tradition? Do any of the traditions appear to be a better or worse fit for the particular situation? (For example, recall that the Ends-Based tradition may overlook human rights). Do the professions involved in the ethical situation differ in their perspectives regarding the contribution from each tradition?

c. Context (Realms and Situation)
Take the perspective of each realm to consider the case. From the standpoint of the individual (self, patient, family members, team members), what are the relevant issues? Can you identify one or more "cardinal" realms (most important realm for the case)(Glaser, 1994)? Glaser (1994) indicates that most ethical issues involve multiple realms but many have a "cardinal" realm. For example, policy issues of healthcare access involve all realms, but the societal realm is cardinal as access cannot be achieved without political action in the societal realm. Note that this does not obviate the need for individuals to act in the individual, team, or organizational realm to fulfill professional obligations. This is also the point in preparation to consider rich contextual information. What are the most unique aspects of the context that illuminate the actions, motives, and values of patients, families, and healthcare professionals? As discussed in the last chapter, the type of ethical situation may also be relevant to team dialogue as true ethical dilemmas may require more time and effort to reach consensus. Recall the discussion of different types of ethical situations (previous chapter) and consider that different situations may require different responses to address that situation. Members of the team should incorporate understanding the type of situation into individual and team plans. For example, a true ethical dilemma may require more individual analysis and team dialogue than a moral temptation. Similarly, moral distress may require attention to the moral "residue" for individual and team members after the fact. Consideration of the context also incorporates the specific clinical roles played by team members. Team roles should be addressed in the team's plan to address the ethical situation. Where there is overlap in clinical roles, the team may want to address those areas.

Learning Point 3.24 Why is context important in the Dialogic Engagement Model?

The second aspect of preparation is to create the moral commons for your team. A moral commons requires the existence or creation of a shared "space" for discussion of moral issues. For some rehabilitation teams, this space might be a regular team meeting (for example, discharge planning). In other cases, team members must be creative in identifying "space" for the moral commons. The moral commons need not be a formal team meeting. It may be informal discussion between several team members via telephone, electronic communication, or in passing. The ultimate goal is to make sure that there is space for rehabilitation team members to discuss ethical issues that arise. Creating the moral commons can be challenging in the current healthcare environment where finance, efficiency, productivity, and reimbursement receive so much emphasis. Creating shared safe space for honest dialogue requires that relevant stakeholders are present, able to trust each other, and free to express their opinions. This requires the following conditions:

a.   Relevant stakeholders are represented.
Everyone with a legitimate stake in the issue at hand should be represented, including team members, administrators, patients, and families. The direct inclusion of patients and families may pose logistical challenges, necessitating more indirect methods of representation. For example, a patient advocate might represent patient interests. Representation does not require that all stakeholders are always present, but that relevant stakeholders have a voice in the decisions.

b.   Collegiality
True dialogue requires collegiality grounded in respect for other group members and is based on recognizing each other as moral equals. Further, this requires group members to put differences in power and status within the organization or team aside for the purposes of the group. Additionally, collegiality involves adopting rules for group interaction that facilitate participation (for example, speaking in turn, listening to one another, responding respectfully).

Learning Point 3.25   Why do you have to put aside power to increase collegiality?

c.   Role assignments
Group members are assigned responsibilities for focusing on one or more of the dimensions and for different aspects of group process (agenda setting, facilitation, recording group insights, summarizing the work of the group, and providing feedback). These roles should rotate so that all group members shape the work of the group. An example of an assignment for a session might be to take responsibility for ensuring that the group addresses all four major ethical traditions (dimension) and serves as facilitator (process). The role assignment process may also be more informal, depending on the organizational setting.

d.   Building moments for review and course setting
The group should set an agenda for moral deliberation and to address the needs of the group. It is important that the group capture the insights of the group, record these insights for further review, summarize learning, and review the progress in light of the group's goals and agenda. Built into this dialogic process should be moments to review and moments to re-evaluate the direction of the conversation. The primary goal would be that the team routinely attends to ethical matters.

Learning Point 3.26   Reiterate what constitutes a moral commons.

Learning Point 3.27   Why do you need an agenda for moral deliberation?

e.   The group determines the pertinent issues based upon prior individual preparation
Each group member should bring a one or two sentence statement summarizing the nature of the ethical issue in non-technical language.

The team uses the shared language and concepts to frame a shared common understanding of the ethical situation. The group will then determine how to frame the goals and agenda for discussion by determining the ethical issue that the group is discussing.

f. Every member of the group has input to the conversation
    Each person in the group has input by expressing opinions and responding to the ideas of others. While amount of time speaking may vary from time to time, no one person should dominate the conversation. The person in the role of facilitator should help "direct traffic" so that quiet members of the group are able to express their views.

g. Active engagement in the conversation (both talking and listening)
    Members of the group should attempt to balance talking and listening. Responding to others requires active and engaged listening in order to appreciate the perspective of others (not simply hearing their words). Group members take responsibility for growing in their ability to listen and speak, based on self-evaluation and feedback from the group regarding their skills.

h. Critical analysis
    Critical analysis involves revisiting the elements considered in preparation within the group from a critical perspective and with feedback from the group. Critical analysis includes consideration of ethical, practice, fiscal, community resources, functional, and human capital issues.

i. Dialogue toward consensus
    Although it may not always be possible to achieve consensus, the intent to work toward consensus promotes mutual respect and reinforces moral community. Reaching consensus is not simply endorsing a majority opinion. Rather, it involves exploring the alternatives of each member of the group. Each member should provide a statement of recommended response to the ethical situation. Following discussion, the group should reach a preliminary agreement on the preferred response. Dissenting group members are then provided an opportunity for a dissenting perspective. The group then works toward reaching agreement regarding a course of action that is acceptable (if not preferred) by all.

Learning Point 3.28   Describe the Dialogic Engagement Model.

j. Emotional and intuitive input – how does it feel?
    Although we often emphasize the rational aspects of ethical decision making, there is growing recognition that emotion and intuition are important considerations (Haidt, 2001; Kidder, 1995; Youssef et al., 2012). Kidder (1995) suggests that ethics should include a "gut check" to consider how the decision feels. Emotion and intuition are also important to consider in developing an action plan and attending to moral residue (Epstein & Hamric, 2009). If group consensus and action are contrary to an individual's strong feelings, these should be addressed.

Learning Point 3.29   How do feelings play a role in the Dialogic Engagement Model?

The desired outcome for dialogic process is that the team reaches consensus on a plan of action to respond to the ethical situation. As indicated in Figure 3.1, the Dialogic Engagement Model should yield a plan for moral agency for individuals and the team as a whole.

The third dimension of the Dialogic Engagement Model is summative reflection. This aspect of the model pertains to examining hidden or implicit assumptions about yourself, culture, worldview, and team roles and making them explicit or visible. Consider how your own personal and cultural background influence your view and that of others regarding this situation. How might your own background cause you to overlook important aspects of the situation? Summative reflection by the team is an iterative response whereby group members revisit the group's decision. Each group member should "sleep on the decision," critically reflect on the decision, and explore intuitions and emotions resulting from the decision. Group members should then check back with other group members in person or via email. This final summative dimension acknowledges the dual process (Haidt, 2001) of reason/emotion and individual/group that constitute individual and team moral agency. Additionally, this summative revisiting supports the development of moral community.

Learning Point 3.30   How is self-reflection used in the Dialogic Engagement Model?

Learning Point 3.31   Explain the role of summative in the Dialogic Engagement Model.

Delany et al. (2010) refer to this kind of reflection as "reflexivity," a term borrowed from qualitative research and previously mentioned earlier. It refers to the researcher's willingness to engage in critical reflection on the impact of the researcher's values and involvement on the research. Cutcliffe (2003) identifies two different aspects to reflexivity: 1) self-reflection on one's beliefs, values, emotions, preconceptions, and social role and 2) the ability to "bracket" or set these subjective experiences aside (p. 137). To be actively engaged is to listen carefully and respond to the perspective of others. An important aspect of reflexivity is to consider the hidden and taken for granted aspects of everyday life that are somewhat obscured by daily routine.

Learning Point 3.32   What is reflexivity? Can you think of an example where you were called on to engage in reflexivity?

Revisit which aspects of individual and team moral agency are most important for the case under consideration. Reflect on how the situation fits your professional development, skills, and weaknesses. How will this affect your response to the case? For example, if the situation most calls for moral courage and your self-assessment is that your personal dislike of conflict presents challenges in moral courage, how might you address this? Revisit these types of considerations for the team, organization, society, and global realms. This requires self-analysis and in depth reflection about one's own self in relationship to the situation.

The desired outcome for the third dimension of the model (summative reflection) is on-going professional development and enhanced moral agency for the individual and the team. This growth is grounded in feedback from one's self and others in relation to the team. **TABLE 3.5** summarizes the Dialogic Engagement Model and provides sample questions relevant to each dimension.

TABLE 3.5 Dialogic Engagement Model: Processes and Sample Questions		
Dimension	**Goal or Process**	**Sample Questions**
1. Preparation	Ethical Analysis: Perform your own ethical analysis – using professional values and tools of analysis. Consider moral commons elements to articulate the ethical values at stake in a brief non-technical statement. Establish the Commons: Identify or create shared space for the commons. Create an atmosphere of trust and collegiality to support honest dialogue. Listen carefully for voice, tradition, and perspective.	• How would you characterize the ethical issue or case in human terms, preferably as narrative? Which voices are predominant or muted? • Are there issues of team or organizational culture that potentially impede dialogue or team moral agency? • What issues of power and status may affect creation of the moral commons? • What is your own preferred ethical tradition? • Can you identify the ethical tradition of others? • What is your initial impression of significant issues from each of the four key elements of the moral commons (ethical tradition, identity, and context/realms)?
2. Dialogic Process (Individual and Team)	The ability to engage in critical dialogue with the goal of reaching mutual consensus, respect for others, professional maturation, and moral community.	• What are the perspectives of stakeholders and those involved? • Are different languages/traditions being used? • What does analysis from each ethical tradition suggest as a course of action for the team? • How do different roles and scopes of practice influence perspectives? • What course of action do you choose? • How will you deal with negative aspects of your decision? • What social structural barriers exist?

(continues)

TABLE 3.5 Dialogic Engagement Model: Processes and Sample Questions
(continued)

Dimension	Goal or Process	Sample Questions
3. Summative Reflection	An iterative revisiting of thoughts and emotions by individuals and the group following reaching a decision or consensus. Critical self-reflection on personal, professional, team perspectives; values, and roles as they affect yourself or others and actively listening and responding to other's experiences.	• How do my personal, professional, and interprofessional identities and history affect others? • How am I affected by the identities of others? • What aspects of moral agency and professional formation represent strengths and weaknesses in this situation? • What social or cultural beliefs or biases (social or organizational) might have influenced perceptions of self and others, or impeded dialogue? • Are there "taken for granted" aspects of everyday life that are hidden from me or other team members? • What needs to be done to support individual or team moral agency? • Do you agree with the decision reached by the group? Why or why not?

▶ Application of the Dialogic Engagement Model

Now that you have learned about the Dialogic Engagement Model, it is time to put the model into action. We have described the Dialogic Engagement Model as a process for moral deliberation, more than a step-by step approach or decision-making framework. Our description assumes that you will be working with other professionals (either student peers, colleagues, or others) to deliberate on an ethical issue important to your team. We realize that you may be a student or professional without immediate access to a team or group. We have outlined instructions for considering two cases taken from rehabilitation practice. We suggest that you find peers for moral deliberation following your individual preparation and analysis. This is consistent with the dialogic emphasis of the model assuming that we learn, refine, and grow in response to the thoughts and values of others. Additionally, practice in moral deliberation is essential for interprofessional rehabilitation ethics.

In the next section, three cases and an instructional worksheet sheet are presented for practical application. Consider the following case taken from the literature:

Case of Mr. and Mrs. Jones

Mr. Jones, a 54-year-old man, was involved in a motor vehicle crash approximately 2 weeks ago and sustained a spinal cord injury (SCI) and mild traumatic brain injury (TBI). He is currently an inpatient on the rehabilitation service and has waxing and waning decisional capacity as a result of mild cognitive impairments. His wife of 23 years is his surrogate decision maker for complex medical decisions. Mrs. Jones has been at his bedside crying, and Mr. Jones has told staff members that he feels guilty. During the course of treatment, it was revealed that Mr. Jones was having an affair and was involved in the accident when he was with his lover, Ann, who sustained minimal injuries and was discharged from acute care. His wife believed he was out of town and was stunned to get a call from the hospital about the accident. While Mr. Jones was in a confused state, he called out for Ann, and his wife has become suspicious. Mrs. Jones has been coming in regularly to visit Mr. Jones and has now been asking the staff about what happened and who he was with when he had the accident. She has restricted his visitors to the immediate family. Their two adult children, Mary and Tim, ages 22 and 20 years, are unaware of their father's affair but have also been asking staff members about what is going on.

This case has caused angst among the staff. Some staff members identify with the wife and are angry at Mr. Jones. Others believe that it is a private situation between spouses and their children and does not have an impact on health care. Still others are worried about asking Mrs. Jones to provide personal care after discharge when, according to some staff members, her marriage may be "based on lies." What are some key ethical issues in this case? What would you advise the team? (Levine et al., 2015)

Use the worksheet in **TABLE 3.6** to analyze the case and develop most important points and considerations. Work with a team or group to determine a plan for the case. How would you characterize the case? What are the major challenges for the team in this situation?

The case of Mr. Jones was discussed at a professional conference (APTA CSM conference, 2018); one participant noted that in a similar situation the intensity of feelings among the team members became problematic. As a result of team dialogue, one team member suggested to another team member that she recuse herself from the case because she was not able to interact in an objective manner. The team members also agreed to discontinue non-productive personal discussion ("gossiping").

TABLE 3.6 Worksheet: Instructions and Resources for Cases

Dimension	Questions and Notes
Preparation Individual analysis Establish the moral commons	Analyze the issue from your own professional perspective. Consider each of the elements of the moral commons (ethical tradition, identity, and context [situation and realms]) in relation to individual and team moral agency.

(continues)

TABLE 3.6 Worksheet: Instructions and Resources for Cases	_(continued)_
Dimension	**Questions and Notes**
	Ethical Traditions: Analyze ethical concerns from the perspective of each of the 4 major traditions. What does each add? Does any have prominence or better fit?
	Identity:
	Context (Situation and Realms):
	Individual moral agency:
	Team moral agency:
	Access additional resources (literature, codes of ethics, mentor advice).
	Summarize in a non-technical sentence or two the ethical issues at stake.
	Questions and notes from preparation
	Team: If you are working with an interprofessional team, determine when you will meet.
	When you meet, review ground rules to ensure a safe zone for moral deliberation.
	Individual reader: If you are working individually, find at least one other person with whom to confer.
	Review the moral deliberation process.
	It can be valuable to act as the hospital ethics committee assigned to determine what to do.
	Questions and notes about the commons
Dialogic Process	Group determines the pertinent issues based upon prior individual preparation.
	Every member of the group has input to the conversation and is able to express their views.
	Active engagement in the conversation (both talking and listening).
	Critical analysis.
	Dialogue toward consensus about individual and team moral agency.
	What is the Team's plan?

Summative Reflection	Reflexive engagement.
	Questioning of assumptions
	Ethical reciprocity: Putting yourself in others' shoes.
	Individuals and group revisit and check back with each other.
	Are there team issues of care and moral community that need attention?
	Next steps? Actions and team processes needed?
	Emotional and intuitive input – how does it feel?
	What are individual and team strengths and weaknesses? What aspects of moral agency require development?
	Questions and notes from preparation

Case of Mr. Smith

Mr. Smith, an 87-year-old shopkeeper, had lived all his life in the apartment above the shop handed down to him from his father. His sister lived with him; neither had children. Mr. Smith was independent in all activities of daily living (ADLs), as well as in tending the shop. Mr. Smith had sustained a fall, leading to hospital admission. He was subsequently diagnosed with uraemia resulting from recurring urinary retention and urinary tract infections, mild cognitive impairment, and degenerating spinal stenosis with significant impairments of his balance, sensation, proprioception, strength, and motor control.

Mr. Smith was transferred to older adult inpatient rehabilitation. Here, he worked for 12 weeks with a team comprising a medical doctor, primary nurse, social worker, physiotherapist, occupational therapist, and pharmacist. Through various formal and informal assessments, the team concluded that Mr. Smith required moderate to maximal assistance to complete his ADLs. He was able to walk with a walker and hands-on assistance for very short distances, but during his stay, he mainly relied on a wheelchair for mobility. Mr. Smith's occupations at home required him to go up and down a spiral staircase several times daily. This was now difficult because of his decreased strength and coordination. His impairments and the physical layout of the bathroom impeded his ability to maintain adequate hygiene and prevent recurring infections. Mr. Smith presented with variable cognitive capacities; for example, he conversed about global impacts of stock market activity, but demonstrated significant difficulty with simple mathematics. This was problematic as he did all financial transactions for his shop manually.

Discharge home placed Mr. Smith at risk of declining medically and sustaining another fall. Team discussions revealed uncertainty as to whether Mr. Smith was capable or not of appreciating the implications of living on his own with these impairments. Mr. Smith did not agree with the team's assessment that he would require assistance upon returning home, nor did he agree that a wheelchair would assist with his mobility. The healthcare team worked extensively with Mr. Smith in an effort to increase his

(continues)

(continued)

understanding of his needs and difficulties he may encounter in his home, as well as to provide information about resources and available assistance. Overall, however, team members reported feeling that he lacked insight into his needs and abilities. Mr. Smith asserted that he wished to return to the only home he had ever known and to tend to his shop. He said that living elsewhere would make him unhappy and be 'meaningless'. Mr. Smith's sister was worried that she and her brother might face risks if they returned to their current living situation. She offered to move with him to long-term care, but Mr. Smith declined her offer. He also declined homecare, stating that it would be 'unnecessary' because he had always taken care of himself and would continue to do so.

Reproduced from Durocher & Gibson (2010).

Case of Jasper

Jasper is a 69-year-old widower* who experienced a right hemispheric cerebrovascular accident and currently is aphasic and has dysphagia. He demonstrates aspiration on his swallow study. Although he has a PEG, his adult daughter continues to feed him orally. When he chokes and coughs, his daughter, who is his durable power of attorney for health care, insists that he would rather die eating than be exclusively tube-fed. The attending physician assessed Jasper for his capacity to make the decision regarding oral feedings, and she determines that he lacks capacity at this time to make this decision. She writes an order requesting the speech pathologist (SP) to also assess his capacity, and to work with the adult daughter to minimize harmful effects from oral feedings. The SP, after assessing Jasper, agrees that he lacks the capacity to decide at this time. She does not believe oral feedings are safe and refuses to be complicit in facilitating any oral feedings. She tells the attending physician that Jasper's case must be transferred to another SP who can comply with the attending physician's order.

*The patient's name and other critical identifying information have been changed.

Reproduced from Savage, Parson, Zollman, & Kirschner (2009).

Set up a team of four to five people to discuss each case. Allow for about one hour of discussion in total. For moral deliberation for each case, consider the following questions:

1. What were the similarities and differences of issues raised in the two cases?
2. Did you emphasize different aspects of the preparation or discussion for the two cases?
3. Are there issues that the team would need to address following the incident described in the case? (For example, moral distress.)
4. What aspects of preparation did you find difficult or challenging?
5. What was your final determination about what team and moral agency would involve in that case?
6. What factors in the case would contribute or detract from the moral commons?

These cases illustrate that ethical issues in interprofessional rehabilitation do not have simple or easy answers, and some degree of moral uncertainty is inevitable.

▶ Summary and Conclusion

In this chapter we have discussed the Dialogic Engagement Model for addressing interprofessional rehabilitation ethics. We described the challenges of organizational and team culture that may shape ethical experiences, create moral distress or moral residue, and contribute to professional burnout. Following an overview of ethical issues commonly encountered by rehabilitation, we explored ethical decision-making models used by rehabilitation professionals. Although ethical decision-making frameworks can be useful to less experienced professionals, they have limitations in addressing complex ethical issues that are encountered in interprofessional rehabilitation ethics. The chapter concluded by outlining and describing the Dialogic Engagement Model that will be the focus of the remainder of this text. Subsequent chapters apply the Dialogic Engagement Model to cases in rehabilitation ethics.

Closing Reflections

Learning Activities

3.1   Personal Conviction and Dialogue
1.   Think of a personal or professional discussion in which you encountered moral indeterminacy? How did you address the situation?
2.   Do you agree that there is no single unitary ethical truth?
3.   What effect does your personal belief about ethical truth (pro or con) have on professional and interprofessional practice?

3.2   Polarized Discussion
1.   Some commentators note that polarized debate has become an increasing problem in the United States. Do you agree?
2.   What role does social media play in polarized dialogue?
3.   What is the effect of polarized debate on professional and interprofessional practice?

3.3   Situational Analysis
Consider the following two situations:

Discharge planning–What are the considerations when the patient wants to return home but it is unsafe ?

Intimate Partner Violence–You have promised not to reveal that your patient is the victim of intimate partner violence but it appears that she/he is in imminent danger.
1.   How would each of the ethical traditions address these situations? Do they lead to different decisions or provide different perspectives?
2.   What is your "natural fit" or "comfort zone" for ethical tradition as a personal individual and as a professional? Which of the four traditions is a "stretch" for you?
3.   Which of the traditions has been most important in your profession?
4.   What is the effect of relying too heavily on just one tradition?
5.   What additional information would the team need to address the situation?

3.4 **Comparing Different Frameworks for Interprofessional Ethics**
Compare the following ethical decision-making models: quadrant of Jonsen et al. (2006). Park's (2012) generic steps, CoreValues (Manson, 2012), and the dialogic model of Irvine et al. (2004). What are the strengths and weaknesses with regard to interprofessional rehabilitation ethics?

 # Take Away Messages

- Rehabilitation professionals often make ethical decisions from a "siloed" perspective, relying on their own profession's ethical guidelines.
- Teams and healthcare organizations may, at times, serve as either barriers or facilitators to interprofessional collaboration regarding ethical situations.
- Rehabilitation professionals must move beyond a focus on the individual professional making ethical decisions to embrace team and organizational processes that support ethical action. The individual professional's ethical judgments are "necessary but not sufficient" for interprofessional ethical behavior because these ethical decisions must be implemented in team and organizational contexts.
- Ethical decision-making frameworks provide a practical process for working through ethical situations. In contrast to this practical goal, ethical theories address deeper and more general ethical questions.
- The plethora of ethical theories, frameworks, and approaches may create conflicts in ethical language and perspectives during moral discussions. This challenge is complicated by the postmodern reality that there may be no single right answer to ethical situations (moral indeterminacy). As a result of this and other factors, rehabilitation professionals may not have a "moral commons" for discussion of ethical situations.
- Three foundations to facilitate creating a moral commons are embracing ethical pluralism, maintaining a practical focus, and acknowledging ethical traditions. This requires professionals to be "multilingual" in ethical theories.
- To facilitate the moral commons, the Dialogic Engagement Model uses four major ethical traditions to classify many ethical theories: Rule-Based, Ends-Based, Virtue-Based, and Narrative-Based. Each of the traditions contributes to our understanding of ethical situations.
- The principles approach (part of the Rule-Based tradition) has been used extensively in medical ethics and represents a type of common ethical language.
- The Dialogic Engagement Model is an ethical decision-making framework and a process for interprofessional moral deliberation that builds on dialogic ethics, active engagement, reflection, and moral deliberation.

References

Abma, T. A., Molewijk, B., & Widdershoven, G. A. (2009). Good care in ongoing dialogue. Improving the quality of care through moral deliberation and responsive evaluation. *Health Care Analysis,* *17*(3), 217–235. doi:10.1007/s10728-008-0102-z
Addams, J. (1902). *Democracy and social action.* New York: MacMillan Press.
Austin, W. (2007). The ethics of everyday practice: Healthcare environments as moral communities. *Advances in Nursing Science, 30*(1), 81–88.
Baker, R. (2014). *Before bioethics: A history of American medical ethics from the colonial period to the bioethics revolution.* New York, NY: Oxford University Press.

Beauchamp, T. L., & Childress, J. F. (2009). *Principles of biomedical ethics* (6th ed.). New York, NY: Oxford University Press.

Betan, E. J. (1997). Toward a hermeneutic model of ethical decision making in clinical practice. *Ethics & Behavior, 7*(4), 347–365.

Burger, K. G., Kramlich, D., Malitas, M., Page-Cutrara, K., & Whitfield-Harris, L. (2014). Application of the symphonological approach to faculty-to-faculty incivility in nursing education. *Journal of Nursing Education, 53*(10), 563–568. http://dx.doi.org/10.3928/01484834-20140922-02

Carrier, A., Levasseur, M., Bédard, D., & Desrosiers, J. (2010). Community occupational therapists' clinical reasoning: Identifying tacit knowledge. *Australian Occupational Therapy Journal, 57*(6), 356–365. doi:10.1111/j.1440-1630.2010.00875.x

Carter, S. M., Rychetnik, L., Lloyd, B., Kerridge, I. H., Baur, L., Bauman, A., . . . Zask, A. (2011). Evidence, ethics, and values: A framework for health promotion. *American Journal of Public Health, 101*(3), 465–472. doi:10.2105/ajph.2010.195545

Clark, P. G., Cott, C., & Drinka, T. J. (2007). Theory and practice in interprofessional ethics: A framework for understanding ethical issues in health care teams. *Journal of Interprofessional Care, 21*(6), 591–603. doi:10.1080/13561820701653227

Cutcliffe, J. R. (2003). Reconsidering reflexivity: Introducing the case for intellectual entrepreneurship. *Qualitative Health Research, 13*(1), 136–148. doi:10.1177/1049732302239416

Delany, C. M., Edwards, I., Jensen, G. M., & Skinner, E. (2010). Closing the gap between ethics knowledge and practice through active engagement: An applied model of physical therapy ethics. *Physical Therapy, 90*(7), 1068–1078. doi:10.2522/ptj.20090379

Durocher, E., & Gibson, B. E. (2010). Navigating ethical discharge planning: A case study in older adult rehabilitation. *Australian Occupational Therapy Journal, 57*(1), 2–7. doi:10.1111/j.1440-1630.2009.00826.x

Epstein, E. G., & Hamric, A. B. (2009). Moral distress, moral residue, and the crescendo effect. *Journal of Clinical Ethics, 20*(4), 330–342.

Ess, C. (2006). Ethical pluralism and global information ethics. *Ethics and Information Technology, 8*(4), 215–226. doi:10.1007/s10676-006-9113-3

Gilligan, C. (1993). *In a different voice: Psychological theory and women's development.* Cambridge, MA: Harvard University Press.

Glaser, J. W. (1994). *Three realms of ethics.* Kansas City, MO: Rowan and Littlefield.

Greenfield, B. H., & Jensen, G. M. (2010). Understanding the lived experiences of patients: Application of a phenomenological approach to ethics. *Physical Therapy, 90*(8), 1185–1197. doi:10.2522/ptj.20090348.

Haidt, J. (2001). The emotional dog and its rational tail: A social intuitionist approach to moral judgment. *Psychological Review, 108*(4), 814–834. doi:10.1037/0033-295X.108.4.814

Hinman, L. M. (2013). *Ethics: A pluralistic approach to moral theory* (5th ed.). Boston, MA: Wadsworth, Cengage Learning.

Hunt, M. R., & Ells, C. (2013). A patient-centered care ethics analysis model for rehabilitation. *American Journal of Physical Medicine and Rehabilitation, 92*(9), 818–827. doi:10.1097/PHM.0b013e318292309b

Irvine, R., Kerridge, I., & McPhee, J. (2004). Towards a dialogical ethics of interprofessionalism. *Journal of Postgraduate Medicine, 50*(4), 278–280.

Jonsen, A. R., Siegler, M., & Winslade, W. J. (2006). *Clinical ethics: A practical approach to ethical decisions in clinical medicine.* New York: McGraw Hill, Medical Pub. Division.

Kenny, B., Lincoln, M., & Balandin, S. (2007). A dynamic model of ethical reasoning in speech pathology. *Journal of Medical Ethics, 33*(9), 508–513. doi:10.1136/jme.2006.017715

Kidder, R. M. (1995). *How good people make tough choices.* New York, NY: Morrow.

Levine, C., Hoffman, J. M., Byron, J., Arnold, R., Kondrat, A., & Mukherjee, D. (2015). Surrogate decision making and truth telling in a rehabilitation case. *PM&R, 7*(7), 762–769. doi:10.1016/j.pmrj.2015.05.021.

Manson, H. M. (2012). The development of the CoRE-Values framework as an aid to ethical decision-making. *Medical Teacher, 34*(4), e258–268. doi:10.3109/0142159X.2012.660217

Molewijk, A. C., Abma, T., Stolper, M., & Widdershoven, G. (2008). Teaching ethics in the clinic. The theory and practice of moral case deliberation. *Journal of Medical Ethics, 34*(2), 120–124. doi:10.1136/jme.2006.018580

O'Rourke, M., & Crowley, S. J. (2013). Philosophical intervention and cross-disciplinary science: The story of the Toolbox Project. *Synthese, 190*(11), 1937–1954. doi:10.1007/s11229 -012-0175-y

Park, E-J. (2012). An integrated ethical decision-making model for nurses. *Nursing Ethics, 19*(1), 139–159. doi:10.1177/0969733011413491

Purtilo, R. B., & Doherty, R. F. (2011). *Ethical dimensions in the health professions* (5th ed.). St. Louis, Mo: Elsevier/Saunders.

Savage, T. A., Parson, J., Zollman, F., & Kirschner, K. L. (2009). Rehabilitation team disagreement: Guidelines for resolution. *Physical Medicine and Rehabilitation, 1*(12), 1091–1097. doi:10.1016/j. pmrj.2009.09.017

Strike, K. A. (1995). Profesional ethics and the education of professionals. *Educational Horizons, 74*(1), 29–36. doi:10.2307/42925139

Tsai, T-C., & Harasym, P. H. (2010). A medical ethical reasoning model and its contributions to medical education. *Medical Education, 44*(9), 864–873. doi:10.1111/j.1365-2923.2010.03722.x

Van Denend, T., & Finlayson, M. (2007). Ethical decision making in clinical research: Application of CELIBATE. *American Journal of Occupational Therapy, 61*(1), 92–95. doi:10.5014/ajot.61.1.92

van der Dam, S., Abma, T. A., Kardol, M. J., & Widdershoven, G. A. (2012). "Here's my dilemma". Moral case deliberation as a platform for discussing everyday ethics in elderly care. *Health Care Analysis, 20*(3), 250–267. doi:10.1007/s10728-011-0185-9

van der Dam, S., Schols, J. M., Kardol, T. J., Molewijk, B. C., Widdershoven, G. A., & Abma, T. A. (2013). The discovery of deliberation. From ambiguity to appreciation through the learning process of doing Moral Case Deliberation in Dutch elderly care. *Social Science and Medicine, 83*, 125–132. doi:10.1016/j.socscimed.2013.01.024

Wall, S., & Austin, W. (2008). The influence of teams, supervisors and organizations on healthcare practitioners' abilities to practise ethically. *Nursing Leadership, 21*(4), 85–99.

Weidema, F. C., Molewijk, A. C., Widdershoven, G. A., & Abma, T. A. (2012). Enacting ethics: Bottom-up involvement in implementing moral case deliberation. *Health Care Analysis, 20*(1), 1–19. doi:10.1007/s10728-010-0165-5

Widdershoven, G., Abma, T., & Molewijk, B. (2009). Empirical ethics as dialogical practice. *Bioethics, 23*(4), 236–248. doi:10.1111/j.1467-8519.2009.01712.x

Youssef, F. F., Dookeeram, K., Basdeo, V., Francis, E., Doman, M., Mamed, D., . . . Legall, G. (2012). Stress alters personal moral decision making. *Psychoneuroendocrinology, 37*(4), 491–498. http:// dx.doi.org/10.1016/j.psyneuen.2011.07.017

CHAPTER 4

Informed Consent, Decision-Making Capacity, and Shared Decision Making

Bruce H. Greenfield and **Gail M. Jensen**

CHAPTER OUTLINE

- Chapter Overview
- Historical, Legal, and Ethical Background

- Summary and Conclusion

CHAPTER OBJECTIVES

At the conclusion of this chapter, the reader will be able to:

1. Delineate the historical, legal, and ethical factors that have shaped the development of informed consent in health care.
2. Discuss ethical approaches that are unique to rehabilitation.
3. Discuss and evaluate different models of informed consent for rehabilitation.
4. Analyze key elements of informed consent appropriate for rehabilitation.
5. Apply models of informed consent to evaluate a case study.

KEY TERMS

Reading these key terms before reading the chapter will introduce you to key concepts which will then be somewhat familiar to you as you read this chapter. This is an important learning technique that will enhance your learning as a multi-step process. You may even wish to make a flash card set of key terms and quiz yourself on them once or twice before reading the chapter. This will better prepare you to immerse in the language of ethics and better prepare you to integrate the content.

Blanket Consent: An all-encompassing consent to the effect "I authorize so and so to carry out any test/procedure/surgery in the course of my treatment" is often not valid for specific procedures. Additional consent should be obtained before proceeding with specific tests and interventions (Rao, 2008).

Competence: Competence is a legal term. All persons are judged competent until legally judged otherwise. Patients who are deemed never competent include newborns, small children, and individuals who have been severely cognitively impaired since birth (Doherty & Purtilo, 2016, pps. 268, 269).

Decisional Capacity: Decision-making capacity includes the ability to make a choice, understand relevant information, appreciate the situation and its consequences, and process information (Menikoff 2001, p. 280).

Documented Consent: Consent that is documented in the healthcare record either as recorded in the record as having occurred (example: "the patient agreed to these goals") or as a formal written consent document (Hall, Prochazka & Fink, 2012).

Explicit Consent: Consent process in which the patient indicates definitive consent to a treatment either verbally or in writing (Rao, 2008).

Implicit Consent: Process in which consent is inferred or implied by the patient either through body language or silent assent (Carlisle, 2002).

Informed Consent: Informed consent is a tradition in the United States based on an individual's right to liberty, self-determination, and privacy (Meisel & Kuczewski, 1996). The basic elements of informed consent include disclosure, delineation of the benefits and burdens of a proposed intervention, cognition (understanding), recommended alternative treatments, and questions and clarifications. In rehabilitation, informed consent is a process of interactive conversations and shared decision making between healthcare professionals and the patient and/or patient's family (Caplan, Callahan, & Haas, 1987).

Paternalism: Healthcare decision process that is driven or determined by the healthcare provider with minimal or no patient participation. It refers to a course of action (including decisions) for the assumed interest of the person, but without or against that person's informed consent (Sjostrand, Eriksson, Juth, & Helgesson, 2013). Some contrast weak paternalism (healthcare provider making decisions to protect from harm) with strong paternalism (decisions made by the provider to promote the best interests of the patient as perceived by the provider).

Shared Decision Making: Shared decision making involves an exchange of ideas between patient/family and healthcare provider in the decision itself. Shared decision making occurs when real choice exists and the healthcare professional involves the patient in the decision (Whitney, McGuire, & McCullough, 2003).

Substituted Judgment: An appointed surrogate makes a statement that reflects what the surrogate believed the patient would have wanted when he or she was competent (Doherty & Purtilo, 2016, p. 269). In a case of substituted judgment the patient does not have an advanced directive or living will.

Surrogate or Proxy: Consent provided when someone is appointed to consent on behalf of an individual who has been deemed legally incompetent (Doherty & Purtilo, 2016, p. 269).

Verbal Consent: A verbal consent occurs if and when a patient states his or her consent to a procedure verbally but does not sign any written form. Verbal consent may be adequate for routine treatment (Kakar, Gambhir, Singh, Kaur, & Nanda, 2014).

▶ Chapter Overview

Much has been written on how to implement informed consent in healthcare practice. Many legal and ethical scholars argue that informed consent is one of the cornerstones of the U.S. healthcare system. The histories of biomedical research informed consent and clinical practice informed consent are distinct but may converge at many points (Kegley, 2004; Meisel & Kuczewski, 1996). The focus of this chapter will be on rehabilitation practice and informed consent.

The basis of informed consent for healthcare decision making is the principle of autonomy. From a healthcare perspective, the principle of autonomy is codified into most codes of ethics. The Code of Ethics of the American Physical Therapy Association, for example, states in principle 2C that "physical therapists shall provide the information necessary to allow patients or their surrogates to make informed decisions about physical therapy care or participation in clinical research" (APTA Code of Ethics, 2018). The American Occupational Therapy Association (AOTA) Code of Ethics obligates practitioners to "respect the right of the individual to self-determination, privacy, confidentiality, and consent" (2015). Similarly, speech-language practitioners are obligated to "obtain informed consent from the persons they serve about the nature and possible risks and effects of services provided, technology employed, and products dispensed" (American Speech-Language Association, 2016). From a practice standpoint, that has come to mean that a patient or surrogate has the right to be apprised of the purpose of a medical intervention, the attendant risks and benefits, and alternative treatments (Beauchamp & Childress, 2009).

Learning Point 4.1 How does the Code of Ethics for your profession address informed consent?

In many instances, the process of informed consent has become routinized to the point that its original intent does not meet its stated goals – to allow patients the appropriate information and time to process that information to make an informed decision (Meisel & Kuczewski, 1996). Consideration about the patient's values, expectations and fears may be recognized but not fully probed. Jones (1999) suggests that some healthcare professionals have become mistrustful of informed consent or view it as a legal obligation. Delany (2003) indicated that this is akin to donning a legal "flak jacket." Although the "flak jacket" approach addresses the legal requirement of informed consent in most states, many view its legal focus as a minimalist and narrow interpretation of informed consent. Delany (2003) argues that the legal approach to informed consent effectively ignores the ethical basis underlying its intent by distancing the action of disclosure from the foundational moral theory and patient-centered approaches.

> **Learning Point 4.2**   Why does Delany use the metaphor of a flak jacket to describe the legal approach to informed consent?

The common tradition of informed consent is derived from a Rule-Based, contractual, or one-time event perspective. In this perspective, informed consent has been obtained when a patient, or patient's family member, signs a consent form. This model of informed consent serves as a legal document, helpful to a healthcare professionals in the defense of a potential law suit (Meisel & Kuczewski, 1996).

Rehabilitation presents a different set of circumstances for patient care than acute care. Based on the ICF model (Jette, 2006) those who present with disabilities are influenced by a dynamic interchange of both physical and psychosocial factors – all of which require a unique, complex, and often long-term approach to care. These unique approaches raise ethical issues that may be different than those raised in acute care. For example, how do we judge what constitutes a quality outcome? Who makes that decision? What is the difference between compensation and cure? How do we address a person's loss of embodiment? What role does technology play? Who pays for intervention? To the extent that persons who suffer life changing diseases or injuries that affect their own sense of self and future, how should we view the process of informed consent to educate the patient/client as to the possibilities available? What ethical approaches to informed consent work best in these situations?

> **Learning Point 4.3**   What other issues may be unique to rehabilitation practice?

The purpose of this chapter is to explore the process of informed consent in rehabilitation. We seek to explore the question: How does the process of informed consent differ in rehabilitation? What ethical imperatives drive those differences? What does informed consent mean for the interprofessional care team when there are common goals accomplished by different team members? Discussion of the process of informed consent in rehabilitation will encompass the following areas: (1) historical, legal, and ethical background, (2) characteristics of rehabilitation, and (3) informed consent in rehabilitation.

▶ Historical, Legal, and Ethical Background

The legal premise of informed consent is fundamental in American jurisprudence. This premise is best articulated in an early legal case in the United States, Schloendorff v Society of New York Hospital by Justice Benjamin Cardozo (Menikoff, 2001). Finding for the plaintiff who did not consent to an operation that the surgeon nevertheless performed, he wrote that all adults have the right to make decisions about procedures on their body (Menikoff, 2001). Without this consent, the healthcare practitioner may be committing battery, the act of touching another without his or her consent (Doherty & Purtilo, 2016, p. 255).

From an ethical and legal standpoint informed consent is an aspect of the fiduciary relationship between a healthcare professional and the patient. In such a relationship, an individual has placed a special trust in a healthcare professional who is required to work for the best interests of that individual (Beachamp & Childress, 2009). The healthcare principle of beneficence codified in most professions code of ethics indicates clinicians should have the welfare of the patient as a goal of care. From a legal standpoint, the physician-patient relationship in the United States was ruled as a fiduciary relationship in a 1974 case, Miller v Kennedy (Menikoff, 2001).

However, it was not until the 1957 court case Salgo v Leland Stanford Board of Trustees that the actual term "informed consent" was first used in legal case law (Katz, 1998). The plaintiff in this case, who became a paraplegic following a procedure for a circulatory problem, alleged that his physician did not properly disclose ahead of time essential information concerning risks. The court found that it was the duty of the physician to disclose relevant information to the patient. "Interestingly, the entire informed consent paragraph was adopted verbatim from the *amicus curiae* brief (friend of the court brief that is unsolicited and offers information that bears on the case) submitted by the College of Surgeons (Meisel & Kuscewski, 1996). Most states have adopted and developed informed consent laws to govern medical and healthcare professional practice, but this varies by state as to who is covered.

Doherty and Purtilo (2016) point out that some legal experts consider informed consent as a legal contract between the patient and health professional. A contract is a legal agreement that binds one party to provide services to another (Menikoff, 2001, p. 153). The concept of health care as a legal contract has been used in some medical situations to justify patient abandonment by a healthcare professional.

Learning Point 4.4   Would it be appropriate from an ethical perspective to abandon a patient?

Whether informed consent serves as a formal contract between provider and patient, the law recognizes several challenges in attempting to elicit informed consent. For instance, some states have different disclosure standards based on providing patients "reasonable information" versus full and "complete disclosure" (King & Moulton, 2009).

The issue of the legality of providing a standardized general consent form when entering a hospital for care may not be appropriate for rehabilitation. Collaborative care necessitates individual consent from different team members, or a different model of collaborative informed consent.

Some argue informed consent that emphasizes legal imperatives is too narrowly construed by ignoring ethical obligations and patient rights (Delany, 2003). Informed consent should be based on principles of respect for patient autonomy, dignity, and beneficence and as part of the caring relationship between the provider and his/her client. From that perspective, the purpose of informed consent, while still a recognizable legal requirement, is also recognized and embraced by practitioners as part of the process of an ethics of care that privileges patient centeredness and shared decision making. The ethos of informed consent is to forge a meaningful relationship of trust between healthcare practitioners and their patients.

Standards of Informed Consent

Currently, three legal standards of informed consent are used in healthcare practice: (1) provider-based, informed consent (the professional practice standard; customary medical language); (2) the reasonable person/patient standard, and (3) the subjective standard (Beauchamp & Childress, 2009). Provider-based standards grant healthcare providers' discretion in determining how much information to provide patients, the amount of disclosure required to meet the legal standards of care defined in reference to the actions of other providers, the degree what a reasonably prudent practitioner in the same field would do. Although half the states in the United States abide by a provider-based standard of consent, those who argue against these standards base their arguments on its assumption that all healthcare providers agree on standards in a given field and in a particular patient case. King and Moulton (2009) argue that providers may not be in the best position to make treatment decisions and should not limit disclosure of alternatives.

Alternatively, patient-based standards place greater emphasis on the patient role in making informed decisions to the extent to which provider expertise would longer subsume objective patient preference. The standard is based on the needs of an objective and reasonable patient and what they would want to know, requiring a provider to disclose all material risks. Of course, the constituted material risk was still left to the judgement of the physician.

Finally, the subjective model judges the adequacy of the information by reference to the specific informational needs of the individual person, rather than by a hypothetical "reasonable person." This standard is more contextual than the other two in that the provision of informed consent is tailored to individual needs, goals, and expectations. Beauchamp and Childress (2009) argue that the subjective standard is the preferable moral standard of disclosure, because it alone meets persons' specific informational needs.

There are a few exceptions to the obligation of providing informed consent, including therapeutic privilege. Therapeutic privilege states that a healthcare professional may legitimately withhold information based on a sound professional judgment, if divulging the information would potentially harm a person who is depressed, emotionally drained or unstable (Beauchamp & Childress, 2009). This approach is somewhat different than a strong paternalistic approach in which the healthcare professional may withhold or downplay alternative treatment options based on his or her belief of the best option.

Informed Consent in Rehabilitation

Four major characteristics distinguish rehabilitation care from acute care. They are the team approach, family context, active versus passive participation, and informed consent (Caplan, Callahan, & Haas, 1987: Kueczewski, 2009).

Team Approach

In order to understand how the team approach works in rehabilitation, it is important to review the current ICF model described in Chapter 2. Recall that the ICF model depicts six domains of changes in normal health status that ultimately can contribute to disability or inability to participate in an identified social role (Jette, 2006). The ICF model makes it evident that caring for patients' with disabilities requires multiple types of expertise contributing to the domain of health. Based on their expertise, education, and clinical training, we can expect healthcare professionals to have primary patient care responsibilities in certain domains while having secondary responsibilities in other domains. For example, it is generally acknowledged that the physician in a healthcare team has the primary responsibility to diagnose and treat disease and pathology. Yet, the physician should also collaborate with other members of the rehabilitation team, most noticeably physical therapy and occupational therapy to help diagnose sensory and movement impairments linked to function and disability. Additionally, the team works closely with neuropsychology and social work to uncover and explore the psychosocial issues of care. As pointed out in Chapter 2, for the team to work seamlessly, it must develop a framework for collaborative communication, respect, and practice. Principles of professional autonomy between individual team members must be balanced with principles of trust, professional integrity, procedural justice, and beneficence toward the patient/client and family.

Pecukonis, Doyle, and Bliss (2008) describe that seamless interprofessional teamwork requires an understanding and appreciation of the roles and contributions that each profession brings to the helping process. Moreover, each rehabilitation team member must incorporate a shared vision of team decision making, planning, and goal setting. What often challenges this seamless process is the concept of professional-centrism based on strong group affiliation that is positively correlated with negative attitudes toward other groups. The author argues that to be successful in developing interprofessional teamwork across the domains of practice, we must develop ways to challenge and dispel notions of professional-centrism, seeking ways of developing a common moral framework (or moral commons). Challenges faced by the team include team dynamics when disequilibrium arises between team decisions and individual professional decisions; lack of respect of one's knowledge contribution to the team; and a hierarchically structured organizational structure (Kvanstrom, 2008). As will be discussed shortly, informed consent processes pose unique challenges in rehabilitation partly due to how individual members of the team share treatment responsibilities with each other and the patient.

Learning Point 4.5   What are the three major challenges of interprofessional teams? Have you experienced these?

Family

The family is often intimately involved as a primary stakeholder in rehabilitation. To the extent to which a patient may lack capacity or competence to make treatment choices (e.g., patients with traumatic brain injury), the family takes on a large role as surrogates to make informed decisions about patient care. This poses challenges to the healthcare team in balancing the needs of the patient with the needs of the family. For example, in patients with severe stroke, spinal cord injury, or closed head injury, where it is often difficult to predict patterns of recovery and outcomes, family members may be confused with the changing status of the patient, and implications for recovery and return to previous levels of function and social role. For family members who face changing treatment options, these choices requiring updated informed consent may be overwhelming. Additionally, team members are sometimes faced with families and surrogates who have different opinions about consenting to a certain course of treatment. Advanced directives focused on end of life do not typically address how individuals who have suffered severe neurologic insult and lost capacity would want to be treated during rehabilitation. As a result, families often struggle to do what they think is in the best interest of their loved one.

Active Versus Passive Participation

Rehabilitation team members expect patients to be active participants in the process of care. Active participation requires genuine participation, including shared aims and desires between the stakeholders and rehabilitation team (Wainapel & Morice 2014). That is, participants are emotionally and motivationally engaged with each other. Chewning and Sleath (1996) point out that in active participation the provider's role is to be a partner in the decision processes influenced by the patient's desires and abilities. Such an approach is consistent with the concept of patient-driven care and the ICF model of health and disability. Therapy and informed consent can be viewed as an iterative planning cycle. In contrast, patients are often viewed as passive participants within the older biomedical model of care.

The challenge for rehabilitation professionals is how best to obtain informed consent that honors both the legal requirements and the ethical obligation to respect patient autonomy. These requirements include patient understanding of the choices being proposed, voluntariness, and any other full disclosure that might impact the patient's decision. The timing of obtaining informed consent is also important (Schenker & Meisel, 2011; Wainapel & Morice, 2014). Often in clinical practice, the consent process occurs immediately before the procedure where the patient may have little or no time to process all the information that is being given. Decisional-capacity of patients may vary based on the time of the day due to medications, pain level, and metabolic status (Wainapel & Morice, 2014). Given these considerations, several ethical traditions of informed consent have been proposed and applied in rehabilitation.

Rule-Based Tradition

Chapter 3 describes four major ethical traditions in health care: Rule-Based, Ends-Based, Virtue-Based, and Narrative-Based. The most common ethical tradition of informed consent is Rule-Based. This is often implemented as a contractual or event "process". In many cases, consent forms are used as a matter of routine, and hospital attorneys see this form as providing protection against liability. The belief is that this approach does have some value, creating an inference that the patient or surrogate at least has an opportunity to read the information on it. Although informed consent as "event" is widespread, this approach has many critics (Meisel & Kuczewski, 1996), largely because of some myths about its process and usefulness.

We cannot assume that signing a consent form is informed consent. The information on the consent form may be inadequate or overly complex, or fails to specify all risks and alternatives, providing the patient with a false sense of security. Second, patients often want more than information. As Meisel and Kuczewski (1996) point out, often they want advice. To the extent that they might want to know what the healthcare professional would do, informed consent is part of a process of human interaction; or of shared decision making. That is, rather than think of informed consent as an event, we should think of it as a conversation or a process related to an ethics of care. In an ethics of care approach, the healthcare professional creates an environment of trust with the patient through a mutual and reciprocal dialogue (Branch, 2000). This approach broadens the focus of informed consent as a communicative practice

(Delany, 2003), or a commitment to a conversation. Critics point out that a prolonged process of informed consent may be ideal, but impractical given the exigencies of clinical practice time, and the immediacy of acute care interventions.

> **Learning Point 4.6**   What are the limitations of viewing informed consent as an event rather than part of a dialogue?

Narrative Tradition

The Narrative-Based tradition is known as the educational approach, ethics of care approach, or shared decision-making approach. This approach emphasizes the critical role of communication, understanding emotions, and empathy (Dohan, Garrett, Rendle, Halley, & Abramson, 2016). In the Narrative-Based tradition, healthcare professionals help patients construct preferences. Shared understanding is key where the healthcare professional is mindful of not only the patient's values, thoughts, and feelings but also self-reflective of what he or she brings forward (Epstein & Street, 2011). Shared knowledge includes the healthcare professional's knowledge of the patient as person – his or her habits, culture, family, and prior behavior under uncertainty. Because this approach is interactional, ideas and perspectives emerge through shared thoughts, feelings, perceptions, and meanings among two or more people.

Given the comprehensive needs of rehabilitation patients, it is clear that the Rule-Based tradition alone is inadequate, and that rehabilitation professionals must rely heavily on the narrative tradition in obtaining informed consent.

> **Learning Point 4.7**   Why is it important to use a Narrative-Based approach to informed consent in the rehabilitation setting?

Persons whose life prospects have dramatically changed due to injury or disease such as spinal cord injury or stroke may have difficulty understanding and appreciating the choices before them. Many patients in rehabilitation are existentially confused as they struggle with how they were before injury, who they are currently, and who they will become (Greenfield, 2011). Psychosocial issues such as depression and emotional trauma may prevent them from properly understanding and evaluating the potential levels of activity and achievement available to them. In such situations, preferences tend to be remarkably sensitive to the subtle effects of framing, ordering, and tone of voice, word choice, and recent experiences (Epstein & Peters, 2009).

Furthermore, because the patient and family become active participants in their care and recovery, shared deliberation involves exploring the degree to which preferences are articulated or tacit, clear or nebulous, stable or unstable, informed and uninformed. Motivation becomes paramount as the healthcare team tries to instill in patients the intrinsic motivation necessary to undergo often long and arduous rehabilitation and recovery (Ryan & Deci, 2000). Although a legally explicit agreement is necessary for informed consent in these circumstances, it should not be conflated with the attunement and collaborative understanding that characterizes shared decision making. When there is shared decision making the healthcare team can better use motivational approaches to promote behavior changes, overcome initial inertia, and promote patient self-management. Shared decision making is facilitated by the Dialogic Engagement Model described in Chapter 3. Disagreements among the team should be addressed without involving the patient or family to avoid creating doubt or conflict. The Dialogic Engagement Model calls for collaboration and ongoing deliberation among the team members, wherein all members are given a voice to state their preferences, goals, concerns, and professional expectations. The key for constructive negotiation is for the team to be morally committed to the welfare of the patient using dialogic engagement.

Learning Point 4.8   How can the Dialogic Engagement Model facilitate shared decision making?

The following cases illustrate the challenges and approaches to informed consent in rehabilitation.

Case of Mr. X

Mr. X is a 70 year-old man with a history of severe back pain for almost a decade. Mr. X was formerly a proud steel worker. This pain contributed to his decision to take to an early retirement buyout from a local company about ten years ago. The pain has increased in recent months and radiates downward from the lower back to the legs.

Since retirement, Mr. X has gained a good deal of weight although two attempts to control it resulted in significant weight losses. He denies that his weight is linked to his back pain but his medical records make it seem likely that it is. Mr. X's lifestyle includes occasional alcohol consumption and he smokes a pack of cigarettes each day. His medical history is also significant for rheumatoid arthritis and chronic obstructive pulmonary disease (COPD).

Mr. X's mood is quite variable. It is observed that when he goes to his various therapies (e.g., physical therapy, occupational therapy) he participates well and seems to make some progress. Unfortunately, every morning Mr. X refuses therapy, stating that it is "[expletive deleted] – awful that he has to be taken care of like a baby," or that his pain is too much that day. When asked by the nursing staff why he's not going to therapy, he sometimes says "What's the use?"

Mr. X has a 33-year-old son, Skip, who is a banker. Skip is married with two children. He says that his father was always a fighter. Skip says that he believes his father can be so again. If Mr. X can get to the point where he can take care of most daily living functions ("if he just doesn't stay in bed all day"), Skip and his wife would like Mr. X to live with them. If not, Mr. X will have to find some sort of structured living situation.

Reproduced from Kusczewski & Pinkus (1999).

This case raises several questions related to informed consent and patient care.

1. When does consent to therapy actually occur? When he was admitted and signed a general consent to treatment form? At weekly reviews of his treatment plan? Each morning?
2. Is it acceptable to enlist the help of others such as family in persuading Mr. X?
3. Is it ethically permissible for the therapists to take a paternalistic approach and be somewhat forceful in getting Mr. X to therapy?
4. Is Mr. X competent to make these choices?

Informed consent is often best conceived as a process in rehabilitation. The rehabilitation team can correctly surmise that Mr. X's initial general informed consent to work toward his rehabilitation goals was part of his informed consent process. Because informed consent always requires (from a team perspective) a blending of overall treatment goals and particular treatment therapies, the team should meet periodically and review treatment goals in light of the changing status of the patient.

Based on the Dialogic Engagement Model, the team should agree on a uniform approach to proceed each morning in getting the patient out of bed to therapy. This could include being more forceful (paternalistic) and, or enlisting family members to help encourage the patient. From the perspective of shared decision making and an ethics of care approach, the rehabilitation team is obligated to gain additional insight into the workings of Mr. X's mind other than what we have already heard. That is, it is not clear why Mr. X is reluctant to attend therapy even though it seems to be helping, and ultimately will help him return home with his family. This conversation should be part of ongoing informed consent.

Learning Point 4.9 Is it ethical to use persuasion, manipulation or coercion in obtaining consent? Would this change at different points of the rehabilitation process?

Learning Point 4.10 What ideas do you have for fostering motivation for this patient?

Rehabilitation is an essential part of burn treatment (Procter, 2010). The rehabilitation for patients with burn injuries requires interprofessional teamwork and care that can last for several years. Depending on the stages of rehabilitation from the acute to the rehabilitation phase, obtaining informed consent is an ongoing process of open dialogue and shared decision making between the patient and members of the interprofessional team.

The following is a case that illustrates the challenges of obtaining informed consent in a burn patient in the acute stages of rehabilitation.

Case of Bill

Bill Flowers, age 21, was admitted three weeks ago to the critical care unit of a major metropolitan hospital with third degree burns over 40 percent of his body. These burns occurred following an explosion at a paint manufacturing company where he works. He is a single and lives alone. His parents and sibling live in another state.

Bill was placed in the burn unit. The burn unit consists of an interprofessional care team specialized in the care of patients with burns. Team members include a surgeon, nurse, physical therapist, occupational therapist, psychologist, and social worker. Bill confessed upon admission to the emergency staff that he did not trust hospitals. To make matters worse, because Bill had a past history of injecting himself with meth, he was deemed by hospital staff a risk for HIV. The Hospital followed the recommendation of the most recent Center for Disease Control (CDC) Guidelines (CDC, Sept 22, 2006 https://www.cdc.gov/mmwr/preview/mmwrhtml/rr5514a1.htm), for patients in

(continues)

(continued)

healthcare settings; separate written consent for HIV testing should not be required: general consent for medical care should be considered sufficient to encompass consent for HIV testing. Although some states have statutes indicating that patents cannot be forced to take an HIV test, Bill was not provided specific informed consent to be tested for HIV. He subsequently tested positive for HIV. When Bill found out that he had been tested for HIV without his specific consent, he became irate at the hospital and hospital care team.

The interprofessional care team meets once weekly to share progress of patients and coordinate updated goals and treatment plans. The team worked well together. Unfortunately, two weeks ago, the team surgeon had to leave his position at the hospital due to personal reasons. An older surgeon took his place on the team- he was grumpy, condescending, and very opinionated. Two weeks after admission the team surgeon planned to apply skin grafts to Bill's burns. Bill was very reluctant to give his consent to the surgeon for this procedure, partly because he did not trust hospitals and was still angry about the HIV test. After some discussion, the surgeon promised Bill that if he agreed to surgery that he would not be bothered by any other healthcare provider to participate in any other activities or interventions. So it was not surprising after surgery that Bill declined to participate in all rehabilitation activities.

This case raises several issues about informed consent and healthcare team dynamics. First, as in the previous case, this case raises the question if a blanket consent form is sufficient for a patient's consent for specific procedures and tests. Rao (2008) argues that an all-encompassing consent, which authorizes a hospital to carry out any procedure or intervention, is not valid. Additional and specific consent should be provided from each member of an interprofessional care team. Clearly, this patient was not aware of the extent of the blanket consent he signed. This reinforced the patient's natural distrust of hospitals. Secondly, communication and team collaboration broke down with the arrival of the new surgeon. In this case, he made an arbitrary promise to Bill that was not realistic given the need for acute rehabilitation in burn patients, and without consulting other members of the team. Kvarnstrom (2008) qualitatively explored interprofessional teams in order to determine major causes of critical incidences that led to breakdown in team functioning. As in this case, a critical incident was identified to occur when team members were not valued equally. Additionally, team members had difficulties when they perceived a member of the team embraced hierarchical values.

As noted, informed consent is often best conceived as a process. This is particularly the case when a patient is recovering from burns and moves through a process of acute and long-term rehabilitation since goals and approaches to treatments change at various stages of recovery. In this situation, informed consent provided by team members required a blending of overall treatment goals and particular treatments and therapies (Kuczewski & Pinkus, 1999). This case demonstrates what can occur when a member of the team takes it upon himself to speak for the rest of the team to selfishly promote his own agenda functioning.

Learning Point 4.11   How might we apply the Dialogic Engagement Model to address the breakdown in team functioning?

▶ Summary and Conclusion

In this chapter, we explored the legal and ethical background of informed consent. We described the components of informed consent and its limitations in shared decision making. Following a discussion of informed consent in acute care, we examined the differences in applying informed consent in acute care versus rehabilitation medicine. Included in that discussion were the elements of rehabilitation that underlie those differences. We finished by presenting two cases that illustrate the challenges of providing informed consent in rehabilitation, and to challenge the readers for thoughtful reflection about how they might navigate through these cases.

In summary, the common tradition of informed consent is Rule-Based, often implemented as a contract, using an event approach. Rehabilitation professionals should view informed consent as a process of ongoing shared decision making, rather than a one-time event. Because rehabilitation often involves patients' actively involved in long-term care, healthcare professionals should help patients construct preferences of care based on their changing functional status through an ongoing collaborative process of communication, mutual understanding and empathy. Because rehabilitation commonly is team-based, to be successful, this process is reflected in the Dialogic Engagement Model.

Closing Reflections

Learning Activities

4.1   Reflective Practice Exercise
1. As a member of a rehabilitation healthcare team, think about how informed consent was provided to a patient by the healthcare team. How does the team address the situation?
2. Do you think a blanket consent form is sufficient for a patient in rehabilitation? Why or why not?
3. As a rehabilitation professional in private practice, do you routinely obtain informed consent? If so, how and when?

4.2   Reflective Practice Exercise
1. Contrast Rule-Based informed consent with the educational model of informed consent. What are the strengths and weakness of both?

4.3   Reflective Practice Exercise
1. Think about the last time you cared for a patient who lacked cognitive capacity. How did you obtain informed consent?
2. What challenges and issues did you face?

 Take Away Messages

- Medical ethics literature has discussed the ethical principle of informed consent extensively. Informed consent has its basis in the ethical principle of autonomy. Informed consent is an aspect of the fiduciary relationship with the patient.

- The legal view of informed consent is a more minimalist and narrower interpretation than the ethical view of informed consent.
- The common medical tradition of informed consent emphasizes a rule-based contractual, one-time event model of informed consent whereby a patient or family member signs a consent form. Because the context and process of rehabilitation are very different from medicine, informed consent for rehabilitation differs from medicine.
- Four characteristics of the rehabilitation setting that influence informed consent are the team approach, family context, and active (versus passive) participation of the patient.
- The purpose of informed consent in rehabilitation is part of the process of an ethics of care that privileges patient centeredness and shared decision making. The ethos of informed consent is to forge a meaningful relationship of trust among healthcare practitioners and their patients.
- Informed consent processes pose unique challenges in rehabilitation partly because of how individual members of the team share treatment responsibilities with each other and with the patient.
- Rehabilitation professionals should view informed consent as a process of ongoing shared decision making, rather than a one-time event.
- The Narrative-Based Tradition is an educational approach to informed consent, consistent with the shared decision making required in rehabilitation settings. The Rule-Based Approach alone may not be adequate for the comprehensive needs of rehabilitation patients and the iterative nature of decision making.
- The Dialogic Engagement Model calls for collaboration and ongoing deliberation among the team members, wherein all members are given a voice to state their preferences, goals, concerns, and professional expectations. Commitment to the patient's welfare through dialogic engagement is key to constructive team negotiation.

References

American Occupational Therapy Association. (2015). Occupational therapy code of ethics (2015). *American Journal of Occupational Therapy, 69*(Suppl 3), 6913410030. http://dx.doi.org/10.5014/ajot.2015.696S03

American Speech Language Association. (2016). *Code of Ethics*. Retrieved from www.asha.org/policyAvailable

APTA. (2018). *Code of Ethics for the Physical Therapist*. Retrieved from https://www.apta.org/uploadedFiles/APTAorg/About_Us/Policies/Ethics/CodeofEthics.pdf

Beauchamp, T. L., & Childress, J. F. (2009). *Principles of biomedical ethics* (6th ed.). New York, NY: Oxford University Press.

Branch, W. T. (2000). The ethics of caring and medical education. *Academic Medicine, 75*(2), 127–132.

Caplan, A. L., Callahan, D., & Haas, J. (1987). Ethical & policy issues in rehabilitation medicine. *The Hastings Center Report, 17*(4), 1–20.

Carlisle, J. R. (2002). Informed consent in physical medicine and rehabilitation: The physician/patient relationship – the doctor as a fiduciary, *Physical Medicine and Rehabilitation Clinics of North America, 13*, 213–224.

Chewning, B., & Sleath, B. (1996). Medication decision-making and management: A client-centered model. *Social Science and Medicine, 42*(3), 389–398.

Delaney, C. (2003). Informed consent: Broadening the focus. *Australian Journal of Physiotherapy, 49*, 159–161.

Dohan, D., Garrett, S. B., Rendle, K. A., Halley, M., Abramson, C. (2016). The importance of integrating narrative into health care decision making. *Health Affairs, 35*(4) 720–725. doi:10.1377/hlthaff.2015.1373

Doherty, R., & Purtilo. R. B. (2016). *Ethical dimensions in the health professions* (6th ed.). St. Louis: Elsevier.

Epstein, R. C., & Street, R. L. (2011). Shared mind: Communication, decision making, and autonomy in serious illness. *Annals of Family Medicine, 9*, 454–461. doi:10.1370/afm.1301

Epstein, R. M., & Peters, E. (2009). Beyond information: Exploring patients' preferences. *Journal of the American Medical Association, 302*(2), 195–197.

Greenfield, B. (2011). Phenomenology as a philosophical orientation for understanding the transformative experience of disabling illness. *Topics in Stroke Rehabilitation, 18*(1), 35–39.

Hall, D. E., Prochazka, A. V., & Fink, A. S. (2012). Informed consent for clinical treatment. *Canadian Medical Association Journal, 184*(5), 533–540.

Jette, M. A. (2006). Toward a common language for function, disability, and health. *Physical Therapy, 86*(5), 726–734.

Jones, M. A. (1999). Informed consent and other fairy stories. *Medical Law Review, 7*, 103–134.

Kakar, H., Gambhir, R. S., Singh, S., Kaur, A., & Nanda, T. (2014). Informed consent: Cornerstone in ethical medical and dental practice. *Journal of Family Medicine and Primary Care, 3*(1), 68–71.

Katz, J. (1998). Reflections on informed consent: 40 years after its birth. *Journal of the American College of Surgeons, 186*(4), 466–474. https://doi.org/10.1016/S1072-7515(98)00045-3

Kegley, J. A. K. (2004). Challenges to informed consent. *EMBO Reports, 5*(9), 832–836. doi: 10.1038/sj.embor.7400246

King, J. S., & Moulton, B. W. (2009) Rethinking informed consent: The case for shared medical decision-making. *American Journal of Law and Medicine, 32*(4), 429–501.

Kuczewski M. G. (2009). Introduction to Rehabilitation Ethics. Clinical Bioethics (BEHP 401), Masters in Bioethics, Loyola University.

Kuczeweski, M. G., & Pinkus, R. L. B. (1999). *This* is consent to therapy? In *An ethics casebook for hospitals: Practical approaches to everyday cases* (pp. 143–147). Washington DC: Georgetown University Press.

Kvanstrom, S. (2008). Difficulties in collaboration: A critical incident study of interprofessional healthcare teamwork. *Journal of Interprofessional Care, 22*(2), 191–203.

Meisel, A., & Kuczewski, M. (1996). Legal and ethical myths about informed consent. *Archives of Internal Medicine, 156*, 2521–2526.

Menikoff, J. (2001). *Law and bioethics an introduction.* Washington DC: Georgetown University Press.

Pecukonis, E., Doyle, O., & Bliss, D. L. (2008). Reducing barriers to interprofessional training: Promoting interprofessional cultural competence. *Journal of Interprofessional Care , 22*(4), 417–428.

Procter, F. (2010). Rehabilitation in the burn patient. *Indian Plastic Surgery, 43* (Suppl), S101–S113.

Rao, K. H. S. (2008). Informed consent: An ethical obligation or legal compulsion? *Journal of Cutaneous and Aesthetic Surgery, 1*(1), 33–35.

Ryan, R. M., & Deci, E. L. (2000). Intrinsic and extrinsic motivations: Classic definitions and new directions. *Contemporary Educational Psychology, 25*, 54–67. doi:10.1006/ceps.1999

Salgo vs Leland Stanford Board of Trustees. Justia US Law. Retrieved from http://law.justia.com/cases/california/court-of-appeal/2d/154/560.html

Schenker, Y., & Meisel, A. (2011). Informed consent in clinical care: Practical considerations in the effort to achieve ethical goals. *Journal of the American Medical Association, 305*(110), 1130–1131. doi.10.1001/jama.2011.333

Sjostrand, M., Eriksson, S., Juth, S., & Helgesson, G. (2013). Paternalism in the name of autonomy. *Journal of Medicine and Philosophy, 38*, 710–724.

Wainapel, S. F., & Morice, K. (2014). Ethical issues commonly managed during rehabilitation. *Physician Medicine and Rehabilitation.* Retrieved from https://now.aapmr.org/ethical-issues-commonly-managed-during-rehabilitation

Whitney, S. N., McGuire, A. L., & McCullough, L. B. (2003). A typology of shared decision-making, informed consent, and simple consent. *Annals of Internal Medicine, 140*, 54–59.

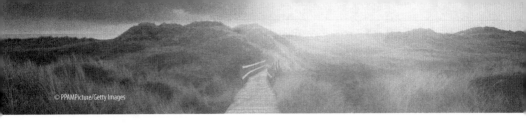

CHAPTER 5

Professional Culture Related to Ethics

Jeffrey Lee Crabtree and **Charlotte Brâsic Royeen**

CHAPTER OUTLINE

- Chapter Overview
- Culture
- Collectivist and Individualist Orientations
- Understanding Ways of Knowing: An Exposition on Ontology, Epistemology, and Axiology
- Application of Ways of Knowing to Interprofessional Ethics: Ontology, Epistemology, and Axiology

- Understanding Ways of Doing: An Exposition on Evidence and Evidence-Based Practice
- Methodology
- Method
- Evidence-Based Practice (EBP)
- Organizational Culture: The Cultural Behavior Continuum Context
- Application of Culture and Interprofessional Ethics with the Dialogic Engagement Model
- Summary and Conclusion

CHAPTER OBJECTIVES

At the conclusion of this chapter, the reader will be able to:

1. Understand that one's world view may influence what collaborators identify as information critical to effective interventions.
2. Recognize personal cultural values that may conflict with colleague and patient cultural values.
3. Judge whether collaborative interventions match the needs of patients based on their collectivist/individualist orientation.
4. Justify the intervention method based on an understanding of the patient's cultural values.
5. Construct a collaborative environment that recognizes cultural differences among professions and leads to effective interventions.

(continues)

CHAPTER OBJECTIVES   (continued)

6. Measure the effectiveness of intervention outcomes based on a proficient understanding of culture.
7. Design collaborative interventions that integrate quantitative and qualitative understandings of evidence.

KEY TERMS

Reading these key terms before reading the chapter will introduce you to key concepts which will then be somewhat familiar to you as you read this chapter. This is an important learning technique that will enhance your learning as a multi-step process. You may even wish to make a flash card set of key terms and quiz yourself on them once or twice before reading the chapter. This will better prepare you to immerse in the language of ethics and better prepare you to integrate the content.

Notice to the Reader: These are primarily philosophical terms with varying meanings depending on the context of use. Consequently, the following definitions are somewhat simplistic. The reader is encouraged to seek more specific meanings from a variety of encyclopedias or dictionaries.

Axiology: Of what is considered knowable, axiology is concerned with classifying what things are good, and what makes them good. For instance, a traditional question of axiology concerns whether subjective feelings are of value.

Collectivism: Cultural term characteristic of cohesiveness among individuals and of placing the group over the individual. Members of collectivist cultures tend to value what supports the group over what supports the individual.

Culture: Socially constructed set of beliefs and values through which we view the world, ourselves, other professions, and our patients.

Epistemology: Attempts to answer the question, what are the sources and necessary and sufficient conditions of knowing something? These are possible justifications of our beliefs, and epistemology addresses issues such as whether these justifications must be internal or external to one's knowing.

Evidence-Based Practice: In the simplest terms, evidence is something knowable like an outward sign that provides proof of something. Evidence-based practice in health care, then, entails making healthcare decisions based on intentional and judicious use of current evidence, individual clinical expertise, and patient values.

Individualism: Cultural term characteristic of emphasizing competition and personal achievement. Members of individualist cultures tend to value what supports the individual over what supports the group.

Methodology: Is concerned with identifying the best approaches, such as systematic observation and experimentation, inductive and deductive reasoning, and the formation and testing of hypotheses and theories, to best gain knowledge or understanding.

Ontology: Is on one hand the study of what there is or what exists. On the other hand, it is the study of the general features and relations of those things that do exist.

Ways of Knowing: Acknowledges that there are many knowledge-based disciplines, such as mathematics, human science, history, and ethics, and within each one there are different "ways of knowing" which include, but are not limited to, emotion, faith, memory, reason, and what is perceived through our senses.

▶ Chapter Overview

This chapter addresses a fundamental challenge related to interprofessional ethics, and one that is only beginning to be addressed (Guess, 2004): The influence of personal and professional culture on the decision-making process that leads to ethical actions in interprofessional collaborations. We may implicitly know how varied culture is in the United States, that each of us has a culture, and that our profession has a culture; yet rarely do we make that awareness explicit and examine our professional and personal cultures or analyze them in relation to decisions about patient care. The typical literature on culture often describes and compares cultures (Axinn, Blair, Herohiada, & Thach, 2004). The purpose of this chapter, somewhat differently, is not to explore culture across race, ethnic group or socioeconomic status, but rather to explore how culture also pertains to professions. Accordingly, traditional multicultural, ethnic, and racial cross cultural issues are not addressed here. Rather, we are focusing on issues of bias or variations of culture across professional cultures.

We examine our many assumptions about cultures by discussing decision-making concepts related to, and influenced by, culture. These include our collectivist and/or individualist orientation; an interactive system of ontology, epistemology, and axiology; what we consider to be evidence pertinent to our patients; what evidence we use to document our effectiveness and patient outcomes; and the cultural behavior continuum context within which we work. Through examples and vignettes, we explore the need for rapprochement or creation of harmonious relationships between professions that have different cultures. We finish with a summary and conclusions.

▶ Culture

According to some, culture is so much a part of the person it ". . . cannot be reified, seen as distinct from the self, nor can it be treated as something objective or subjective; and, second, agency and culture are intertwined and distributed across levels of knowing (Christopher & Bickhard, 2007, p. 259–295). Furthermore, in a comprehensive review of core issues in neuroanthropology, Domínguez, Juan, Lewis, Turner, and Egan (2009) found that:

> . . . the extent and breadth of the influence of culture on the brain: literally all brain areas, cortical and subcortical, respond to regularities in the cultural stream of experience. Furthermore, culture not only shapes preexisting patterns of neural activity, but it may also determine whether a pattern is at all present. In addition to influencing brain function culture also changes the structure of the brain. . . . [and]. . . . cultural regularities can modulate cognitive function both implicitly and explicitly. (p. 43)

Culture is neither a facilitator nor a barrier to interprofessional ethics. It is a socially constructed framework through which we have developed our institutional structures (Greif, 1994; Uschold & Gruninger, 1996). It is, therefore, a perspective through which we view the world, ourselves, other professions, and our patients. The concept of culture is complex. Even commonly understood differences in an individual's culture can cause consternation in a collaborative team. Classic examples in health care include cultural variations in worship practices. For example, patients' days of worship or religious holidays do not always match those of the healthcare organization and cultural holidays of particular religious groups of any sort can appear intrusive or difficult to accommodate.

The Webster online dictionary includes a number of characteristics that describe culture from the beliefs of formal religious groups, to shared attitudes and values that characterize social groups, to specific values and practices that are shared by people in a particular field or profession (Culture, n.d.). Our approach to looking at culture across professions is relatively novel and may take a different slant to which you are accustomed. Most consideration of culture concerns ethnicity or racial group. Our look at culture, by contrast, looks at professional affiliation as a cultural group.

Cultural differences among interprofessionals or between professionals and patients are common.

> **Learning Point 5.1**   Can you think of an instance in which you realized that cultural difference was an important dynamic?

The holy month of Ramadan provides a good example. For one thing, the obligations of Muslims to fast during Ramadan have obvious dietary implications for the patient and collaborative team, but those obligations extend beyond what members of the team might understand. For example, any number of missed days of fasting may need to be made up during the year (Taheri & Jackson, n.d.). Also, while not directly related to health care, the collaborative team in an outpatient setting, for example, might find that providing a room in the clinic for prayer during Ramadan could improve outpatient attendance during the month of Ramadan (Taheri & Jackson, n.d.).

The literature is rich with studies and examples of the effect of culture on individuals and ranges from neurological evidence that culture may influence a person's inclination or disinclination to affective disorders, self-judgments, or decisions and values (Chiao & Blizinsky, 2009; Chiao et al., 2009). Professional cultures influence how individuals view other professions (Almas & Odegard, 2010; Austin & Martin, 2007), and culture can influence how each of us perceives our patients.

The literature often organizes cultures on a continuum between collectivism and individualism, but such a conceptual model is not without controversy. As Schwartz (1990) has pointed out, the collectivism and individualism continuum tends to exclude some common values that serve both individualism and collectivism. Controversy aside, to better understand how culture influences interprofessional ethical decision making, we provide a brief explanation of the continuum between collaboration or individuals in the next section.

▶ Collectivist and Individualist Orientations

Concepts of cultural collectivism and individualism are discussed together because they can be seen, in their pure forms, as two opposing points on a continuum of personal obligations we have to others. For example, Oyserman, Coon, and Kemmelmeier (2002), suggest "[t]he core element of individualism is the assumption that individuals are independent of one another" (p. 4) while "[t]he core element of collectivism is the assumption that groups bind and mutually obligate individuals" (p. 5). Typically, the United States and most of "western culture" is considered to embrace an individualistic model whereas countries of the eastern part of the world tend to operate as a more collective culture.

Learning Point 5.2 Does your cultural background value individualism or collectivism more heavily?

Japan and the United States are contrasting examples in which Japan is generally understood to value group harmony and the common greater good over the individual's needs, while the United States is generally understood to support what is good for the individual over the group. Furthermore, evidence from a significant study of 83 meta-analysis and 170 other studies suggests ones' individualism or collectivism orientation has an influence over basic psychological domains (Oyserman, Coon, & Kemmelmeier, 2002). In summary they found:

1. Not everyone makes sense of the self in terms of high self-esteem or positive self-views, as Americans do.
2. Far from being universally tied to [individualism] or to [collectivism], well-being is related to attaining culturally valued outcomes.
3. In terms of attribution and cognitive style, not everyone spontaneously and persistently ignores contextual influence on human behavior as Americans do.
4. Finally, people are likely to differ in what they understand to be reinforcing and rewarding and how they treat in-group as opposed to out-group members.
5. Further, the body of cultural evidence does make clear the need to include relationality and desire for closeness to others as components of self-concept, well-being, and intergroup relations, whether considering these parts of a single psychology or as multiple psychologies (p. 45).

Learning Point 5.3 What is meant by in-group and out-group?

The variable influence that psychological domains have on practitioners assures that within any interprofessional collaboration, there will be varying senses of obligation to the patient, to the interprofessional team, and to society.

A look at the extremes of this continuum in American society can further help explain the concept of individualism versus collectivism. In 1980, after President Regan abolished the draft to help the country transition from a conscript to a fully volunteer army, the U.S. Army developed the recruiting slogan: "Be All You Can Be" that was used until 2001. It was believed that this slogan and accompanying advertisements were instrumental in making this military transition from conscript to volunteer army possible (Evans, 2015). In essence, this slogan was an appeal to be the best individual you can be (individualism), not the best team member you can be (Bailey, 2009), presumably without any particular obligation to others (collectivism).

From a collectivist perspective, perhaps the best known example of collectivist culture is the kibbutzim of Israel, known as collective community centered farms. Even in the United States there are communes sprinkled throughout the country that similarly embrace the collectivist end of the continuum. For example, the Acorn

Farm in Mineral, Virginia (Fellowship for Intentional Community, 2017), which is affiliated with the Fellowship for Intentional Community (http://www.ic.org), espouses collectivist values. According to Acorn Community Farm site (Fellowship for Intentional Community, 2017):

> We live on a working farm which means there is always plenty to do. Everyone is expected to contribute 42 hours of labor a week. . . .We grow herbs and food for our kitchen & seeds for our business, care for lots of livestock (chickens, cows, goats, & pigs!), cook two community meals daily, educate our children, maintain our land & buildings, and do office jobs like accounting, seed packing and order picking/shipping. . . . Members may also work outside jobs to fulfill their labor quota. All of this work is valued equally.

Two vignettes regarding the continuum of individualism to collectivism from the healthcare perspective are presented for consideration.

VIGNETTE ONE

Consider the case in a healthcare setting in which the team is discussing discharge planning after an elderly woman has been in the hospital for four weeks. When considering the patient's required level of independence for discharge, the U.S. born occupational therapist may push hard for the patient to be independent in bathing and toileting, which also requires independent transfers. The occupational therapist offers an extensive justification based on the concepts of functional independence. The physical therapist, born in Taiwan, believes independence is not an appropriate goal and wants to train the family caregivers to assist with needed transfers based on the concept of interdependence and filial obligation to care for the mother.

From your perspective, what should be the outcome recommendation and why?

VIGNETTE TWO

This case is focused on the interprofessional collaboration process. One practitioner expresses frustration about how team meetings take precious time away from treatment. In this instance, she views her time allotment from an individualistically-oriented perspective while team meetings reflect a collectivist viewpoint. From your perspective, is this therapist correct? Should she minimize team meetings and put more time into direct treatment? From your perspective, what is the correct outcome and why?

▶ Understanding Ways of Knowing: An Exposition on Ontology, Epistemology, and Axiology

This section will explore an integrated and interactive system that helps explain the complexities of ways of knowing. This system is composed of ontology (what we know), epistemology (how we know what we know), and axiology (the value we place on what we know). Each part of the system is interdependent with the other and together form the basis of ways of doing because to take action, we need a methodology. That methodology explains and supports a particular method or methods we use to confirm or explain what we know. Especially in the context of interprofessional practice and ethics where there can be multiple, and sometimes competing, ways of knowing and doing, this integrated and interactive system needs to be made explicit.

Of the many possible variations of what the system looks like, a physical therapist's world view might include the idea that human movement in the physical world is knowable (ontology) and that it is measurable (epistemology) through our senses. Furthermore, movement is valuable (axiology). In practice, because physical therapists can "know" a human's movement and because people value movement, their movement is an important part of physical therapy, interventions, and outcomes. From a somewhat different perspective, an occupational therapist's world view (ontology) might include the idea that we can know humans' subjective emotions, and that their emotions can be described and measured (epistemology) and are valued (axiology). In practice, because occupational therapists can "know" other humans' emotions and because people value emotions, emotions are considered measurable and an important part of occupational therapy interventions and outcomes.

Learning Point 5.4   What is your personal ontology, epistemology and axiology?

The concepts of ontology, epistemology, and axiology come directly from philosophy. Accordingly, in the interprofessional practice arena, any system that hopes to explain ways of knowing is also fraught with disagreement and controversy. We review the system here because sound interprofessional rehabilitation and decision-making processes that lead to ethical actions are informed, in part, by the results of science and research. So in a sense, this section is best described as the application of what researchers and scientists believe to be a useful explanation of the complexities of ways of knowing.

FIGURE 5.1 depicts the interrelationships between the elements of this interactive or interrelated system and suggests that the individual interprofessional practitioner and her profession exist at the intersections of ontology, epistemology, and axiology. Thus, this chapter is not a philosophical treatise, but provides the reader with a foundational understanding of professional domains. We encourage the reader to explore the meanings and application of this system with your own collaboration team.

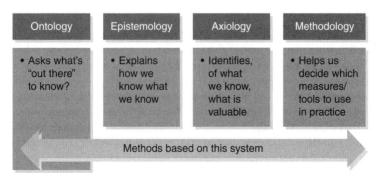

FIGURE 5.1 Interrelationships between the elements of the interrelated system.

▶ Application of Ways of Knowing to Interprofessional Ethics: Ontology, Epistemology, and Axiology

Making the ways of knowing explicit is necessary to understand why professionals view situations differently, interpret patient conditions and challenges differently, and sometimes make decisions that lead to ethical actions with which others in the collaborative team disagree.

Ontology

Ontology is generally defined as: "a branch of metaphysics concerned with the nature and relations of being" ("Ontology", n.d.). The second Merriam-Webster definition, however, "a particular theory about the nature of being or the kinds of things that have existence" ("Ontology", n.d.), suggests just how complicated and diverse ontology can be. An individual's or profession's ontology, just like culture, may be particular to a profession or may have common elements among several professions. Professional ontology is often taken for granted, and in many cases, if articulated at all, is over simplified.

> **Learning Point 5.5**   What are the implications of professional ontology being taken for granted? What are the potential consequences of professions not self-consciously examining ontology?

Often a person's ontology is also considered a person's world view, or apprehension and conception of the world ("Worldview", n.d.).

Epistemology

Epistemology overlaps with ontology and axiology and generally explains how we know what we know within each profession or discipline. This level of understanding takes interprofessional education and training to a deeper level of understanding. Simply put, examples of different, but likely familiar, epistemological stances are post-positivism and constructivism—often associated with quantitative and qualitative types of research, respectively, and somewhat overlapping views of how we know what we know (Trochim, 2006). With post-positivism, typically what we know of reality is fallible and based on conjecture, but an objective reality does exist. With this perspective, the researcher would make every effort to control confounding variables, but still acknowledge that the results of the study may be flawed. The practitioners would be conscious of the fact that evidence they used to support an intervention could be flawed. Constructivist (Mallon, 2014) researchers would not likely believe an objective reality exists or expect to gain knowledge that was independent of their or of other's inquiries. Constructivists would expect no universal laws to apply to their area of research. Likewise, constructivist practitioners would likely acknowledge that they will never truly know, in any object sense, their patient.

> **Learning Point 5.6**   Is there an implicit epistemology of EBP?

Axiology

As stated earlier, axiology sometimes called value theory, has to do with what value we place on what we know. As Schroeder says: "Axiology can be thought of as primarily concerned with classifying what things are good, and how good they are. For instance, a traditional question of axiology concerns whether the objects of value are subjective psychological states, or objective states of the world" (Schroeder, 2016). In the context of this chapter, it is important to acknowledge that all professions implicitly, if not explicitly, have an axiological stance. This is an awareness of what it knows to be the good, bad, or ugly and makes value-based judgments in the context of multicultural collaborative teams providing services. Value-based medicine (VBM) provides a good example of the challenges and the potential solutions to these value-laden circumstances. For example, Little, Lipworth, Gordon, Markham, and Kerridge (2012) explain that:

> A clinical practice based on values is practice that remains constantly aware of cultural interpretations of the foundational values. By recognizing that different cultures and different groups within societies play out foundational values in different ways, VBM recognizes and respects the common needs that all people have for survival, security and flourishing. (p. 8)

▶ Understanding Ways of Doing: An Exposition on Evidence and Evidence-Based Practice

As stated at the beginning, our intention is to render explicit the many assumptions we have about our personal and professional cultures and their impact on ways of knowing. To do that, we have explored culture, collectivistic and individualistic orientations, and the interactive system of ontology, epistemology, and axiology. In the following section we explore ways of doing that by-and-largely emerging from our beliefs about ways of knowing. Common emergence of evidence can be seen in our everyday language. For example, thinking back on observing a person who raised his voice to a waitress and gestured menacingly, we are likely to think: Evidently he was angry at the waitress; such a strong assertion of a "fact" will likely elicit the question: How do you know that?

Evidence

Common notions of evidence, outward signs or something that provides proof ("Evidence", n.d.), of course, have been around as long as humans. Sackett and colleagues in 1996 narrowed the definition for healthcare professions of evidence to:

> . . . the best available external clinical evidence. . . [from]. . . clinically relevant research, often from the basic sciences of medicine, but especially from patient centred clinical research into the accuracy and precision of diagnostic tests (including the clinical examination), the power of prognostic markers, and the efficacy and safety of therapeutic, rehabilitative, and preventive regimens. (pp. 71–72)

As a member of a collaborative team we work through the elements of a particular case, and are influenced by what we believe to be knowable (ontology); our theory that guides how gain knowledge (epistemology); and our understanding of what is important about what we know (axiology). Whether consciously or not, to answer questions about what we know about our patients or their needs, we choose strategies we think best organize and represent data about our patients (methodology), and we choose tools, or measures, we believe best collect needed information and data (method). The products of that process are the acceptable or unacceptable evidence upon which to act and to document patient outcomes.

There is much disagreement across and within professions about what constitutes acceptable evidence and the best actions to take that yield ethical practice. These disagreements can be traced to differences between a profession's cultural beliefs about its ontology, epistemology, and methodology. However, there is unanimity about the need to base our professional decisions and actions on evidence (Aarons, Hurlburt, & Horwitz, 2011; Satterfield et al., 2009; Weisz, Jensen-Doss, & Hawley, 2006).

The healthcare literature abounds with evidence of authors and professions wrestling with ways of knowing and ways of doing. Examples of such include those from speech and language pathology (Ratner, 2006; Zipoli & Kennedy, 2005), mental health practitioners (Lehman & Steinwachs, 2003; Tanenbaum, 2005), physical therapy (Landsman, 2006; Menon, Korner-Bitensky, Kastner, McKibbon, & Straus 2009), art therapy (Clift, 2012; Slayton, D'Archer, & Kaplan, 2010), music therapy (Abrams, 2010; Ellis, Koenig, & Thayer, 2012), occupational therapy (Bennett et al., 2003; Kinsella & Whiteford, 2009; Yerxa, 1990), and nursing (Arslanian-Engoren, Hicks, Whall, & Algase, 2005; Banning, 2005).

Learning Point 5.7 What is your profession's view of evidence-based practice?

Scott and McSherry (2009), in their review of the nursing literature, exemplify discussion about the relationship between evidence and practice that are common in the healthcare literature. In their critical review of 83 nursing articles, they state:

> The review clearly shows that for evidence-based nursing to occur, nurses need to be aware of what evidence based nursing means, what constitutes evidence, how evidence-based nursing differs from evidence-based medicine and evidence-based practice and what the process is to engage with and apply the evidence. (p. 1085)

To paraphrase their conclusions, for evidence-based practice to occur in collaborative teams, all healthcare professionals need to be aware of what evidence means in their profession as well in other professions, what constitutes evidence, how one profession's evidence differs from another, and the best process with which to engage and apply evidence.

Learning Point 5.8 Consider the questions posed in the text for your profession.

▶ Methodology

To better understand the concept of evidence-based practice it is useful to make explicit the role methodology and method play in the process of clinical, ethical, decision making. According to the *Stanford Encyclopedia of Philosophy*, methodology, which they call the scientific method:

> . . . is an enormously successful human enterprise. The study of scientific method [methodology] is the attempt to discern the activities by which that success is achieved. Among the activities often identified as characteristic of science are systematic observation and experimentation, inductive and deductive reasoning, and the formation and testing of hypotheses and theories. (Andersen & Hepburn, 2016, n.p.)

Methodology is an extension of epistemology in that it explains, supports, and informs the methods used in an area of study, anything from the disciplines of philosophy and history to health care. And depending on the area of study, the methodologies may be very few or very numerous. To continue with the examples described previously, post-positivism research methodologies may be quantitative in nature, in the hopes of being able to separate as much objective information as possible from inevitable subjective information. Examples would be to use double-blinded randomly controlled trials to control for as many variables as possible. Practitioners would be conscious of the fact that what evidence they used to support an intervention could be flawed, but would use assessments or evaluations that met the highest standards of reliability and validity as possible.

The constructivist researcher would use methodologies that meet the rigorous standards of qualitative research such as credibility, transferability, auditability, and confirmability (Creswell & Poth, 2017). Constructivist practitioners might well use methodologies from the post-positivist tradition but would likely also seek information about their patient or patient's condition through observation of the patient, through dialectical reasoning and interactions with their patient (Creswell & Poth, 2017).

▶ Method

Finally, method, in the most simplistic sense of the word, is both a way of doing something and a way of quantifying or qualifying something. Method as a way of doing, for example, includes the Suzuki (1898–1998) method of teaching violin (Kendall, 1973); the value added method of marketing in which you get a free appraisal, and with the purchase of the item, a free meal; and the minimally invasive total hip replacement method which, according to its advocates, causes less pain and allows for physical therapy the same day of the surgery (Berger et al., 2004).

Method is also a way of measuring, quantifying or qualifying, something. If you wanted to better understand how graduates of the Suzuki method felt about the method, you could use a descriptive methodology and survey graduates about what they think about the Suzuki method. If you wanted to evaluate the effectiveness of the minimally invasive total hip replacement, you could use an experimental methodology, a randomized control trial study, to compare the posterior and anterior approaches to hip replacements to ascertain which is most effective.

Method in the healthcare practice arena, as the saying goes, is where the organizing of information meets the road. Now more than ever, we seek evidence upon which to make healthcare decisions and to maximize the chances of these decisions being ethical. The evidence we use often comes from results of our evaluation and assessment methods. Without going into the fine distinctions between evaluation and assessment, the choices of which evaluation or assessment we choose depend on our beliefs about what is knowable (ontology); our theories of knowledge that guide how we go about gaining knowledge (epistemology); what we think is worth knowing, its validity and scope, and the worth of that knowledge (axiology); and the methods that best yield the evidence we need to make treatment decisions.

Choosing which method in health care that would yield the best results and provide the best documentation of outcomes and or value of care is a culturally charged process with potentially very high stakes to the patient and the collaborative interprofessional team. And this is where methodology comes into the picture. What is the best method of learning whether the Suzuki method or the minimally invasive total hip replacement is effective? At this point, health care is in a state of flux but numbers and quantitative measurement have been the dominant model in the past. As we move to value versus volume-based health care, we may see changes.

▶ Evidence-Based Practice (EBP)

As we have suggested, there is little agreement among healthcare professions about what is the best or most valuable evidence that answers critical questions about our patients or that best supports a claim. This acknowledgement underscores why there are so many specialties within medicine, for example, or why there are so many different healthcare professions. Each specialty and profession brings to the healthcare field and to patient interventions different ways of knowing and of doing all of which are influenced by culture.

In their review of the concepts and controversies of evidence-based practice in rehabilitation, Dijkers, Murphy, and Krellman (2012) conclude:

> . . . rehabilitation professionals will have to oversee and facilitate the next major paradigm shift in the rehabilitation sciences: the redefinition of evidence from an inconsistent combination of basic science research findings and the experientially derived opinions of individual professionals, to findings derived from clinical research conducted using designs appropriate to answer the question(s) at hand. Only then will rehabilitation researchers and clinicians truly be engaging in EBP. (p. S172)

It is interesting to note, however, that these authors neglected the even more complicated paradigm shift of redefining evidence from not only ". . . an inconsistent combination of basic science research findings and the experientially derived opinions of individual professionals. . . ," but additionally, redefining or finding common ground from among the multiplicity of interprofessional perspectives that must be acknowledged and addressed ". . . to answer the question(s) at hand. Only then will rehabilitation researchers and clinicians truly be engaging in EBP" (Dijkers, Murphy, & Krellman, 2012, p. S172).

To meet the requirement of "truly engaging in EBP", several authors explored ways of refining and expanding the concepts included in EBP. For example, Satterfield et al. (2009) conclude "…environment and organizational factors to create a cultural context that moderates the acceptability of an intervention, its feasibility, and the balance between fidelity and adaptation that is needed for effective implementation" (p. 382). They acknowledge that the influence of the practice environment and organizational context may vary considerably depending on the professions involved. For example,

> . . . some disciplines, such as nursing, social work, and public health, may be more likely to choose or modify evidence-based interventions based on context. Nursing's practices are organizational, and the feasibility of its practice recommendations is modified by governing policies, purchasing agreements, and affiliations. Because it is a social science, social work naturally incorporates attributes of the client's environment into the plan of care. (p. 382)

Others have both expanded the content of the traditional EBP model and expanded the rationale for making evidence-based decisions to better fit the epistemological concerns of a profession. For example, Tomlin and Borgetto (2011) claim that the typical EBP model contains a single hierarchy of primarily quantitative levels of evidence. This kind of evidence tends to have high levels of internal validity, but lack generalizability to real world situations. They further maintain that this model ". . . fails to incorporate at parity all types of research evidence that are valuable in the practice of occupational therapy" (p. 189) and suggest that additional dimensions of qualitative evidence must be included in EBP models. This sort of expanded EBP rationale suits the need for evidence needed to inform, for example, the demands facing people with disabling conditions of living and working in the community.

We recommend that the reader explore her or his professional literature for information about the evidence controversies and leading edge evidence-based practice in their profession. You may discover "cross cultural" or cross professional variation in what is accepted as evidence-based practice. In the following section, we discuss the context in which interprofessional collaboration or cross cultural transactions take place, everything from the acute rehabilitation inpatient setting to home care.

Learning Point 5.9   How should interprofessional teams negotiate potential disagreements about the meaning and use of evidence?

▶ Organizational Culture: The Cultural Behavior Continuum Context

When speaking of culture as a dimension of human behavior, it is useful to describe the entire range of possible individual and organizational responses to cultural and ethnic diversity explained by one's culture. For this purpose we use a concept articulated by the late Bob Hallowell (personal communication, 2001), a colleague from the Omaha Indian Tribe of Nebraska. He described a range of cultural contexts for behaviors. This range includes overt cultural destructiveness, covert cultural destructiveness, cultural blindness, cultural sensitivity, cultural competence, cultural proficiency, and institutionalized cultural proficiency. We use these more to describe the spoken or unspoken collective context of a work setting, rather than to describe individual biases. These points along the cultural behavior continuum context are described in detail in **TABLE 5.1**.

TABLE 5.1 Cultural Behavior Continuum Context of Bob Hallowell	
Context	**Collective Behavior**
1. Overt Cultural Destructiveness	Describes organizational attitudes and beliefs that support intentional and militant actions to intentionally kill or subdue people in the name of cultural beliefs and values.
2. Covert Cultural Destructiveness	Describes subtle, non-lethal, organizational attitudes and beliefs that limit access to social and economic resources, and prevent an individual or group of people from acting in their values and beliefs and from practicing cultural-specific rituals and ceremonies and from speaking their native language.
3. Cultural Blindness	Describes when the organizational setting does not recognize, acknowledge, or validate cultural values and differences of other ethnic or cultural groups. Those differences, regardless of their potential value to the observer, are not allowed to exist.
4. Cultural Sensitivity	Indicates an organizational setting that supports awareness, understanding, or appreciation of others' differences, values, beliefs, and the like. But as used in this continuum, cultural sensitivity, at its worst is superficial and condescending, and at its best falls short of any meaningful effort on the part of a person of one culture to examine and understand a person of another culture.
5. Cultural Competence	Describes a setting in which reflecting on one's own culture, values, beliefs, and experiences with people from different ethnic groups and cultures with the ability to apply what is learned from those reflections to make everyday practice with patients of different cultural backgrounds as fair and caring as possible.
6. Institutionalized Cultural Proficiency Context	Describes the circumstance in which an organization, hospital, or rehabilitation clinic includes in their mission and organization strategies, the expectation that all employees exhibit culturally competent behaviors resulting from self-examination and efforts to understand and appreciate different culture's beliefs, values, etc., and that these stated goals are truly operationalized.

Table 5-1 depicts the continuum of behavior when considering culture. It is useful to self-assess or to assess others in terms of where they may fall within this continuum.

Learning Point 5.10   What examples of the cultural behavior continuum described in Table 5-1 have you experienced?

VIGNETTE THREE

Vignette Three incorporates use of Table 5-1 in the following: You work in a setting in which there is an unwritten rule that people keep their personal values to themselves in order to be culturally neutral in the workplace. This "rule" is meant to foster neither acceptance nor rejection of all cultures and peoples' values and to encourage fair treatment of fellow practitioners and patients. You are all right with that; you do not push your values on anyone, and you would just as soon no one pushes his/her cultural values on you. You have heard about terms like collectivism, individualism, autonomy, and nonmaleficence, but are not really sure what they mean or especially how they might apply in your setting with your patient.

This vignette represents the "cultural sensitivity" point on the continuum of what Hallowell (Crabtree, Royeen, & Benton, 2006) called the cultural behavior continuum seen in Table 5-1. On the surface cultural sensitivity seems to support awareness, understanding, or appreciation of others' differences, values, and beliefs. But at its worst is superficial and condescending, and does not facilitate the needed discussion among members of the interprofessional collaboration or between professionals and patients—discussions that would help clarify each stakeholder's values and begin the process of rapprochement needed for effective and ethical interventions.

We maintain that to be effective and ethical interprofessional practitioners, one must perform in at least the "cultural competence" point along the continuum and be working toward "institutionalized cultural proficiency." At the cultural competence point on the continuum practitioners reflect on their experiences with people from different ethnic groups and cultures. They apply what they learn (both what might be discomforting or comforting) and apply what is learned from those reflections to make everyday practice with patients of different cultural backgrounds as fair and caring as possible. At the institutionalized cultural proficiency point on the continuum, practitioners guide, support, and encourage inclusion of cultural competence in organization's mission statements, policies and procedures, strategic goals, and the like to help assure institutionalized cultural proficiency.

Learning Point 5.11   Where would you place your work setting on the cultural behavior continuum?

Both intuitively and scientifically it seems clear that individuals in interprofessional practice are cultural beings. Furthermore:

1. We work in settings that can be placed along an *ethical behavior continuum*
2. Each of us can be identified as having a particular cultural collectivist-individualist orientation

3. Each of us has a world view that helps us organize and understand ourselves and our patients as cultural beings

4. Each of us has different kinds and levels of evidence we believe are critical for our understanding of our patients' needs and interventions, and finally

5. Professions have their own unique cultures, and

6. While it is likely there are matches between the cultural orientation of interprofessional teams and the cultural orientation of patients, there are many occasions when no match occurs.

With this variety of sometimes conflicting views and orientations, how do we assure that our final, collective decisions support sound interprofessional ethics? This text offers a strategy for rapprochement using the Dialogic Engagement Model among the many professions involved in the patient's interprofessional care and later we explore this rapprochement strategy in detail, but first it will be useful to explain why and justification of rapprochement is necessary.

Recalling the discussion about culture, the collectivist-individualist orientation, levels of evidence, the cultural behavior context, and ways of knowing and doing, imagine you received a letter from the executor of your long-lost great-uncle's estate. Sort of a "Back to the Future" scientist, he left you a computerized machine that collects all possible data from everything around it, within the range of a typical human being's senses. The computer is without culture; it has no world view. It has no collectivist or individualist orientation, and functions outside of any context such as the cultural behavioral context. This computer collects nanometers of light; the absorbance or percent transmittance of light for color; hertz and decibels of soundwaves; degrees of temperature; vibration frequencies; units of force; discrete aromatic compounds for smell; and the like. This machine also collects animal heart rates, body temperature, posture, body mass, volume of speech and other noises, and all sorts of motion from the rise and fall of a person's chest to the wagging of a dog's tail.

So what? Well, this computer does not have an ontology, epistemology, or axiology. It does not sort received data based on a particular methodology, or method, and does not have an evidence hierarchy with which to organize information or document outcomes. It does not put names or ascribe meaning or values to the data it collects. It does not equate 12°F to being cold; a motorcycle traveling 60 mph on a residential street as traveling fast or dangerously; it does not distinguish between the chemical compounds of smoke coming from a barbeque grill or from a cigarette, and it does not discriminate between a screeching smoke alarm or a television storm warning. Furthermore, this computer does not interpret the crouch and slow methodical tail switching of a cat preparing to attack, or the tears flowing from a child's eyes indicating physical or emotional pain. Finally, this computer does not make meaning-based or value-based decisions about the information it reports and does not take action on those decisions.

As practitioners, we are our own "Back to the Future" computers, only with a world view. In the practice setting we identify what is important about the information we collect, we interpret and make sense of the information, and we figure out the best way to understand and measure the information. Based on our assessment of value of the information; we postulate a way of applying the information;

we watch for signs that our application of the information worked; and then we document evidence of the patient outcomes. All of this is done through the lens of culture, and this is one of the most important interprofessional ethics challenges we face: Do the efforts of say six professionals, each with their own cultural orientation, using six different perspectives, working in an influential context, yield the hoped for outcome for a unique individual?

In interprofessional collaborations, groups of people collect all sorts of information from our patients, their family and caregivers, service providers, and the environment, before, during, and after our interventions. We may collect information independently, sometimes in parallel with other practitioners, or sometimes sequentially. Information is sometimes gathered informally and other times formally. And the information has been gathered by way of multiple perspectives, yet all of that information must make sense every step along the way to the conclusion of an intervention for one person. Similar to the proverbial four blind men touching a unique part of the elephant, we mean to describe a fully functional elephant, yet all practitioners bring to the process their own unique understanding of: 1) what can be known about the patient (ontology); 2) how best can the information be known (epistemology); 3) what is most valuable or useful about that information (axiology); and 4) what is the evidentiary worth or value of that information.

Why is it important to analyze and explore culture related to interprofessional rehabilitation ethics? From the patient's perspective, one should expect ethical, effective care resulting from any interprofessional collaboration whether the practitioners were born in different countries, matured in different cultures, or subscribe to different ways of thinking and doing.

▶ Application of Culture and Interprofessional Ethics with the Dialogic Engagement Model

Brigandt's (2010) explanation of the need for integration of quantitative and qualitative (or reductionistic and pluralistic) understanding of evidence in biology beautifully expresses what rapprochement between professions in complex, collaborative, interprofessional practice might look like:

> Integration (or unification) is not a regulative ideal or an aim in itself, but is usually needed to solve a particular scientific problem. The nature of such a problem (complex explanation or epistemic goal) determines the amount and . . . kind of integration required. These philosophical considerations—especially the notion of a problem or epistemic goal pursued by scientists—are a central part of an epistemology of explanatory integration that amounts to neither reduction nor mere pluralism. (p. 24)

Considering all of this, we believe that rapprochement – or the commitment to harmonious relations – is the best way to begin to work through the Dialogical Engagement Model. For only through respect, active listening, paraphrasing, identifying points of dissension and points of agreement, and understanding each other, i.e., the tools of rapprochement, can we begin to develop and act as effective teams in service to others.

▶ Summary and Conclusion

This chapter attempted to make explicit many of the beliefs we have about culture, ways of knowing, and ways of doing that are typically only known implicitly. To do so, the authors walked the readers through a complex array of ideas that undergird understanding of professional culture as it pertains to working in teams and using the Dialogic Engagement Model. We have reviewed what constitutes culture. Subsequently, we highlighted collectivism and individualism orientations. We explored a system for understanding ways of knowing including ontology, epistemology, and axiology and ways of doing based upon evidence (evidence-based practice). A conceptual model of variables affecting clinical decisions was presented. Three short vignettes were presented to foster critical thinking and reflection related to concepts presented herein. A short section on the application of culture and interprofessional ethics using rapprochement was presented. Finally, a summary was given.

Closing Reflections

Learning Activities

5.1   **Culture**: How would you describe your profession's world view and what it considers valuable information about patients? What sorts of ethical conflicts have you seen between your profession's world view and the world view of other professions?

5.2   **Collectivism and Individualism Orientations**: Do you consider your profession more collectivist or individualistic in orientation and what are examples of practice ethical conflicts that could arise based on that orientation? What are examples of how collaborative practitioners can overcome cultural differences to create positive, ethical, patient outcomes?

5.3   **Ontology, Epistemology, and Axiology**: What are examples in your profession of how these three concepts are interconnected? How do these concepts influence your profession's beliefs about how best to measure treatment outcomes?

5.4   **The Cultural Behavior Continuum Context**: Of the various points along the cultural behavioral continuum, which ones are likely to foster ethical patient outcomes and why?

5.5   **Methodology**: What is the relationship between epistemology and methodology? How is it that epistemology and a profession's culture influence its preferred methods?

5.6   **Method**: Why might using multiple kinds of method in research or practice be critical to ethical patient outcomes?

5.7   **Evidence-Based Practice:** Why base practice on evidence? What different kinds of evidence can be effectively used to support ethical, effective, practice?

Take Away Messages

- Culture is a socially constructed perspective or worldview.
- Consideration of culture extends beyond race, socioeconomic status, and other aspects of cultural differences.
- Professions, organizations, and institutions are cultural groups, but we rarely examine the effect of professional culture on patient care decisions.
- Personal and professional culture are not inherently either barriers or facilitators for interprofessional ethics.
- One key indicator of culture is represented by the individualist versus collectivist orientation.
- Epistemology, axiology, and ontology are interdependent aspects of professional culture that may not be explicitly articulated or examined.
- Method represents the way in which epistemology, axiology, and ontology are integrated into practice.
- Rehabilitation professions do not agree about the best method for integrating evidence-based practice into use, and this will be a significant issue for interprofessional practice in the future.
- To be effective and ethical interprofessional practitioners, one must perform at least at the "cultural competence" point along the cultural behavior continuum and be working toward "institutionalized cultural proficiency."
- Rapprochement (commitment to harmonious relationships) is a necessary step in implementing the Dialogic Engagement Model and effective interprofessional collaboration.

References

Aarons, G. A., Hurlburt, M., & Horwitz, S. M. (2011). Advancing a conceptual model of evidence-based practice implementation in public service sectors. *Administration and Policy in Mental Health and Mental Health Services Research, 38*(1), 4–23. doi: 10.1007/s10488-010-0327-7

Abrams, B. (2010). Evidence-based music therapy practice: An integral understanding. *Journal of Music Therapy, 47*(4), 351–379.

Andersen, H., & Hepburn, B. (2015). Scientific method. In E. N. Zalta (Ed.), *The Stanford encyclopedia of philosophy* (Summer 2016 Edition). Retrieved from https://plato.stanford.edu /archives /sum2016/entries/scientific-method/

Arslanian-Engoren, C., Hicks, F. D., Whall, A. L., & Algase, D. L. (2005). An ontological view of advanced practice nursing. *Research and Theory for Nursing Practice, 19*(4), 315–322.

Axinn, C.N., Blair, E., Heorhiadi, A., & Thach, S. V. (2004). Comparing ethical ideologies across cultures. *Journal of Business Ethics, 54*(2), 103–119.

Audi, R. (2003). *Epistemology: A contemporary introduction to the theory of knowledge.* (Vol. 2). New York: Routledge.

Austin, Z., Gregory, P. A., & Martin, J. C. (2007). Negotiation of interprofessional culture shock: The experiences of pharmacists who become physicians. *Journal of Interprofessional Care, 21*(1), 83–93.

Bailey, B. L. (2009). *America's army: Making the all-volunteer force.* Cambridge, MA: Harvard University Press.

Banning, M. (2005). Conceptions of evidence, evidence-based medicine, evidence-based practice and their use in nursing: Independent nurse prescribers' views. *Journal of Clinical Nursing, 14*(4), 411–417.

Bennett, S., Tooth, L., McKenna, K., Rodger, S., Strong, J., Ziviani, J., & Gibson, L. (2003). Perceptions of evidence-based practice: A survey of Australian occupational therapists. *Australian Occupational Therapy Journal, 50*(1), 13–22.

Berger, R. A., Jacobs, J. J., Meneghini, R. M., Della Valle, C., Paprosky, W., & Rosenberg, A. G. (2004). Rapid rehabilitation and recovery with minimally invasive total hip arthroplasty. *Clinical Orthopaedics and Related Research, 429*, 239–247. doi:10.1097/01.blo.0000150127.80647.80

Brigandt, I. (2010). Beyond reduction and pluralism: Toward an epistemology of explanatory integration in biology. *Erkenntnis, 73*(3), 295–311.

Campbell-Meiklejohn, D., Simonsen, A., Frith, C. D., & Daw, N. D. (2016). Independent neural computation of value from other people's confidence. *The Journal of Neuroscience, 37*(3). doi:10.1523/jneurosci.4490-15.2016

Chiao, J. Y., & Blizinsky, K. D. (2009). Culture-gene coevolution of individualism-collectivism and the serotonin transporter gene. *Proceedings Biological Science.* doi:10.1098/rspb.2009.1650

Chiao, J. Y., Harada, T., Komeda, H., Li, Z., Mano, Y., Saito, D., & Iidaka, T. (2009). Dynamic cultural influences on neural representations of the self. *Journal of Cognitive Neuroscience.* doi:10.1162/jocn.2009.21192. [pii]

Clift, S. (2012). Creative arts as a public health resource: Moving from practice-based research to evidence-based practice. *Perspectives in Public Health, 132*(3), 120–127.

Clifton-Soderstrom, M. (2003). Levinas and the patient as other: The ethical foundation of medicine. *The Journal of Medicine and Philosophy, 28*(4), 447–460.

Cook, J. A., & Fonow, M. M. (1986). Knowledge and women's interests: Issues of epistemology and methodology in feminist sociological research. *Sociological Inquiry, 56*(1), 2–29.

Corazzon, R. (2000). *Theory and history of ontology* (pp. 1–5). Retrieved from www.ontology.co

Crabtree, J. L., Royeen, M., & Benton, J. (2006). Cultural proficiency in rehabilitation: An introduction. In M. Royeen & J. L. Crabtree (Eds.). *Culture in rehabilitation: From competency to proficiency* (pp. 1–16). Upper Saddle River, NJ: Pearson Prentice Hall.

Creswell, J. W., & Poth, C. N. (2017). *Qualitative inquiry and research design: Choosing among five approaches* (4th Ed.). Thousand Oaks, CA: Sage Publications.

Culture. (n.d.). Merriam-Webster online. Retrieved from https://www.merriam-webster.com /dictionary/culture

Dijkers, M. P., Murphy, S. L., & Krellman, J. (2012). Evidence-based practice for rehabilitation professionals: Concepts and controversies. *Archives of Physical Medicine and Rehabilitation, 93*(8), S164–S176. doi:10.1016/j.apmr.2011.12.014

Domínguez, D., Juan, F., Lewis, E. D., Turner, R., & Egan, G. F. (2009). The brain in culture and culture in the brain: A review of core issues in neuroanthropology. In J. Chiao, Y. (Ed.), *Progress in brain research* (pp. 43–64). New York, NY: Elsevier.

Edwards, A., Elwyn, G., Hood, K., & Rollnick, S. (2000). Judging the 'weight of evidence' in systematic reviews: Introducing rigour into the qualitative overview stage by assessing Signal and Noise. *Journal of Evaluation in Clinical Practice, 6*(2), 177–184. doi:10.1046/j.1365-2753.2000.00212.x

Ellis, R. J., Koenig, J., & Thayer, J. F. (2012). Getting to the heart: Autonomic nervous system function in the context of evidence-based music therapy. *Music and Medicine, 4*(2), 90–99. doi:10.1177/1943862112437766

Evans, T. (2015). All we could be: How an advertising campaign helped remake the army. Retrieved from https://armyhistory.org/all-we-could-be-how-an-advertising-campaign-helped-remake-the-army/

Evidence. (n.d.). Merriam-Webster online. Retrieved from https://www.merriam-webster.com /dictionary/evidence

Fellowship for Intentional Community. (2017). Acorn Community Farm. Retrieved from http:// www.ic.org/directory/acorn-community-farm/

Fristedt, S., Areskoug-Josefsson, K., & Kammerlind, A. (2016). Factors influencing the use of evidence based practice among physiotherapists and occupational therapists in their clinical work. *The Internet Journal of Allied Health Sciences & Practice, 14*(3).

Greif, A. (1994). Cultural beliefs and the organization of society: A historical and theoretical reflection on collectivist and individualist societies. *Journal of Political Economy, 102*(5), 912–950.

Guess, C. (2004). Decision-making in individualistic and collectivistic cultures. *Online Readings in Psychology and Culture, 4*(1). http://dx.doi.org/10.9707/2307-0919.1032

James, D. (2015). How to get clear about method, methodology, epistemology and ontology, once and for all. Paper presented at the Economic and Social Research Council First Year Student Conference, Cardiff, Wales. YouTube. Retrieved from https://www.youtube.com /watch?v=b83ZfBoQ_Kw and http://www.walesdtc.ac.uk/conference/programme/how-to-get -clear-about-method-methodology-epistemology-and-ontology-once-and-for-all/

Kendall, J. (1973). The Suzuki® Violin Method in American Music Education. Van Nuys, CA Alfred Music.

Kinsella, E. A., & Whiteford, G. E. (2009). Knowledge generation and utilisation in occupational therapy: Towards epistemic reflexivity. *Australian Occupational Therapy Journal, 56*(4), 249–258.

Landsman, G. H. (2006). What evidence, whose evidence? Physical therapy in New York State's clinical practice guideline and in the lives of mothers of disabled children. *Social Science and Medicine, 62*(11), 2670–2680. doi:S0277-9536(05)00618-0[pii]10.1016/j.socscimed.2005.11.028

Lehman, A. F., & Steinwachs, D. M. (2003). Evidence-based psychosocial treatment practices in schizophrenia: Lessons from the patient outcomes research team (PORT) project. *Journal of the American Academy of Psychoanalysis and Dynamic Psychiatry, 31*(1: Special issue), 141–154.

Little, M., Lipworth, W., Gordon, J., Markham, P., & Kerridge, I. (2012). Values-based medicine and modest foundationalism. *Journal of Evaluation in Clinical Practice, 18*(5), 1020–1026.

Mallon, R. (2014). Approaches to social construction. In E. N. Zalta (Ed.), *The Stanford encyclopedia of philosophy* (Winter 2014 Edition). Retrieved from https://plato.stanford.edu/archives /win2014/entries/social-construction-naturalistic/

Menon, A., Korner-Bitensky, N., Kastner, M., McKibbon, K. A., & Straus, S. (2009). Strategies for rehabilitation professionals to move evidence-based knowledge into practice: A systematic review. *Journal of Rehabilitation Medicine, 41*(13), 1024–1032. doi:10.2340/16501977-0451

Meyer, A. (1957). *Psychobiology: A science of man.* Springfield, IL: Charles C. Thomas, Publisher.

Orchowsky, S. (2014). An introduction to evidence-based practices. Rockville, MD: National Criminal Justice Association. Retrieved from https://www.ncjrs.gov/App/Publications/abstract .aspx?ID=268582

Ontology. (n.d.). Merriam-Webster online. Retrieved from https://www.merriam-webster.com /dictionary/ontology

Oyserman, D., Coon, H. M., & Kemmelmeier, M. (2002). Rethinking individualism and collectivism: Evaluation of theoretical assumptions and meta-analyses. *Psychological Bulletin, 128*(1), 3–72.

Oyserman, D., & Lee, S. W. S. (2008). Does culture influence what and how we think? Effects of priming individualism and collectivism. *Psychological Bulletin, 134*(2), 311–342. doi:2008-01984-007[pii].10.1037/0033-2909.134.2.311

Poli, R. (2003). Descriptive, formal and formalized ontologies. In D. Fisette (Ed.), *Husserl's logical investigations reconsidered* (pp. 183–210). Rotterdam, Netherlands: Springer.

Ratner, N. B. (2006). Evidence-based practice: An examination of its ramifications for the practice of speech-language pathology. *Language, Speech, and Hearing Services in Schools, 37*(4), 257–267.

Reed, P. G. (1997). Nursing: The ontology of the discipline. *Nursing Science Quarterly, 10*(2), 76–79. doi:10.1177/089431849701000207

Rubenstein-Montano, B., Liebowitz, J., Buchwalter, J., McCaw, D., Newman, B., Rebeck, K., & Team, T. K. M. M. (2001). A systems thinking framework for knowledge management. *Decision Support Systems, 31*(1), 5–16.

Sackett, D. L., & Rosenberg, W. M. C. (1995). The need for evidence-based medicine. *Journal of the Royal Society of Medicine, 88,* 620–624. Retrieved from http://pubmedcentralcanada.ca /picrender.cgi?accid=PMC1295384&blobtype=pdf

Sackett, D. L., Rosenberg, W. M. C., Muir Gray, J. A., Haynes, R. B., & Richardson, W. S. (1996). Evidence based medicine: What it is and what it isn't. *British Medical Journal, 312,* 71–71. Retrieved from http://pubmedcentralcanada.ca/picrender.cgi?accid=PMC2349778&blobtype=pdf

Satterfield, J. M., Spring, B., Brownson, R. C., Mullen, E. J., Newhouse, R. P., Walker, B. B., & Whitlock, E. P. (2009). Toward a transdisciplinary model of evidence-based practice. *Milbank Quarterly, 87*(2), 368–390.

Schroeder, M. (2016). Value theory. In E. N. Zalta (Ed.), *The Stanford encyclopedia of philosophy* (Fall 2016 Edition). Retrieved from https://plato.stanford.edu/archives/fall2016/entries/value -theory/

Schwartz, S. H. (1990). Individualism-collectivism: Critique and proposed refinements. *Journal of Cross-Cultural Psychology, 21*(2), 139–157. http://dx.doi.org/10.1177/0022022190212001

Scott, K., & McSherry, R. (2009). Evidence-based nursing: Clarifying the concepts for nurses in practice. *Journal of Clinical Nursing, 18*(8), 1085–1095.

Slayton, S. C., D'Archer, J., & Kaplan, F. (2010). Outcome studies on the efficacy of art therapy: A review of findings. *Art Therapy, 27*(3), 108–118.

Steultjens, E. M. J., Dekker, J., Bouter, L. M., Leemrijse, C. J., & van den Ende, C. H. M. (2005). Evidence of the efficacy of occupational therapy in different conditions: An overview of systematic reviews. *Clinical Rehabilitation, 19*(3), 247–254.

Taheri, N., & Jackson, J. C. (n. d.). *Clinical pearl: Ramadan - Reminder to health care providers*. Ethnomed. Retrieved from https://ethnomed.org/cross-cultural-health/religion/ramadan-practitioners

Tanenbaum, S. J. (2005). Evidence-based practice as mental health policy: Three controversies and a caveat. *Health Affairs, 24*(1), 163–173.

Tomlin, G., & Borgetto, B. (2011). Research Pyramid: A new evidence-based practice model for occupational therapy. *American Journal of Occupational Therapy, 65*(2), 189–196. doi:10.5014/ajot.2011.000828

Tomlin, G. S., & Dougherty, D. (2014). Decision-making and sources of evidence in occupational therapy and other health professions. Evidence-informed practice/Entscheidungsfindung und evidenzquellen in der ergotherapie und weiteren gesundheitsberufen. evidenzinformierte praxis. *International Journal of Health Professions, 1*(1), 13–19.

Trochim, W. M. (2006). *The research methods knowledge base* (2nd ed.). Retrieved from http://www.socialresearchmethods.net/kb/positvsm.php

Uschold, M., & Gruninger, M. (1996). Ontologies: Principles, methods and applications. *The Knowledge Engineering Review, 11*(2), 93–136. doi:10.1017/S0269888900007797

Weisz, J. R., Jensen-Doss, A., & Hawley, K. M. (2006). Evidence-based youth psychotherapies versus usual clinical care: A meta-analysis of direct comparisons. *American Psychologist, 61*(7), 671.

Worldview. (n.d.). Merriam-Webster online. Retrieved from https://www.merriam-webster.com/dictionary/worldview

Yerxa, E. J. (1990). An introduction to occupational science, a foundation for occupational therapy in the 21st century. *Occupational Therapy in Health Care, 6*(4), 1–17.

Zipoli, R. P., & Kennedy, M. (2005). Evidence-based practice among Speech-Language Pathologists: Attitudes, utilization, and barriers. *American Journal of Speech-Language Pathology, 14*(3), 208–220.

CHAPTER 6

Ethical Issues in the Rehabilitation of Children and Adolescents

Clare M. Delany

CHAPTER OUTLINE

- Chapter Overview
- Section 1: Ethical Values in Pediatric Rehabilitation
- Section 2: The Dialogic Process in Pediatric Rehabilitation Practice
- A Model of Clinical Ethics Consultation
- Summary and Conclusion

CHAPTER OBJECTIVES

At the conclusion of this chapter, the reader will be able to:

1. Identify elements of the Dialogic Engagement Model within the context of pediatric rehabilitation.
2. Describe common ethical challenges encountered in the pediatric rehabilitation context.
3. Have an understanding of how rehabilitation professionals engage in ethical deliberation and decision making.
4. Be aware of the potential role of multidisciplinary clinical ethics consultations for supporting the development of professional moral agency.

KEY TERMS

Reading these key terms before reading the chapter will introduce you to key concepts which will then be somewhat familiar to you as you read this chapter. This is an important learning technique that will enhance your learning as a multi-step process. You may even wish to make a flash card set of key terms and quiz yourself on them once or twice before reading the chapter. This will better prepare you to immerse in the language of ethics and better prepare you to integrate the content.

Community of Practice: In health care, this refers to a group of people who work alongside each other and share common professional interests and goals. In pediatric rehabilitation practice, there are a range of practitioners bringing different practice paradigms, but sharing a common interest in order to provide a benefit to a child both within, and separate to, the family unit.

Interprofessional Collaborative Practice: Refers to health professionals from different disciplinary backgrounds working together with patients, families, carers [sic], and communities to deliver the highest quality of care" (WHO, 2010).

Moral Authority: Refers to the scope of authority a person has to make moral decisions on behalf of and in the interests of themselves or another. In the pediatric context, parents have moral authority to make decisions on behalf of their child. However, this authority does not extend to causing harm to their child.

Moral Commons: A safe zone for ethical deliberation characterized by mutual respect for personal and professional identity, common language, inclusion of relevant stakeholders, and the dialogic process. The three key elements of the moral commons are identity (personal and professional), ethical tradition, and context.

Moral Deliberation: This refers to the process of conversation, reflection, and dialogue focused on weighing ethically relevant considerations. In the pediatric rehabilitation context, it includes consideration of the interests of the child, the child's family, and the interprofessional team.

▶ Chapter Overview

In this chapter pediatric rehabilitation is used as a clinical backdrop to situate the three dimensions of the Dialogic Engagement Model. The first section focuses on foundational ethical principles and concepts which underpin pediatric rehabilitation, and which resonate with the 'prepare' dimension of the Dialogic Engagement Model. In the second section, data from a qualitative research project mapping ethical issues in pediatric rehabilitation are presented to illustrate how individual clinicians engage in the 'dialogic process' dimension of the model. In the final section, a clinical ethics consultation service is described as an example of workplace-based support which effectively enacts the third dimension of the Dialogic Engagement Model, 'reflection leading to growth in moral agency'.

The Dialogic Engagement Model introduced in this text, extends the three steps of a previously developed model of ethical reflection and decision making (Delany, Edwards, Jensen, & Skinner, 2010). In the 'Active Engagement Model', the three steps proposed were for individual practitioners to actively listen, to be reflexive about their professional values and goals and to think critically about ethical principles and norms (Delany, Edwards, Jensen, & Skinner, 2010; Nesbit, Jensen, & Delany, 2018). The Dialogic Engagement Model shifts the emphasis from individual processes of thinking, to the importance of developing a shared language around ethical concepts that can be understood and accessed by different health professionals working within rehabilitation teams. This shift is significant. The key goal of this chapter is to show how the Dialogic Engagement Model can be used to analyze, frame, and guide ethical reflection and action in a specific area of rehabilitation practice.

▶ Section 1: Ethical Values in Pediatric Rehabilitation

(a) Acting in a Child's Best Interests: Providing Beneficial Care and Avoiding Harm

In the pediatric rehabilitation context, acting in a child's best interests is a fundamental underpinning ethical value. However, clinicians and parents may hold differing views about what counts as best interests for a child. Each health professional brings a particular disciplinary perspective regarding treatment goals and clinical paradigms of practice (Delany, Edwards, Jensen, & Skinner, 2010). These translate to different values and perspectives about what is in the best interests of a child and/or their family in different stages of a child's illness or development (Flett & Stoffell, 2003; Koch, 2001). For example, in the ongoing treatment of children with conditions such as cystic fibrosis or cerebral palsy, a social worker will be concerned with ensuring that the child and their family has sufficient supports to cope with the emotional and physical toll from the condition; a physical therapist will focus on maintaining or improving function in a physical sense; an occupational therapist will be concerned with the child's ability to participate in a range of activities and a physician may be concerned with ongoing drug management.

> **Learning Point 6.1**   How might different professional foci converge or diverge in team planning to bring about the child's' best interests?

Further complexity in rehabilitation contexts may arise because of limited evidence from published research of the effectiveness of rehabilitation-based treatments (Leong, 2002; Reilly, Douglas, & Oates, 2004). Despite this, rehabilitation practitioners are often required by either the family or other healthcare disciplines to provide ongoing care and management for children particularly where other avenues of acute medical care and treatment are considered to be futile (Delany & Gibson, 2016b; Guedert & Grosseman, 2012). This may lead to moral concern and conflicting views about whether the treatment being requested is potentially harmful rather than beneficial.

A further facet of determining which rehabilitation goals are the most appropriate to ensure a child's life goes as well as it can in the context of their health condition and family situation is to be open to, and be prepared for, 'change'. Children's needs and values change as they develop and grow, and the nature and impact of acute and chronic injury and disability also changes over time. Parents' needs, understanding, and responses to rehabilitation goals change as they experience their child's illness or disability journey (Delany & Gibson, 2016b; Piggot, Paterson, & Hocking, 2002).

This facet of rehabilitation has particular relevance with the Dialogic Engagement Model. Health professionals need to be prepared to adjust their goals and expectations of treatment and they need to be alert as to how their goals and professional assumptions about what matters for a child, intersect with the child's interests, the parents' values and goals, and the wider treating team. Gibson et al. (2009) have previously discussed how treatment directed at 'fixing' or 'normalizing' an aspect of a child's problem such as a focus on supporting walking through aids or exercise programs, may conflict with or diminish other developmental needs of a child, for example to participate with others (by using a wheelchair). Being aware of, and distinguishing between which interests are being emphasized and targeted in rehabilitation is an important component of developing a shared set of values among clinicians and represents the ethical work required in the 'prepare' dimension of the Dialogic Engagement Model.

Awareness of treatment goals and the possibility that parents or members of the treating team may hold different views is illustrated in the empirical cases discussed later. In the case of the educational play therapist, the ethical concern was not only to ensure that a specific clinical goal was obtained (a clear image from the medical resonance imaging) procedure, but also to promote some control for the child within the testing procedure and to avoid short-term harms of anxiety and longer-term harms of a child associating MRI procedures with discomfort and lack of control. Giving children some control over decision making within health care is an example of a second foundational ethical value in pediatric rehabilitation. Balanced against the important value of respecting the moral authority of parents to make decisions for their child, the ethical goal of respect for a child's developing autonomy involves providing age appropriate information and opportunities to contribute.

(b) Respecting Child and Parental Autonomy

Influenced by the 1989 United Nations Convention on the Rights of the Child (United Nations, 1989), children's rights to information have been recognized as an important principle in the ethical delivery of pediatric health care and in rehabilitation. Although there is wide consensus that children should be presented with "honest" information delivered in a "developmentally appropriate" manner (Masera et al., 1997), decisions about how much information to give are based on assessing developmental stages and may be challenging to interpret and implement in practice since people can still disagree about their moral weight and significance (Bluebond-Langner, DeCicco, & Belasco, 2005). Children develop at different rates. They experience and understand illness individually and are influenced by the culture and communication patterns within their family.

The legal concept of the mature minor (Alderson, 2017) recognizes that for certain clinical decisions, a child may be mature enough to receive information, to reflect on the options available and to provide their view, give their assent or in some circumstances provide their informed consent (Alderson, 2017; Gillick, 1985; United Nations, 1989).

Learning Point 6.2   What is meant by the term mature minor?

Learning Point 6.3   What is the difference between assent and informed consent?

The ethical concept of assent gives independent ethical weight to a child's agreement, and requires information to be tailored to their capacities to understand (Spriggs & Gillam, 2008). However, again, deciding what to say and how to best communicate with a child directly or through his/her parents can be ethically contentious.

In the pediatric setting, parents or a child's legal guardians have primary responsibility to decide what is in the interests of their child and to make health decisions on their child's behalf. However, this legal position and moral authority is not absolute. Parents do not have an ethical entitlement to cause suffering or injury to their child, and especially when this could be avoided by a different medical pathway (McDougall, Delany, & Gillam, 2016, p. 17). An example of differences in values about what is ethically and clinically important for a child is in the case of Lucy (Delany & Gibson, 2016a, p. 98) described at the end of this chapter. In this case, there is a clear difference between parents' and the therapists' views of the scope and limits of physical therapy treatment.

In the next section, empirical examples are used to demonstrate how individual clinicians encounter and respond to other examples of moral uncertainty and conflict. This section shifts the focus to the second dimension of the Dialogic Engagement Model and uses empirically derived data about individual and team dialogic processes in the area of pediatric rehabilitation practice. The examples are drawn from data about ethical challenges encountered by rehabilitation professionals. They highlight differing moral standpoints and perspectives, and illustrate how rehabilitation professionals go about establishing common moral ground between team members, children, and parents.

▶ Section 2: The Dialogic Process in Pediatric Rehabilitation Practice

The data is drawn from a study conducted at the Royal Children's Hospital, a large tertiary pediatric teaching hospital, in Melbourne, Australia. Ethical approval for this project was provided in 2009 by the hospital human research ethics committee (Ref. no. 29082 D). The goals of the project were to document the ethical dimensions of the everyday experiences of rehabilitation professionals working in a large pediatric setting in both rehabilitation and acute clinical contexts. Phenomenology was the guiding methodology (Greenfield & Jensen, 2010) and semi-structured interviews aimed to elicit detailed descriptions of participants' lived experiences (Rice & Ezzy, 1999) (**FIGURE 6.1**).

1. Are there ethical issues that are unique to your area of practice?
2. ·Can you describe them?
3. What types of issues are ethical issues in your everyday work?
4. What makes them ethically important?
5. How do you react to ethical issues in your practice?
6. What sources of knowledge help you in your encounters with ethical dilemmas or issues?
7. What do you regard as the features of a good ethical decision?
8. What are the main challenges to good ethical decisions in your clinical practice experience?

FIGURE 6.1 Interview questions.

Findings from this research have been separately published in three papers (Delany & Conwell, 2012; Delany & Galvin, 2014; Delany, Richards, Stewart, & Kosta, 2017). The first example derives from a single interview with an educational play therapist who describes how she prepares a child to undergo magnetic resonance imaging (MRI) (Delany & Conwell, 2012). This scanning procedure requires a child to lie very still under a large and noisy machine for at least 15 minutes. Play-based interventions emphasize language that derives from and supports the child's perspective, and enables the child to act out and develop a sense of primary and/or secondary control over the situation. A key goal for educational play therapy is to build on each child's individual coping style, by gaining an understanding their developmental behavioral tendencies under stress.

The therapist describes how she negotiated with team members and parents to ensure that a child has a positive experience when undergoing an MRI. This dialogic process is an example of the need to establish common clinical and ethical values about what is best for a child. This type of interprofessional communication requires high levels of collaboration and coordination within a team (Edwards, 2009; Radomski & Beckett, 2011).

The play therapist described three main ethical dimensions of her role:

1. To maximize benefits and minimize harms associated with a child undergoing an MRI procedure. Benefits included providing a child with opportunities to exercise some control of their own coping mechanisms and required assessing their readiness to undergo the procedure.

Learning Point 6.4   Which ethical principles provide a basis for maximizing benefits and minimizing harms?

2. To develop a relationship with other members of the team to ensure they are also aware of the child's readiness and triggers for stress. This involved ensuring all clinicians had the same goals about what matters for this child both in the short term – obtaining the necessary image from the MRI procedure – and in the long-term – ensuring the child is not traumatized by the experience. The therapist described how it was not always possible to achieve the latter, and she highlighted that if this teamwork is not in place, the experience for the child can become highly stressful:

    "I find that if things don't go well it is either because I haven't worked with particular nurses or [physicians] before and they don't understand my role, or it's something that they've asked me to come in ad hoc and when you come it is too late [after the examination has already started] and you might already have a distressed child."

3. To have a clear understanding of her own clinical and moral role so that she could recognize when the interprofessional team worked well together and when it did not:

    "So in medical imaging, I know when to step in because they'll look at me and give me a nod of... "we need you now", or I know by their actions that they don't need me at all, they're handling the situation really well so I just step back. So it's about that 'give and take' that you don't own what you do as a play therapist. You want to be able to give those skills across to other colleagues so that when you're not there, they're utilizing it and I think you need to respect it enough that if something is going well, you don't need to jump in."

Articulating these three ethical values provides concrete examples of both 'preparing' and 'establishing a moral commons.' This dialogic work is grounded in the imperative of the interprofessional team to work together and to be dynamic, responsive, and non-hierarchical to achieve both short- and long-term goals centred around creating a positive experience for the child. A key goal for the therapist was to ensure that all team members had an opportunity to discuss the best approach, or were sufficiently familiar with each other's work and were able to develop shared goals for the child.

The second example (Delany & Galvin, 2014) is an occupational therapist working with Sophie, a five-year-old child with a dense hemiplegia affecting her dominant left side. The therapist describes feeling uncertain about whether to retrain Sophie's non-dominant hand for writing or whether to wait until her stroke-affected and dominant hand showed signs of recovery. The therapist's ethical concern was how and when to provide Sophie's parents with factual information about the benefits and risks of retraining a non-dominant hand in a young child, especially given the uncertainty about prognosis and response to therapy. Switching to the non-dominant hand would enable Sophie to participate more at her school and would also reassure the parents who were keen to see some progress in Sophie's capacities to participate in some way. However, it may not have been the best long-term clinical outcome. The occupational therapist was particularly concerned that giving parents too much information might cause the parents to become anxious and might impact on their hope and optimism about Sophie's recovery (Kearney & Griffin, 2001).

Learning Point 6.5   Is it possible to "over-inform" as part of informed consent? How does one determine how much information to provide?

In the interview the occupational therapist expressed three main ethical concerns:

1. The first was a concern about the potential harms of "making the wrong decision and disadvantaging Sophie in the future…[because], the decision to train her non-dominant hand has profound implications for her later proficiency in writing and other hand functions."

2. The second was a concern about "how much to involve Sophie in this process…[because] I know she can make active choices about which hand she prefers right now, but is not able to think into the future."

Learning Point 6.6   How can rehabilitation professionals best approach balancing long and short-term considerations for children and adolescents?

3. The third ethical concern related to respecting her parents' involvement in this therapeutic decision, which was described as not wanting to "leave the parents behind."

The ethical challenges raised in this case study were not based on conflicting values and perspectives held by different people. Instead, they were more nuanced.

They concerned how and when to communicate short and long-term goals so that Sophie's parents were able to understand the complexity and potential consequences of treatment decisions, and how to support them to be actively involved in these types of decisions. These challenges strongly resonate with the first dimension of the dialogic engagement model because they provide an example of a therapist striving to find some common moral ground and language to use to assist Sophie's parents to understand their daughter's clinical situation and to be in a position to express their preferences and share some of the treatment decisions.

The third paper reports findings from interviews with nine pediatric social workers. Participants described two main roles. The first was to be a collaborative member of the interprofessional team caring for a child, and the second was to advocate for and empower children and their families. Specific ethical concerns raised across all of the interviews included: identifying priorities for discharge; how much and when to follow up with families; how to distribute limited resources; how to best respond to parents' concerns (through direct support or more indirectly via advocacy within the interprofessional team); how to communicate information sensitively for each family situation; when and how to speak up in interprofessional team meetings; how to situate and advocate for the needs of families among differing perspectives held by members of the interprofessional team, and how to support parents without undermining physicians. These ethical issues are grouped into five themes which reinforce the significance of the dialogic process of interprofessional communication in facilitating ethical outcomes associated with patient and family involvement in clinical decision making.

Theme 1: Troublesome Knowledge Challenge

Participants described having knowledge or information which they perceived to be ethically troubling because it had the potential to either benefit or harm families. For example, as members of the interprofessional team, they had access to information about a child's diagnosis, prognosis, and treatment plans before the family knew this information. This was ethically troubling because it sometimes prevented or delayed them from supporting and empowering parents to participate in and develop coping strategies to deal with their child's condition. At other times, they received information from the family which was critical of the health team, and juggling responsibilities to both the family and the team was challenging.

> **Learning Point 6.7**   Have you ever experienced having "troublesome knowledge"?

Theme 2: Diplomacy Challenge

This theme was closely related to the first. It arose as a consequence of the hierarchical nature of hospital work, and concerned how to best communicate information within the health team so as to respect different professional knowledge and decision making, while also advocating on behalf of the patient and the patient's family. An example quote is:

> Well it's the [physicians'] assessment in the end, well it's whether I guess we can influence them in trying to balance up social and medical... So yeah, we have social workers listening to them [families] about the way things are, but I don't feel confident pushing a [physician] to do something they don't feel completely happy about...

Theme 3: Conciliation Challenge

The third theme describes the active communication processes used to respond to the diplomacy challenge including how social workers addressed misunderstandings and differing expectations between health professionals and the families. The participants described having to explain a clinician's meaning or intention, and having to interpret a family's reality and circumstances. This often involved seeking common ground (moral commons) so that mutual respect and understanding between the family and other clinicians could flourish.

Theme 4: Every Man and His Dog Challenge

Expressed colloquially, the fourth theme describes the ethical consequences of large team meetings or ward rounds where many members of health teams attended. Each person provided slightly different aspects of clinical care and as a consequence, they each emphasised different aspects of treatment. This was reported as highly stressful for parents who found it overwhelming to be 'the minority' in the room and who found information to be conflicting rather than helpful in building their understanding.

Theme 5: Brick Wall Challenge

This final theme referred to the system, the procedures and aspects of hospital bureaucracy acting as an immovable barrier for parents. The ethical concern for social workers was how to best assist parents to negotiate these systems and processes without overtly criticizing them, and how to manage the available resources to meet each family's needs.

The social work data highlights that recognizing ethical issues in rehabilitation represents only the first step in interprofessional ethical practice. Further steps required to address ethical challenges in everyday practice, require a capacity to actively prepare and engage in dialogue which focuses on seeking mutual understanding about ethical decisions. In the third section of the chapter, a clinical ethics consultations service is briefly described to show how health professionals might be supported to engage in solution-focused and meaningful ethics dialogue with other members of the rehabilitation team and to promote continued growth in their moral agency and development.

▶ A Model of Clinical Ethics Consultation

Clinical ethics committees function as "a multi-disciplinary group of healthcare professionals within a healthcare institution that has been specifically established to address the ethical dilemmas that occur within the institution," (Cranford & Doudera, 1985, p. 2687). Key goals of ethics consultation committees are to resolve conflict, facilitate communication, and ease moral distress in health care (Kesselheim, Johnson, & Joffe, 2010).

The clinical ethics consultation service of which the author is a member, at the Royal Children's Hospital (RCH) in Melbourne, is called the Clinical Ethics Response Group (CERG). The CERG draws from approximately 20 physicians, nurses, rehabilitation professionals, ethics and legal representatives, and the hospital clinical ethicist. In any one case, there are usually eight to 12 members present, depending on their availability. A key aim of the group is to reach a consensus with the treating team about the range of ethically appropriate options in a situation. The discussion and recommendations are documented, and records of the committee's deliberations are provided to the referring clinician and stored in CERG files (Gold, Hall, & Gillam, 2011).

The goals of the CERG, to identify ethical dimensions of a clinical decision and to facilitate discussion and reflection, are all realized through a process of dialogue and recognition of ethical pluralism. **TABLE 6.1** lists the types of questions posed by the ethicists in the CERG committee and how they represent the dimensions of the dialogic model.

TABLE 6.1 The Dialogic Model and Ethics Consultation Question	
Dimensions of the Dialogic Model	**Clinical Ethics Consultation Processes**
1. PREPARE	The goal of the ethics consultation is to bring health professionals together to facilitate common understandings of an ethical issue. The aim is not to achieve conformity with a particular clinical management plan, but to foster a level of understanding, tolerance, and respect about different clinical and ethical views.
2. DIALOGIC PROCESS	Within the consultation meeting, clinicians are encouraged to discuss how they discern the ethical issue and to articulate their views and perspectives:
	This is achieved by inviting clinicians to:
	• Articulate the nature of the ethical issue/s or question/s involved
	• Identify the range of possible options for treatment and management
	• Identify and weigh up the ethical pros and cons of each option
	• Identify options which are clearly ethically appropriate, or not
	Specific questions which encourage this dialogue are:
	• Can you describe in more detail about what you mean by…
	• What does (will) it feel like for this child to have this (treatment)
	• What is the likely outcome of the treatment
	• How certain/uncertain are you about this outcome
	• What do the parents want/feel/understand/hope for
	• What does the child want/feel/understand/hope for
3. SUMMATIVE REFLECTION	Key goals of the ethics consultation process are to draw out the range of values and ethical perspectives about a clinical scenario. The discussion actively canvasses participants to share and reflect on their professional views and perspectives.
	A further explicit goal is to create opportunities to deepen clinicians' self understanding and to reflect on what they would regard as common sense assumptions that typically frame their daily decisions and practices.

▶ Summary and Conclusion

The three sections of this chapter show how the Dialogic Engagement Model can be used to frame and shed light on specific areas of clinical practice – in this case, pediatric rehabilitation work. Mapping the three dimensions of the model against empirical data drawn from pediatric rehabilitation practice, demonstrates the relevance of the model and highlighted the importance of clinicians working within interprofessional teams, to see themselves as a community of people working together in a 'community of practice' (Eraut, 2002). Within such a community, each rehabilitation professional has their own individual moral identity and agency but they also require a strong sense of belonging to the group.

> **Learning Point 6.8**   What are some approaches you can use to establish common moral ground between different health professionals and parents?

This sense of belonging and engaging with each other discussed here provides rich examples of the value and relevance of the Dialogic Engagement Model. It also provides a guide for analyzing and better understanding other areas of clinical practice where health professionals work together as an interprofessional group in the interests of the patient.

Closing Reflections

Learning Activities

Case of Lucy

Lucy is a 13-year-old girl with a brain tumor and new metastases to her spine. She is undergoing active chemotherapy. During her in-patient admission Lucy experienced neurological progression resulting in an incomplete tetraplegia due to multiple spinal lesions. In order to prevent Lucy from losing further mobility and to avoid developing lower limb contractures, the recommended physical therapy intervention involved stretching of lower limb muscles that had started to contract, transfer practice, wheelchair skills, and aquatic therapy. It is unclear if Lucy will ever regain the ability to walk, but there is certainly a possibility.

Lucy is experiencing a significant amount of neuropathic pain which makes it very difficult for her to tolerate having her legs or feet touched. She is very upset about her rapid deterioration and often refuses to engage with physical therapy. She shouts and cries or completely ignores physical therapy staff if she does not want to engage.

Lucy's parents are very keen for Lucy to engage with physical therapy, but they cannot bear to see Lucy distressed within physical therapy sessions. They realize that if she does not participate in physical therapy, there will be a significant increase in the care they need to provide to lift her, push her in a wheelchair and transfer her in and out of the car. They are both over 60 years old and they believed that if Lucy lost any more

(continues)

(continued)

mobility, they would be at risk of injuring themselves. They also want to avoid the need for Lucy to have orthopedic surgery in the future because of worsening lower limb contractures. However, these concerns are always trumped by Lucy's protests; when the physical therapist arrives they always agree with Lucy and cut short the physical therapy session.

Lucy's main therapist, Jill, is an experienced rehabilitation physical therapist, and has worked in the pediatric setting for 15 years. She is becoming very frustrated with Lucy's parents. Their refusal to allow her to work with Lucy and include a full routine of stretches and postural strengthening work means that Lucy is de-conditioning rapidly. Jill believes that Lucy's interests are not well served by cutting short her physical therapy treatment.

Based on Delany & Gibson (2016).

Key Questions

Drawing from each of the steps of the dialogic model:

1. Identify what type of challenges this ethical problem represents.
2. Plan how your 'community of rehabilitation professionals' could respond to the ethical challenges in this case.

 # Take Away Messages

There are two key take away messages from this chapter. The first is that the fundamental ethical value of acting in a child's best interests within pediatric rehabilitation can be contested as clinicians and parents may hold differing views about what matters for a child. The second is that the Dialogic Engagement Model provides a useful framework to assist in developing a shared language around ethical differences and ethical concepts relevant to this area of clinical practice.

-   Acting in the child's best interest is a fundamental ethical underpinning of pediatric rehabilitation. Patients, families, and professionals may not agree as to what constitutes the best interest of the child.
-   Children's needs and values change as they grow and mature. At the same time, the condition or disability and its impact may also change.
-   Rehabilitation goals are developed at the intersection between the child's interests, parent and family values, and the values of the members of the interprofessional team.
-   Focusing on fixed or "normal" development goals (such as, walking) may result in overlooking other important social developmental goals (such as, participation in social interaction or play).
-   Although parents have the legal and moral authority to provide informed consent for the child's health care, children have the right to receive developmentally appropriate information. Mature minors may also provide assent or even informed consent for rehabilitation based on individual development and maturity.

- Balancing the changing values and interests of parents, children, and rehabilitation professionals requires that rehabilitation professionals have the ability to address ethical uncertainty and conflict by creating the moral commons.
- In pediatric rehabilitation, timing and amount of information to provide may be as important an ethical issue as conflicting ethical values.
- Themes of the ethical issues encountered in pediatric rehabilitation include troublesome knowledge, challenging diplomacy, "every man and his dog" composition of team meetings, communication, and the brick wall challenge of organizational bureaucracy.
- Ethics consultation committees may be helpful in resolving conflicts, facilitating communication, and decreasing moral distress. Within pediatric rehabilitation, a key goal of ethics consultation is to define the range of ethically appropriate options.

References

Alderson, P. (2017). Children's consent and the zone of parental discretion. *Clinical Ethics, 12*(2), 55–62. https://doi.org/10.1177/1477750917691887

Bluebond-Langner, M., DeCicco, A., & Belasco, J. (2005). Involving children with life-shortening illnesses in decisions about participation in clinical research: a proposal for shuttle diplomacy and negotiation. In E. Kodish (Ed.), *Ethics and research with children* (pp. 323–344). London, UK: Oxford University Press.

Cranford, R., & Doudera, E. (1985). Hospital ethics committees. *Journal of the American Medical Association, 2,* 2687.

Delany, C., & Conwell, M. (2012). Ethics and teamwork for pediatric medical imaging procedures: Insights from educational play therapy. *Pediatric Radiology, 42*(2), 139–146. doi:10.1007/s00247-011-2271-4

Delany, C., Edwards, I., Jensen, G., & Skinner, E. (2010). Closing the gap between ethics knowledge and practice through active engagement: An applied model of physical therapy ethics. *Physical Therapy, 90*(7), 1068–1078.

Delany, C., & Galvin, J. (2014). Ethics and shared decision-making in paediatric occupational therapy practice. *Developmental Neurorehabilitation, 17*(5), 347–354. doi:10.3109/17518423.2013.784816

Delany, C., & Gibson, B. (2016). The rehabiliation context: the ZPD and ongoing care questions. In R. McDougall, C. Delany, & L. Gillam (Eds.), *When doctors and parents disagree. Ethics, paediatrics and the zone of parental discretion* (pp. 96–112). Sydney, Australia: The Federation Press.

Delany, C., Richards, A., Stewart, H., & Kosta, L. (2017). Five challenges to ethical communication for interprofessional paediatric practice: A social work perspective. *Journal of Interprofessional Care,*(1469-9567 (Electronic)), 1–7. doi:10.1080/13561820.2017.1296419

Delany, C., Spriggs, M., Fry, C. L., & Gillam, L. (2010). The unique nature of clinical ethics in allied health pediatrics: implications for ethics education. *Cambridge Quarterly of Healthcare Ethics, 19*(4), 471–480. doi:10.1017/S0963180110000368

Edwards, A. (2009). Relational agency in collaborations for the well-being of children and young people. *Journal of Children's Services, 4*(1), 33–43.

Eraut, M. (2002). Conceptual analysis and research questions: Do the concepts of "Learning Community" and "Community of Practice" provide added value? Retrieved from https://eric.ed.gov/?id=ED466030

Faden, R. R., & Beauchamp, T. L. (1986). *A history and theory of informed consent.* New York, NY: Oxford University Press.

Flett, P., & Stoffell, B. (2003). Ethical issues in paediatric rehabilitation. *Journal of Paediatric Child Health, 39,* 219–223.

Gibson, B. E., Darrah, J., Cameron, D., Hashemi, G., Kingsnorth, S., Lepage, C., & Menna-Dack, D. (2009). Revisiting therapy assumptions in children's rehabilitation: Clinical and research implications. *Disability and Rehabilitation, 31*(17), 1446–1453.

Gold, H., Hall, G., & Gillam, L. (2011). Role and function of a paediatric clinical ethics service: Experiences at the Royal Children's Hospital, Melbourne. *Journal of Paediatric Child Health, 47*, 632–636.

Greenfield, B. H., & Jensen, G. M. (2010). Understanding the lived experiences of patients: Application of a phenomenological approach to ethics. *Physical Therapy, 90*(8), 1185–1197. doi:10.2522/ptj.20090348

Guedert, J. M., & Grosseman, S. (2012). Ethical problems in pediatrics: What does the setting of care and education show us? *BMC Medical Ethics, 13*(1), 2.

Hadsell, N. A. (2001). Ethical thinking in music therapy. *Journal of Music Therapy, 38*(2), 165–167.

Kearney, P. M., & Griffin, T. (2001). Between joy and sorrow: Being a parent of a child with a developmental disability. *Journal of Advanced Nursing, 34*(5), 582–592.

Kesselheim, J. C., Johnson, J., & Joffe, S. (2010). Ethics consultation in children's hospitals: Results from a survey of paediatric clinical ethicists. *Paediatrics, 125*, 742–746.

Koch, T. (2001). Disability and difference: Balancing social and physical constructions. *Journal of Medical Ethics, 27*, 370–376.

Leong, B. (2002). The vegetative and minimally conscious states in children: Spasticity, muscle contracture and issues for physical therapy treatment. *Brain Injury, 16*(3), 217–230.

Masera, G., Chesler, M. A., Jankovic, M., Ablin, A. R., Ben Arush, M. W., Breatnach, F., & Bellani, F. F. (1997). SIOP Working Committee on psychosocial issues in pediatric oncology: Guidelines for communication of the diagnosis. *Pediatric Blood & Cancer, 28*(5), 382–385. https://doi.org/10.1002/(SICI)1096-911X(199705)28:5<382::AID-MPO12>3.0.CO;2-D

McDougall, R., Delany, C., & Gillam, L. (Eds.). (2016). *When doctors and parents disagree.* Sydney, Australia: Federation Press.

Nesbit, K. C., Jensen, G., & Delany, C. (2018). The active engagement model of applied ethics as a structure for ethical reflection in the context of course-based service learning. *Physiotherapy Theory and Practice, 34*(1), 1–12.

Piggot, J., Paterson, J., & Hocking, C. (2002). Participation in home therapy programs for children with cerebral palsy: A compelling challenge. *Qualitative Health Research, 12*(8), 1112–1129.

Radomski, N., & Beckett, D. (2011). Crossing workplace boundaries: Interprofessional thinking in action. In S. Kitto, J. Chesters, J. Thistlethwaite, & S. Reeves (Eds.), *Sociology of interprofessional health care practice: Critical reflections and concrete solutions.* Hauppauge, NY: Nova Publishers.

Reilly, S., Douglas, J., & Oates, J. (Eds.). (2004). *Evidence based practice in speech pathology.* London, UK: Whurr Publishers.

Rice, P. L., & Ezzy, D. (1999). *Qualitative research methods: A health focus.* Melbourne, Australia: Oxford University Press.

Spriggs, M. P., & Gillam, L. H. (2008). Consent in paediatric research: An evaluation of the guidance provided in the 2007 NHMRC National statement on ethical conduct in human research. *Medical Journal of Australia, 188*(6), 360. https://www.mja.com.au/system/files/issues/188_06_170308/spr10740_fm.pdf

United Nations. (1989). Convention on the Rights of the Child. Retrieved from https://www.ohchr.org/en/professionalinterest/Pages/InternationalLaw.aspx

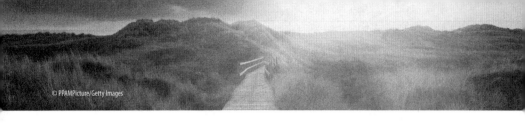

CHAPTER 7

Ethical Issues in the Rehabilitation of Older Adults

Mary Ann Wharton

CHAPTER OBJECTIVES

At the conclusion of this chapter, the reader will be able to:

1. Recognize that older adults' ability to make ethical decisions about health care may be compromised by frailty, recent surgery, illness, medications and/or cognitive decline.
2. Differentiate competence from capacity.
3. Define relational autonomy and describe the effect of an individual's support network on autonomy.
4. Discuss the issue of deception in rehabilitation of persons with cognitive decline.
5. Analyze conflicts in decision making by surrogates, including substituted judgment or best interest standards.
6. Describe ethical concerns related to refusal of care, discharge decisions, in long-term care, end-of-life, and reimbursement.

KEY TERMS

Reading these key terms before reading the chapter will introduce you to key concepts which will then be somewhat familiar to you as you read this chapter. This is an important learning technique that will enhance your learning as a multi-step process. You may even wish to make a flash card set of key terms and quiz yourself on them once or twice before reading the chapter. This will better prepare you to immerse in the language of ethics and better prepare you to integrate the content.

Autonomy: The right of self-determination. In ethics, the right of autonomy allows an individual to make choices and decisions about his or her life, and to have those choices honored as respected by others.

Best Interest Standard for Decision Making: A standard for decision making that may be used by surrogates when the preferences of that individual are unknown.

Capacity: The ability to make an informed decision. Capacity is linked to informed consent. According to Applebaum (2007), capacity includes the ability to communicate choices; the ability to understand information necessary for the specific decision at hand; and the ability to appreciate the implications and significance of the information provided or the choice being made; and the ability to reason by weighing and comparing options and consequences of the potential decision.

Competence: The ability of an individual to consent to or refuse treatment. Competence to make a medical decision must be legally determined. While there is no universal agreement about a legal definition, all agree that one necessary element for competence to be valid is that the patient must understand the factual information that has been given that is relevant to the decision the individual is being asked to make. Therefore, medical competence is rooted in informed consent (Paola, 2010).

Guardian: A person, generally appointed by a judge, who is responsible for making decisions for a person who is incapciated.

Informed Decision: The capacity to provide valid informed consent about a healthcare choice.

Relational Autonomy: The ability of healthcare professionals, family members, and friends to support individuals to make choices that are consistent with that person's sense of what is important to him or her and what makes sense for his or her life. Guided by the principle of beneficence, healthcare professionals and family should seek to promote the well-being of the individual, and endeavor to minimize the likelihood of harm (Kaizer, Spiridigliozzi, & Hunt, 2012).

Substituted Judgment Standard for Decision Making: Decision making that is based on what the person would have decided for him or herself if competent to do so.

Surrogate Decision Maker: A person authorized to participate in or make decisions on behalf of an incapacitated individual.

Therapeutic Lying: A response to an individual with an altered sense of reality that involves validating that individual's own reality by acknowledging the truth of that person's experience, and is used with the intent to bring about good and minimize harm.

▶ Chapter Overview

This chapter focuses on ethical issues faced in the rehabilitation of older adults. The premise is that ethical concerns are complicated by issues associated with aging, including frailty, cognitive impairment, social support systems, and living environment. Specific emphasis is on supporting autonomy, especially as it is compromised by cognitive decline resulting in diminished capacity for decision making. Reflection is provided for using traditional and contemporary ethical theories, codes of ethics, and compassionate care.

▶ Introduction to Ethical Issues in the Rehabilitation of the Geriatric Patient

The percentage of older Americans that report disability and activity limitations increases with age, with 35% reporting difficulty with one or more activity of daily living (Administration on Aging, 2016). Rehabilitation professionals must not only be prepared to meet the clinical needs of these individuals, but they must also have the expertise to address ethical concerns. Ethical issues faced in the rehabilitation of geriatric patients are complex. In addition to age-related changes and chronic conditions that affect activities of daily living, older patients are frequently vulnerable. They may be experiencing cognitive impairment or dementia, which compromises their ability to make autonomous decisions. Rehabilitation professionals must deal with the impact of ethical decisions on families, caregivers, and society. Discharge placement and end-of-life decisions for patients with cognitive deficits are challenging for all members of the rehabilitation team: patients, rehabilitation professionals, family members and other decision makers. As a result of the inherent complexity of these issues, conflict may occur between members of the team. **FIGURE 7.1** summarizes some of the most commonly encountered ethical issues in caring for older patients.

1. Decision-making capacity and competency
2. Surrogate decision making
3. Informed consent
4. Patient autonomy
5. Patient's right to refuse
6. Conflicts in moral and legal rights of patients and families/caregivers
7. Disclosure
8. Truth-telling
9. Discharge Decisions
10. Safety
11. Risk-taking
12. Palliative and end-of-life care
13. Research

FIGURE 7.1 Commonly identified ethical issues in care of geriatric patients.

Learning Point 7.1 What are some of the factors that complicate ethical decisions in the care of geriatric patients?

Other ethical concerns in care of the elderly patient, include choice, truthfulness, and privacy.

Traditional bioethics theories and codes of ethics may provide guidance, but they do not account for the complex issues involved in geriatric rehabilitation. For that reason, rehabilitation professionals should employ other tools for ethical decision making to account for the effect of decisions on the older person's support network, quality of life, and vulnerable status. This chapter will focus on ethical issues related to the rehabilitation of older adults.

▶ Ethics Codes and Theories: Guidance for Rehabilitation Practitioners Providing Care for Older Adults

Traditionally, rehabilitation professionals rely on their respective codes of ethics to provide guidance in dealing with ethical concerns. It is important to recognize that such documents provide general guidance but they do not provide specific answers to an ethical concern. Codes of ethics do not typically account for the complex issues associated with providing care for older adults. Codes of ethics should be used for guidance in the reflective process of moral agency (Jensen, Randall, & Wharton, 2012). For example, situations encountered when caring for older adults may require balancing beneficence and non-maleficence with autonomy when older individuals make risky choices or refuse needed care.

Rehabilitation professionals may find more meaningful guidance from contemporary ethical approaches that focus on life narratives. These approaches advocate consideration of the decision-making context as well as the inter-relationships with others as important aspects of ethical care. They use stories, narrative, biographies, and active engagement to emphasize the importance of the values and virtues. Epstein (1991) advocated mindful practice as one way for clinicians to attend in a nonjudgmental way to their own physical and mental processes during ordinary, everyday tasks with clarity and insight. As such, mindfulness is an extension of reflective practice. Inherent in mindfulness is the ability to listen attentively, recognize bias and judgment, and act with compassion based on insight (Epstein, 1991). In turn, mindfulness integrates a phenomenological approach into clinical reasoning and ethical decision making. It is based on probing, interpreting, and understanding the experiences of how a person lives from that individual's perspective. It also takes into account the needs of all involved stakeholders. Trigger questions (**FIGURE 7.2**) are used to provide an analytical and interpretative response that promote the ability of clinicians to think more deeply and facilitate ethical engagement (Jensen, Randall, & Wharton, 2012; Greenfield & Jensen, 2010).

Active engagement is another related approach that can be helpful when faced with ethical dilemmas involving older adults. Active listening is more than an exchange of information. Active engagement entails listening to the patient's perspective and story, and connecting patient's circumstances, beliefs, values, and assumptions. Thinking reflexively is being aware of one's own perspective and voice in the patient's situation. As such, it increases the practitioner's awareness of their

1. What are the relevant ethical principles?
2. How do they relate to one another?
3. How has the story been cast or framed?
4. What are the ethically important moments?
5. Who is telling the story?
6. What has been left out?
7. Whose voice is not being heard?
8. What is ethically at stake?
9. What does the story tell us that would otherwise not be visible or heard?
10. How does this story lead to ethical mindfulness?

FIGURE 7.2 Trigger questions for facilitating ethical engagement.

Based on Jensen, Randall, & Wharton (2010).

personal values, emotional reactions, and practices, and allows the practitioner to see how these personal reactions may influence the patient's choices. Finally, critical reasoning is incorporated in order to examine assumptions about practices and connections between the professional and social contexts, including critical examination of the meaning and values of the biomedical principles. It also requires the health professional to be aware of the nature and effect of the patient/practitioner relationship within the broader realms of the institution and cultural and societal influences (Delany, Edwards, Jensen, & Skinner, 2010).

The Dialogic Engagement Model, as proposed in this text, will provide healthcare providers with another tool to reflect on the complex ethical problems that are part of everyday ethics in geriatric care. The process of dialogue between all participants involved in a patient's care, the value placed on narrative accounts and on listening and engaging with others, and the mutual learning that are part of this model provide a framework for rehabilitation practitioners to uncover the nuances and complexities encountered in the care of older adults.

Learning Point 7.2 Consider an ethical concern involving rehabilitation care of an older adult. Reflect on how using contemporary ethical theories and creating a moral commons will provide insight to enhance problem-solving.

▶ Autonomy: Special Considerations When Working with Older Adults

The concept of autonomy is fundamental to rehabilitation ethics and has been well-defined in ethics literature. In essence, autonomy allows an individual to make choices and decisions about his or her life, and to have those choices honored and respected by others. As such, autonomy in decision making is essential to self-determination, vital to maintaining self-identity, and linked to quality of life.

Importance of Patient Education

To the extent possible, healthcare professionals should respect autonomy and provide competent care in a way that is not forced or coerced but collaborative. Rehabilitation professionals use a variety of strategies to facilitate the ability of the older individual to make a justifiable and ethical choice. A cardinal strategy is patient education. Rehabilitation professionals should know standards and resources to ensure that patients can receive and understand information about their care when provided verbally or in writing. Effective communication is essential, as healthcare professionals are morally responsible to evaluate the patient's readiness to learn, and to consider their learning styles and preferences, and consider the patient's health literacy as it relates to education material. Health literacy is linked to the patient's capacity to obtain, process, and understand basic health information in order to make appropriate health decisions (Doherty & Purtilo, 2016).

Paternalism and Autonomy

Paternalism may be defined as coercion, or interference with another person's freedom of action.

> **Learning Point 7.3** What is paternalism? Is acting paternalistically ever justified in rehabilitation?

It is rooted in the healthcare professional's understanding coupled with the duty of beneficence and the desire to bring about the best outcome. Paternalism is used when the health professional perceives a need to protect the patient from harm. It is grounded in the values held by the professional, which may conflict with values held by the patient. When a health professional makes a paternalistic decision, he or she, in essence, is acting as a "parent" with all the negative and positive connotations. As such, paternalism limits patient autonomy because the health professional makes the decision "for" the patient instead of "with" the patient. The healthcare professional may justify paternalism by reasons related to the welfare and happiness of the individual.

Contemporary healthcare values may permit healthcare providers to use "gentle paternalism", or "soft paternalism" which combines gentle persuasion with informed consent to achieve patient adherence. The intended purpose is to protect individual patients from making poor choices with potentially harmful consequences. "Hard paternalism" involves using interventions to prevent or mitigate harm even when the person's risky choices and actions are informed, voluntary, and autonomous. In this case, others impose their beliefs about the person's best interest, and deny the person the opportunity to make their own decisions. In its extreme, paternalism can result in a violation of autonomy, which is not considered acceptable in western society (Wharton, 2014; Doherty & Purtilo, 2016; Brauner, 2016; Smebye, Kirkevold, & Engedal, 2016).

Competence and Capacity Defined

Inherent in autonomous decision making is the understanding that the individual has both the competence and capacity to make an autonomous decision. Competence is defined as the ability of an individual to consent to or refuse treatment. While there is no universal agreement about a legal definition, all agree that one necessary element for competence is that the individual must understand the factual information that has been given relevant to the decision the individual is making (Paola, Walker, & Nixon, 2010). Healthcare providers should recognize that questions of patient competence are determined legally, and should not be based on assumptions by the professional, family, or caregiver. Legal determination of competency is typically sought when a person insists on performing beyond his/her capacities, and as a result, may be at risk for harming him/herself or others.

While competence is defined legally, capacity of the individual to make informed decisions may be assessed in clinical settings outside of the legal context. One example of a clinical tool is the Fairfield Guideline (Post & Whitehouse, 1995) for determining decisional capacity for people with Alzheimer's disease. This tool outlines three fundamental criteria: (1) the individual must appreciate that he/she has a choice; (2) the individual must understand the medical situation and prognosis, including the nature of the recommended care and the risks, benefits, alternatives, and likely consequences; and (3) the individual must maintain sufficient decisional stability over time. Other valid assessment tools that are used to determine capacity include the Mini-Mental Status Examination, the Alzheimer's Disease Assessment Scale-cognition, the Global Depression Scale, and the MacArthur Competence Assessment Tool-Treatment (Applebaum, 2007; Rosin & van Dijk, 2005).

The capacity for an individual to make an informed decision is linked to informed consent. Sher outlines three critical elements that comprise the individual's capacity to provide valid informed consent. These elements are: full disclosure, decisional capacity, and voluntary capacity or the ability to make a decision free from coercion (Sher, 2014). Applebaum further clarified that four standards are necessary for valid capacity. These standards include: the ability to communicate a choice; the ability to understand information necessary for the specific decision at hand; the ability to appreciate implications and significance of the information provided or the choice being made; and the ability to reason by weighing and comparing options and consequences of the potential decision (Applebaum, 2007).

Learning Point 7.4   What factors would you consider to determine if a patient had decisional capacity?

Even when the individual's capacity to participate in decision making has been determined, it is frequently challenging for healthcare professionals and caregivers to balance respect for the individual's autonomy with the beneficent notion of avoiding and protecting that person from harm. Caregivers may find themselves in direct conflict with patient wishes. When caregivers perceive that the patient is incapable of making or contributing to decisions about his/her life, they may conclude that beneficence or non-maleficence from their perspective outweighs or overrules the patient's autonomy. A risk is that the caregiver may force a decision that is contrary to the person's preference and choice. Alternately, the caregiver may err on the side of autonomy and allow a risky or unsafe decision.

Learning Point 7.5   Consider how you would distinguish between capacity and competence when providing rehabilitation care to an older adult who is experiencing mild cognitive decline.

Relational Autonomy: Recognizing the Effect of an Individual's Network on Autonomous Decisions

Situations in which older adults that have the capacity to make a decision and wish to make a choice that clinicians and family assess as unduly risky or burdensome create sources of distress. These decisions may even generate division among family members who have different views on the best course of action. The situations can be further complicated by the fact that respect for autonomy also places a negative duty on others to not interfere in the individual's right to autonomy without identifying compelling reasons for such interference.

> **Learning Point 7.6**   Consider the situation where a patient insists on returning to their home even though it is not safe and will require family hardship to facilitate the return.

In these situations, the broader concept of relational autonomy, espoused by feminist bioethicists, may be helpful. Relational autonomy recognizes the interdependences between the individual and that person's network. Therefore, a relational concept of autonomy is based on the understanding of persons as inter-connected, and not as isolated rational thinkers. The context and influences that shape options, choices, and relationships are taken into account in evaluating the patient's reality. Relational autonomy suggests that healthcare professionals, family members, and friends should, to the extent possible, support individuals to make choices consistent with that person's sensibilities. However, those decisions should not conflict with the effect on others in the relationship, including family members, healthcare providers, and society. The healthcare professionals and family should seek to promote the well-being of the individual, guided by the principle of beneficence, and endeavor to minimize the likelihood of harm. Care should be exercised to assure that the professionals provide appropriate education regarding the implications of varying options, with the goal of guiding the individual toward a decision that is likely to benefit the person and also minimize risk (Hunt & Ells, 2011; Kaizer, Spiridigliozzi, & Hunt, 2012).

> **Learning Point 7.7**   Consider why relational autonomy is an important concept when dealing with older adults. Discuss how focusing on the individual's network may influence an ethical decision regarding rehabilitation goals and plans.

▶ Ethical Issues with Older Adults Experiencing Cognitive Decline

Acknowledging Personhood

Ethical concerns when caring for older adults experiencing cognitive decline as a result of degenerative conditions, including Alzheimer's disease and other pathologies, can be particularly challenging to healthcare providers, families, and caregivers. However, it is imperative for rehabilitation professionals to recognize and understand that, even though working with older adults with cognitive decline poses multiple ethical dilemmas, an ethical response demands that we provide compassionate care at the highest level of professional competence. In order to provide ethical and compassionate care, the focus should be on the individual's current strengths and abilities, and not solely on the person's cognitive pathology. Rehabilitation professionals must recognize that the decision-making capacity of a person living with cognitive decline or dementia is dependent on the stage or severity of the disease. It is well established that the decision-making capacity of a person living with dementia decreases as the severity of the dementia increases. In spite of this decline in mental status, it is essential that ethical concerns do not go unrecognized or ignored as the disease progresses, the individual's mental capacity declines, or the person experiences difficult behaviors, undergoes changes in personality, loses language skills, becomes unable to manage activities of daily living, and socially withdraws from family and friends. In spite of these challenges, rehabilitation professionals should strive for optimal care that, as much as possible, includes respecting autonomy, preserving decision-making abilities, upholding confidentiality, and offering meaningful participation in everyday activities of daily living. The focus must not be limited to extraordinary issues such as life or death decisions. Rather, the emphasis of care should consider the everyday experiences that affect the individual's quality of life in order to protect vulnerable individuals from abusive practices. By reflecting on ethics in everyday living, the rehabilitation professional strives to enhance the dignity of the individual.

Current best practices in contemporary dementia care advocate a focus on abilities addressing the individual's current strengths, and not based solely on the person's cognitive pathology (Criss, Heitzman, & Wharton, 2016; Nuffield Council on Bioethics, 2009; Daly & Fahey-McCarthy, 2014). The ethical framework developed by the Nuffield Council on Bioethics is one tool that clinicians can use to guide ethical decision making when dealing with patients experiencing cognitive decline. The value in this framework is that it does not emphasize any particular ethical perspective. Rather, it reflects contemporary ethical and dementia-practice thinking. **FIGURE 7.3** delineates the five components of ethical care for patients with cognitive decline.

The first component of this framework emphasizes a case-by-case approach that fosters an attempt to look at the details of each case from various perspectives. The second and third components stress that dementia is a brain disorder, but that it is possible for a person to live with dementia provided they have the right support system. The fourth component emphasizes promoting autonomy of the individual, and also emphasizes that autonomy must be considered in relational terms since family members and other caregivers are also involved. The fifth component of this model recognizes that individuals with dementia are fellow citizens, and therefore, healthcare providers should act with solidarity, while acknowledging the mutual interdependence and responsibility to support the individual with dementia, their families, and society as a whole. Finally, this framework stresses the importance and value of personhood, which emphasizes that dementia care requires that we value the person throughout the course of their illness, even as the illness progresses and cognitive and other functions decline. In addition to the recommendation that ethical dilemmas be approached on a case-by-case basis, this framework directs rehabilitation professionals to consider potential harms and benefits; to reflect on how the person with dementia would best be helped to live well; and to consider the wishes and well-being of the person with dementia and those involved with their care. The framework takes into account respect for the broadest possible view of personhood, including

Component 1: Care-based approach: three-stage process
- Identify relevant facts
- Interpret and apply ethical values to the facts
- Compare the situation to similar situations

Component 2: Beliefs about nature of dementia
- Brain disorder that is harmful to the individual

Component 3: Belief about quality of life with dementia
- People with dementia can expect to have a good quality of life throughout the course of illness with good care and support.

Component 4: Importance of promoting the interests of the person with dementia and their caregivers
- People with dementia have interests in their autonomy and well-being
- Promoting autonomy involves enabling and fostering relationship that are important to the person and supporting them in maintaining their sense of self and expressing their values
- Autonomy is not simply equated with ability to make rational decisions
- Well-being includes both moment-to-moment experiences of contentment and pleasure, and more objective factors such as level of cognitive functioning.
- The interests of carers must be recognized and promoted

Component 5: Requirement to act in accordance with solidarity
- Recognize the citizenship of people with dementia
- Acknowledge mutual interdependence and responsibility to support people with dementia, both within families and in society as a whole.

Component 6: Recognizing personhood, identity, and value
- The person with dementia requires the same, equally valued, person throughout the course of their illness, regardless of the extent of the changes in their cognitive and other functions

FIGURE 7.3 Ethical framework in dementia care.
Reproduced from Nuffield Council on Bioethics (2009).

the biological, psychosocial, social, spiritual, moral, and legal considerations that apply when providing care for a person with dementia (Nuffield Council on Bioethics, 2009; Hughes & Common, 2015).

Learning Point 7.8   Apply the Nuffield Council ethical framework to an ethical concern involving a patient with dementia. Reflect on how using this tool can enhance your respect for that individual's personhood.

Validation and Therapeutic Lying

An important part of acknowledging personhood is validating a person's reality. The world of an individual experiencing cognitive decline changes as facts about their life, friends, and family are forgotten. Responding to the altered reality of this individual poses ethical concerns for rehabilitation professionals. Questions and anxiety may arise when determining how to respond to a patient's frantic search for a deceased spouse, or when that individual insists on returning home, when in reality, they have lived in a long-term care setting for many years. Literature suggests that many providers resort to deception to ease the distress experienced in these circumstances. However, deception in the form of a lie violates essential ethical principles. Truth-telling is a cardinal virtue that is embedded in both traditional and contemporary ethical theories and is included in professional codes of ethics. In fact, the Principles in the American Physical Therapy Association Code of Ethics for physical therapists and Standards of Ethical Conduct for Physical Therapist Assistants (American Physical Therapy Association, 2010a, 2010b), the Occupational Therapy Code of Ethics (American Occupational Therapy Association, 2015), and the American Speech-Language-Hearing Association Code of Ethics (American Speech-Language-Hearing Association, 2015) all include reference to truth-telling. Arguments for truthfulness include generating trust, encouraging compliance, and preserving autonomy. Care providers who use deception base their choice on the premise that deception that has the welfare of the patient at heart. They believe that the deception is made in the context of the individual experiencing dementia, and is justified by the end result of minimizing harm by reducing anxiety and stress. In this respect, the context of the "lie" aligns itself with the view that intention is central to truth-telling, and the "lie" is therapeutic.

Learning Point 7.9   Which of the four traditions could support therapeutic lying?

Rehabilitation professionals may also view therapeutic lying in the context of compassion and a form of benevolence, or acting for the good of the patient. In essence, this therapeutic lie is a way of validating the patient's own reality. The intent to bring about good and minimize harm causes some to comment that, although lying is prima facie wrong, it is not absolutely wrong in all instances. When the response to a patient with an altered sense of reality involves validating this reality by acknowledging the truth of that person's experience, they argue that it is an ethically mindful response. They believe that refraining from speaking actual truth is not deception and that there is no obligation to tell the truth because the individual did not specifically ask about the falsehoods in their world. They use validation to comfort, and not to purposefully mislead or gain cooperation. Even the Alzheimer's Organization recognizes the use of validation therapy as ethically permissible (Criss, Heitzman, & Wharton, 2016; Tuckett, 2012).

Learning Point 7.10   Consider whether it would ever be permissible to "lie" to a patient. Does your perception change if you frame the "lie" in terms of "validation"?

Effect of Mild Cognitive Impairment (MCI) on Decision-Making Ability

As stated previously, the literature suggests that even mild cognitive decline has a detrimental effect on the individual's decision-making ability, and that this ability decreases with the severity of the dementia. However, it is also acknowledged that cognitive decline is not uniform, and people with dementia may be able to make choices about some aspects of their care while they are incapable in other areas. An example would be an individual who is capable of deciding whether or not to follow the recommendations of the therapists to use a rollator walker for safe community ambulation, but may no longer be able to manage his or her checkbook and finances, or follow a recipe to put together a family meal. This example, and other similar examples, demonstrates that a diagnosis of dementia does not always imply incapacity. In fact, evidence suggests that individuals with mild to moderate cognitive impairment may still be able to respond to preferences and choices about daily living, and may also want to participate in decisions about their treatment and care for as long as possible. Ethically, these wishes should be honored rather than denied or ignored. Using an ethical approach in which the caregivers delve into the meanings of the decision may provide the caregiver with insight to ultimately honor the individual's decision. Seeking to understand the individual's perspective can guide the caregiver to acknowledge the essence of the concept that "I am still here" and may facilitate the caregiver's ability to implement strategies to support the individual in their decision-making capacity (Fetherstonhauge, Tarzia, & Nay, 2013).

Ho, Pinney, and Bozic (2015) discuss concerns related to caring for older adults with mild cognitive impairment that affect attention, language, judgment, memory, reading, or writing, even if such impairment has not reached the threshold for dementia. They state that some older patients with mild cognitive impairment may demonstrate a questionable understanding and/or desire to make healthcare decisions, exhibit lower decisional engagement, and have a higher tendency to defer to family members or other caregivers than younger patients. They note that cognitive impairment, coupled with complex medical and socioeconomic challenges, may cause daunting ethical dilemmas. However, they also caution that healthcare providers must not presume or stereotype all elderly patients as being incapable of making medical decisions, and stress the need to clarify and determine the intellectual capacity and decision-making ability of each patient individually.

While recognizing the relevance of the biomedical principles of beneficence, non-maleficence and justice, the authors of this study cite respect for autonomy as most relevant when determining appropriate decision making with older adults experiencing mild cognitive impairment. Specifically, they cite that physicians may have difficulty respecting the autonomy of patients with mild cognitive impairment who lack the capacity to understand information relevant to treatment decision making. The four criteria that they identify as necessary for demonstrating capacity include the patient's ability to (1) understand information relevant to treatment decision making; (2) appreciate the importance of information for the given situation; (3) reason through relevant information and weigh treatment options; and (4) communicate the treatment decision. They state that the physician/provider may consider a higher threshold for capacity when the patient's decision poses a substantial risk of harm and low benefits, and a lower threshold when the risk is low and benefits are substantial.

Learning Point 7.11 How would you facilitate safe appropriate, and effective decision making when dealing with a patient with mild cognitive decline?

Shared Decision Making

In situations where the patient with mild cognitive impairment meets these four criteria for decision making, they suggest using a shared decision-making approach to foster respect for the patient's autonomy. This approach includes three cardinal features: (1) presenting patients with relevant information regarding the nature of their condition, including risks and benefits of available treatment options; (2) inviting patients to participate in the process through discussion of relevant values, goals, and concerns; and (3) encouraging patients to voluntarily choose the most appropriate alternative.

Learning Point 7.12   How does shared decision making expand traditional notions of informed consent?

Shared decision making focuses on providing high quality information to inform patients and also corresponds with the patient's values, preferences, and life goals. Including family or caregivers to support the decision making can also improve both health literacy and outcomes for these patients. Strong social support has been noted as a significant predictor of key outcome measures for surgical patients. "Teach-back" methods, where patients are asked to restate information or demonstrate knowledge or techniques that were taught, have also been shown to improve health outcomes. The bottom line is that communication and support are integral to ascertain the decision-making capacity and facilitate clinically and ethically appropriate care for individuals with minimal cognitive impairment (Ho et al., 2015).

▶ Decision Making by Surrogates

The fact that the decision-making capacity of an individual with dementia decreases as the severity of the dementia increases poses significant challenges for all involved, and may lead to healthcare providers, family members, and caregivers failing to respect the autonomy of the individual to be involved in making a decision. One solution is using surrogates to participate in, or make decisions on behalf of, the individual. However, it is imperative that rehabilitation providers recognize the appropriateness of involving another individual to make a decision for the person whose capacity is challenged. Far too often, healthcare providers assume that family members have the legal authority and expertise to make decisions on behalf of loved ones, and turn to family members to make decisions without regard for the wishes or ability of the individual with cognitive impairment to participate in the process. The end result is that family members may assume the role of surrogate decision makers without the legal authority or the expertise to do so.

When considering the use of surrogate decision makers, there is a need to assess whether the views of the surrogate accurately reflect the patient's preferences. Studies have shown that the predictions made by surrogates regarding treatment preferences are often mistaken. To minimize this risk, clinicians should evaluate how confident a surrogate is that a particular decision reflects the patient's wishes, and should explore the basis for the surrogate's views about what decision the patient would make. Probing the surrogate about whether he or she had an explicit discussion with the patient to determine what was discussed and what the patient actually said is a strategy that could be used to ascertain the probability that a surrogate is making a valid decision (Brock, Park, & Wendler, 2014). One problem that can occur with any surrogate decision maker is that they may rely on their own values, morals, and beliefs to make decisions on behalf of the individual with cognitive impairment. For example, the surrogate decision maker may follow their own religious beliefs, even though these beliefs may be different from those of the patient. Another problem is that the surrogate decision maker may make decisions that are based on the burden that the caregiver may need to assume rather than consider the patient's wishes. Additionally, the surrogate decision maker may make decisions based on their ability to accept a predictable outcome of medical care, and choose to ignore a "do not resuscitate" order or follow through with a natural death request (Philipsen, Murray, Wood, Bell-Hawkins, & Setlow, 2013).

Rosin and van Dijk (2005) reported on a type of surrogate decision making that is based in the role reversal that may occur between a parent and child when a parent has diminished decision-making capacity. These authors note that the appearance of dependency in older adults is often incorrectly interpreted as loss of autonomy, resulting in a role reversal whereby the child assumes the functions of the parent, including the responsibility for making decisions. They caution that when a son or daughter unnecessarily undertakes responsibility for choices, the ultimate decision could be interpreted as unethical. These authors further discuss that dealing with an infirm parent's personal affairs requires a delicate balance between what the child thinks is best to meet the parent's needs, and what the parent personally needs or wants. In particular, they state that the dilemma is determining a balance between the patient/parent's needs and his or her ability to provide those needs independently on one hand, and the family's concerns that the parent will receive the needed attention and support to meet those needs on the other hand.

In situations where there is a question about the patient's ability to make safe and autonomous decisions, Rosin and van Dijk (2005) state that the healthcare providers must determine whether the patient or the family is the accountable decision maker. Generally, the patient is the priority, but in complex situations, the impact on others must be considered. It is important to acknowledge the burden placed on the older person by the illness, but it is also important to consider the burden on the family.

As the dementia progresses, family members and caregivers find themselves in a position of gradually taking on more decision-making responsibility, especially for decisions about lifestyle, healthcare medical treatments, and end-of-life care. These decisions are complex, and pose significant ethical issues for family members and others in order to make a decision that supports the person's wishes and promotes quality of life. The decision makers at this point are referred to as proxy or surrogate decision makers. Legislation varies from country to country, and even within countries, as to who qualifies as an appropriate surrogate decision maker.

Learning Point 7.13   Reflect on potential problems that may occur when the rehabilitation team relies on surrogates to make decisions for patients with cognitive decline.

Substituted Judgment and Best Interest Standard

Surrogate decisions are generally made using either the substituted judgment standard or the best interest standard. Substituted judgment bases decision making on what the person would have decided for him or herself when competent to do so.

An example would be a daughter making a decision to admit her father to a nursing home when he had become extremely frail and dependent. She based her decision on recalling that her father expressed that he would not want his daughter to have to assume the burden of caring for him if he became disabled. The decision, then, is dependent on the surrogate decision maker knowing or accurately predicting what the person with dementia would have wanted when they were competent to make a decision. This approach can be problematic if the surrogate decision maker has not had a conversation with the person with dementia. If the surrogate decision maker is a spouse or family member, studies suggest that judgment may additionally be clouded by emotional attachment to the person, thereby fostering a more aggressive treatment option. An example would be a husband refusing to transition his wife, who is nonresponsive and diagnosed with end-stage dementia, to a hospice program and instead chooses to direct the care team to continue all possible medical procedures to keep his wife alive even though the interprofessional team recommends that hospice would be a more compassionate decision.

An alternate standard for making surrogate decisions is the best interest standard. This standard is based on determining what would be in the best interests of the now incompetent person when their preferences are unknown. In the case of the terminally ill wife, the husband using the best interest standard may be inclined to make a decision to admit his wife to hospice rather than pursue care that is deemed no longer viable (Fetherstonhaugh et al., 2017; Phillipson et al., 2013).

Some surrogate decision makers may use both the substituted judgment and the best interest standard when making decisions for persons with dementia. This can also prove to be difficult, because it involves balancing what the person with dementia's "past self" would have wanted with what the "now self" might want if they had capacity and access to all available information. The surrogate decision maker must then determine how to reconcile the person's past preferences with current ones, and these preferences may be inconsistent. Also, holding the individual to past preferences does not afford the opportunity for that individual to change their mind or gain a different perspective when faced with the reality of their current situation (Fetherstonhaugh et al., 2017).

Fetherstonhaugh et al. (2013) investigated how surrogate decision makers made important decisions on behalf of persons with dementia. This study revealed three main themes associated with the process of surrogate decision making in dementia: knowing the person's wishes, consulting others, and striking a balance. The researchers found that surrogate decision makers fell into two groups with respect to knowing the person's wishes: those who knew the prior wishes of the person with dementia and those who did not. Those who knew the prior wishes identified a variety of means for knowing the wishes, including formal documentation that was drafted before or at the time of receiving the dementia diagnosis, and informal written directives. In the absence of written directives, surrogate decision makers cited that they were guided by prior conversations about that person's wishes regarding future care needs. The surrogate decision makers reported that knowing the prior wishes could be helpful, but also stated that this knowledge did not always clarify the decision-making process because of uncertainty over whether or not the person with dementia still held the same wish. Several studies have supported this concept and have noted that an older individual's preferences regarding life-sustaining treatments often change over time.

The same study found that most surrogate decision makers consulted with other family members when they were faced with uncertainty or felt the need for a second opinion to make an important decision. Some reported that challenges occurred when there was disagreement among family members. Conversely, other surrogate decision makers reported that consulting with family members strengthened family bonds when the family worked through a decision together. The authors concluded that collaboration with trusted health professionals to seek reassurance is crucial in dementia care.

Of importance to surrogate decision makers in this study was the need to strike a balance between respecting the known wishes of the person with dementia and looking after their perceived "best" interests by keeping the individual safe, comfortable, and receiving good care. Surrogate decision makers noted that disagreements within families arose when the surrogate decision maker placed more weight on independence than on safety.

The surrogate decision makers in this study reported that they acutely felt the enormity of the responsibility of serving as a surrogate decision maker or a person with dementia, especially when making end-of-life decisions. Some surrogate decision makers found it easier to respect the wishes of a person with dementia if they were of advanced age, if they no longer recognized family members, or if the surrogate decision maker perceived that the person no longer had a good quality of life.

Advanced care planning is also critical to facilitate ethical decisions and promote the autonomy of individuals, especially as dementia progresses and the person approaches end-of-life. Advanced care planning may include discussions about wishes and values; discussions and plans for future treatment and care; appointment of surrogate decision makers; and development of written advance care directives. To be most effective, the advanced care planning should preferably start at the time of diagnosis and anticipate the patient's impending cognitive decline. The advanced care plan should also include end-of-life decisions, recognizing that dementia is ultimately a terminal illness. Lastly, the study acknowledged that interpreting and honoring an advanced care plan can be complex for the surrogate decision maker, so health professionals need to recognize the challenges and support the surrogate decision maker in their role (Fetherstonhaugh et al., 2017).

> **Learning Point 7.14**   Differentiate key differences between the substituted judgment and best interest standards used in surrogate decision making.

Role of Guardians, Physicians, Ethics Committees, and the "Same Community Preference" in Decision Making

In situations where older persons do not identify a surrogate decision maker before losing capacity, most states have laws allowing a default surrogate to be selected. This individual may be a family member, but in instances where no family member is available, the courts generally allow a judge to appoint a guardian of person or conservator of person, referred to as a professional guardian. In these situations, the professional guardian is a paid official with no knowledge of the impaired individual before appointment. The number of professional guardians is expected to rise dramatically as the incidence of dementia increases with the aging population.

Professional guardians have unique ethical challenges when making determinations for individuals. The professional guardian may not be able to exercise substituted judgment, since he or she had no prior relationship with the older person. As a result, the professional may rely on the best interest standard. A perceived problem with the professional guardian is that this individual may have no specific training in medical decisions. As a result, they may be reluctant to give orders that limit treatment, opting instead for the perceived safer path of aggressive care or deferring to judicial process. This situation is further complicated because state statues differ, and there is generally a lack of instructions for professional guardians. The lack of standards may provide legal basis to avoid making a decision, put the decision in the hands of judges (Cohen, Wright, Cooney, & Fried, 2015).

Alternatives to current practice have been proposed for shared decision making for an incapacitated person. One approach would be to allow the physician to make decisions in an incapacitated person's best interests in the absence of an identifiable decision maker. However, physicians are less accurate than surrogates at predicting patient treatment preferences, and this process may pose a potential conflict of interest for the physician (Cohen et al., 2015).

Another alternative is to have hospital ethics committees or voluntary surrogate decision-making panels make the decisions using patient preference predictors. Rid and Wendler (2010) report that strangers predict a person's preferences more accurately than family members. One disadvantage to this proposal is the time required for the committee to meet.

Another alternative for decision making is the "same community preference" approach. In this case, the treatment decision is based on the preference of patients in the same community (Rid & Wendler, 2010).

Cohen et al. (2015) discuss the option of establishing formal roles for physicians and guardians to collaborate and make decisions on behalf of the incapacitated person. In this model, the physician would suggest a plan of care that would be in the individual's best interest, and the guardian would ask clarifying questions that consider all perspectives in order to make the best possible ethical decision. Ethics committees and courts would serve as a last resort, when necessary to resolve disagreements. To be successful, this approach requires the availability of in-depth training for the guardians to enable them to work optimally with the physicians. The authors also discuss a model that uses voluntary guardians. In this model, qualified volunteers are recruited to represent incapacitated individuals. These volunteers may include medical students and home health aides (Cohen et al., 2015).

Finally, a model of decision making that is widely endorsed is for the clinician and surrogate decision maker to share responsibility for the decision. While this may relieve some of the stress experienced by surrogate decision makers, it may not provide the goal of providing treatment that is consistent with the values and preferences of the patient. In fact, this model may in essence combine two inaccurate decision makers and not facilitate carrying out the wishes of the incapacitated person (Rid & Wendler, 2010).

Learning Point 7.15   Discuss pros and cons for the various approaches used in decision making.

Conflicts in Surrogate Decision Making

Using surrogate decision makers for incapacitated older adults is complex and may be fraught with conflicts. Eves and Esplen (2015) discuss some of the presumptions and complexities that affect the medical team, the surrogate decision maker, and the patient. They acknowledge that there can be tension between the substitutive judgment standard and procedural decision-making autonomy. Using the substituted judgment standard is based on the presumption that the patient has consistent, unambiguous values and preferences, and that they disclose those preferences in the same way to each person they know and trust. On the other hand, the choice of a surrogate decision maker is a procedural decision that presumes that the surrogate decision maker is chosen because that person can best communicate information that respects the choices of the patient when that individual no longer has the capacity to communicate those choices. The presumption is that the choice of the individual to be the surrogate decision maker is based on merit. Conflict occurs when there are differences of opinion between family members and the surrogate decision maker, or even between the surrogate decision maker and the medical team. Such conflict is not unusual, especially when decisions involve end-of-life choices about medical care. The authors suggest that one viable solution to resolve these complicated ethical situations is through an ethics consultation. The goal of the consultation is to address the uncertainty or conflict among the stakeholders. Strategies employed may include shifting the focus of the conflict by supporting the medical team, attending to the relationships among all stakeholders, and facilitating respectful discourse. In this consultative role, the ethicist does not search for unequivocal truth. Rather, the ethicist assumes the role of a navigator who reserves judgment, but explores inconsistencies and motivations of all stakeholders, including the medical team. In essence, the ethicist serves as a neutral party who is responsible for creating a "safe space" for stakeholders to engage in reflection and address moral distress through focused and facilitated ethics discussion. This environment facilitates the ability of the stakeholders to explore a range of values, beliefs, and alternative ways to consider the facts and to reconcile differences. Ultimately, this safe discourse may lead to mitigation of the emotional burden of the conflict (Eves & Esplin, 2015).

> **Learning Point 7.16**   Reflect on how you would resolve a conflict that could occur with surrogate decision making.

▶ Special Considerations in Geriatric Care

Refusal of Care

Successful rehabilitation of older adults is based on the premise that the patient and rehabilitation professional have similar goals, and that the patient will cooperate and adhere to the rehabilitation plan. Occasionally, there are instances where that is not the case and even a competent patient may refuse to participate in the proposed plan. The professional is then placed in the ethical position of either respecting and accepting the patient's values and autonomous right to refuse care, or employing another strategy to encourage the patient to adhere to treatment. An optimal strategy would be for the therapist to use shared decision-making to collaborate with the patient and integrate that patient's view of rehabilitation into the plan of care. When that strategy fails, therapists may ponder whether to use persuasion, incentives and inducements, threats or coercion, or may even consider explicitly overriding the patient's autonomy. In these situations, the therapist must use ethical reasoning to balance his or her therapeutic view of what is in the patient's best interest with the ethical responsibility to respect the patient's autonomy in refusing care. The therapist must recognize that the older patient's ability and freedom to make a valid choice may be diminished by their health status. Factors including pain, frailty, fear about their prognosis and uncertainty of recovery, and concerns about adequate reimbursement to pay for their medical care all contribute to their vulnerability and may influence their decision to refuse care.

Persuasion, as defined by Anderson and Delany (2016), may be seen as a form of paternalism. It is premised on the notion that when a patient understands the benefits and risks of the treatment goals in terms that are consistent with their values, that patient may be more inclined to participate rather than refuse. It is based on the ethical ideal of shared decision making and patient-centered care. When using persuasion, the therapist treats the patient as a competent adult who is capable of understanding and making a decision based on the projected outcomes of the plan, and the patient's autonomy is respected. An example of persuasion would be for the occupational therapist to encourage a patient to work on putting on a shirt and slacks so that they can learn to be more independent and be discharged back to their own home.

Inducements, or using "incentives" or "rewards" in order to encourage a patient to participate in the rehabilitation plan may be used when efforts to persuade a patient are unsuccessful provided that the reward does not leave the patient worse off, is easy to avoid, and does not involve deception, concealment, or misrepresentation. An example of an inducement would be when a physical therapist offers a patient a cup of tea provided he or she walks from their hospital room to the lounge area at the end of the hall. When using inducements, therapists must recognize whether the inducement diminishes that person's capacity to make an autonomous decision. To be ethical, the person must able to review the inducement objectively and determine whether the inducement is consistent with his or her values.

Inter-personal leverage is another technique that may be used by rehabilitation professionals to get a patient to comply with therapy. One example of inter-personal leverage, mentioned by Anderson and Delany (2016), would be telling a patient that you would be disappointed if he or she didn't participate in a treatment session. These authors view interpersonal leverage as more ethically problematic than persuasion or inducement because it is a form of manipulation of an already vulnerable patient. The patient, desiring to be a "good patient", may find it difficult to say "no" and may not be consciously aware of the impact of the therapist's statement on their decision. This type of treatment pressure that leverages a patient's desire to please and plays on the patient's guilt to effect a behavioral change may rise to a violation of the trusting relationship between the patient and therapist.

Threats are a form of coercion that may result in harm if the patient does not comply. Threats are ethically unacceptable because they are coercive. It is important to differentiate an inducement from a threat. One important moral distinction is the outcome.

Learning Point 7.17   How does an inducement differ from a threat?

An inducement, in which a reward is given in return for a favor, does not leave the person worse off if they continue to refuse treatment.

An important moral consideration of a threat is whether the statement is true or not. The example of a threat cited by Anderson and Delany (2016) is a statement by a therapist that a patient may have to go to a nursing home if the patient doesn't comply with the rehabilitation program. If the statement is reasonable and true, it is an example of an unwelcome prediction rather than a coercive threat. If the statement is not true, it is a coercive threat. If the therapist knows the statement is not true and fails to correct the false belief, that therapist is engaging in deception.

Some healthcare practitioners view deception as benign because it promotes a beneficial outcome for the patient. However, deception diminishes that patient's ability to weigh information and make an informed decision. It is ethically important for rehabilitation professionals to provide accurate and transparent information to enable a patient to be aware of the clinician's goals and values, to voluntarily consider personal values and goals and make an informed decision. Another form of deception is when the professional limits choice to a minor aspect of care but has not obtained consent for the central treatment. The example cited by Anderson and Delany (2016) is giving a patient a choice of where to walk to without obtaining the patient's consent to get out of bed and go for a walk. The authors also cite more troubling forms of deception such as telling a patient an action won't hurt, when in reality, the treatment will result in considerable discomfort. These examples of deception all override the patient's capacity to make a voluntary, informed choice and diminish the trusting relationship between the patient and professional (Anderson & Delany, 2016).

The most disturbing type of patient engagement is compulsion in which the rehabilitation professional overrides a patient's expressed wishes and forces a competent patient to participate in an activity. The example cited is physically pulling a patient out of bed after a patient refuses treatment. This activity may not only be perceived as unethical, but may rise to a criminal charge of assault and battery.

Anderson and Delany (2016) conclude that the use of treatment pressures may be ethically acceptable when it involves persuasion and inducements because these techniques ultimately preserve and respect the autonomy of the patient. They suggest that threats and coercion are ethically problematic, and may be even be unethical, and that compulsion is generally unethical. Rehabilitation professionals need to recognize where their actions fall along the spectrum of the pressures from persuasion to compulsion; be aware of how their actions may limit patient autonomy; have sound ethical justification; and keep interventions that limit patient autonomy limiting to a minimum (Anderson & Delany, 2016).

Carrese (2006) suggests approaches and considerations that rehabilitation professionals can consider when dealing with a patient who refuses care. He identifies assessing the patient's capacity for decision making is an important step. He also recommends that the professional consider the refusal as an opportunity for dialogue with the patient to examine the patient's reason for refusal. Key influences for refusal may include such factors as religious beliefs, cultural background, previous interactions with the healthcare system, and the preferences of family members. He also stresses the importance of determining whether the patient's refusal is consistent with that individual's goals for care, and emphasizes the need to explore whether patient autonomy in refusing care can be reconciled with the patient's welfare (Carrese, 2006).

Discharge Decisions

Complex ethical concerns can be identified with respect to discharge planning in geriatric rehabilitation. A factor that complicates the ethics of discharge plans is competing obligations may affect the rights of many stakeholders, including the

patient, family, and rehabilitation professionals. Traditional bioethics has historically largely ignored the rights of families; however, families are traditionally obliged
to care for each other in ways not expected from friends, neighbors, and strangers.
Therefore, the burden of care associated with the prolonged life of individuals with
chronic and debilitating illnesses is an important consideration, and the obligation
to care for family members must be balanced against the obligation of family members to care for their own physical and emotional needs (Haddad 2000, Wharton,
2014). While the rights of family members must be factored into discharge plans,
they must not have more influence on the plan than the rights of the older patient.
One current temptation is to consult and address the needs of family members while
virtually ignoring the decision-making right and ability of the older individual, even
when that individual is capable of involvement in the process.

A significant discharge challenge may be encountered when a frail, but
cognitively-capable elderly client chooses to live at risk. In this situation, the frail
older adult is deemed capable of understanding the information relevant to making a decision about his or her living situation, appreciates the reasonable and
foreseeable consequences of a decision, and nevertheless makes a decision that the
interprofessional healthcare team deems risky. When confronted with an ethical situation, the clinician should consider using mindful reflection and narrative, in light
of autonomy, non-maleficence, beneficence, and advocacy. Consideration must be
given to the risk of harm to the patient as well as to others, and an attempt must be
made to achieve a balance between respect for individual freedom and the welfare
of all. Considerations should also include the degree of risk versus the probability
of harm and the amount of risk the individual is willing to assume. Clinicians must
avoid ageist viewpoints and take care to avoid questioning the rights and behaviors
of older adults in ways that would never be acceptable when dealing with younger
adults. A question that should be asked when an older adult wants to live at risk is
whether there would be the same degree of worry if the patient were 25 or 55. The
clinician should also consider why it is more concerning that a competent 85 year
old at risk for falling wants to stay at home than it is for a 16 year old wanting to
drive a car or a 25 year old wanting to rock climb. The end result of the ethical
decision-making process may be that clinicians respect the individual's choice, and
set up a plan to support that decision in spite of their personal concerns and fears
for the older individuals' safety. Ultimately, the clinician may come to terms with the
fact that there is no challenge, possibility of triumph, or real aliveness without risk
(Baker, Campton, & Gillis et al., 2007).

Learning Point 7.18 What community resources would you recommend to a
patient who has the legal competence and the capacity to make a decision and yet
chooses a risky discharge destination?

From an administrative standpoint, discharge involves balancing the good of
the patient against other goods, including the needs of the hospital and of society.
Conflicts may arise between the financial interests of the institutions and society
and the welfare of the patients. These are especially evident when financial considerations are viewed in light of the mission of the institution and its administrative
obligations to the staff and the community. An underlying motivation in effecting
the discharge or transfer of a patient from an institution may be the administrative
obligation to ensure that the institution remains viable. This obligation may be seen

to supersede the obligations of the institution to the community, the medical staff, and even the patient. As a result, the needs of individual patients may play a relatively minor role in ethical frameworks espoused by some administrators. Rather, in this context, a patient's needs are balanced against the needs and interests of others. Such conflicts may pose an ethical dilemma for those caregivers directly involved in effecting an appropriate discharge plan for an individual patient (Spielman, 1988).

Typically, discharge involves transition from a hospital to home or to a site of continuing care, and can be viewed as a transition from illness to rehabilitation and health. The question of autonomy, especially when the patient has cognitive impairment, can create ethical conflicts and pose multiple challenges. This can be especially true when a person with mild cognitive impairment or dementia wishes to live at home. These individuals are perceived to be at risk for falls as well as problems with nutrition, drug management, personal hygiene, and safety. They may be targets for fraud and experience social isolation. In spite of these challenges, these individuals may have risk awareness and may recognize that they have limited time to remain in their own homes. As a result, the healthcare professionals and families involved in their care are often faced with the choice between balancing the individual's autonomy, minimizing harm, promoting safety, and well-being. Strategies that promote adherence to ethical standards and serve to minimize harm, promote safety, and support independent living in these situations include referrals to available community agencies that provide both skilled and non-skilled services, recommending home modifications, working with social services to arrange for home-delivered meals, and identifying support groups for family members.

Smeby, Kirkevold, and Engedal (2016) looked at the ethical dilemmas concerning autonomy when individuals with cognitive impairment wished to live at home. This study identified three main ethical dilemmas. First, the autonomy of the person with dementia could conflict with the family and professional caregivers need to prevent harm. Second, the autonomy of the person with dementia could conflict with what family and professional caregivers believe would be best to promote the well-being and interests of the person. Third, the autonomy of the person with dementia could conflict with the autonomy of the family caregiver.

When the situation involved security, both family and professional caregivers were aware of the vulnerability of the person with dementia. On one hand, they wanted to respect that person's autonomy, but they also saw it as essential to take safety measures. They felt the need to provide a safety-net surrounding the person, and to assess the home situation on a regular basis to make necessary adjustments to prevent physical, emotional, and mental harm. They also recognized that it is important to utilize varied services and tailored care as the dementia progresses in order to enable the person with dementia to remain at home as long as possible.

The second ethical dilemma concerning beneficence and the autonomy of the person was most common. In this situation, as the individual's dementia progressed, it became difficult for the person with dementia to determine their best interests and their decision-making capacity became more impaired. They needed to rely more on informal care from family members and formal care from professional caregivers who had the skills to help them. Problems occurred when differences in assessment and understanding of the person's needs hampered continuous negotiation and collaboration between involved parties. The result was a diminished ability to adjust to what the person had to relinquish and hold on to what he or she could still do.

In situations where autonomy of the person with dementia conflicted with the autonomy of the caregiver, no satisfactory solution was identified. It became even more difficult when strained family relations resulted from a conflict of the autonomy of the patient with the autonomy of the caregiver. However, in situations where the family member had affection and feelings of being responsible for the well-being of the patient, conflicts were lessened. In both of these situations, the person with dementia appeared to think that it was reasonable for them to remain living in their home, but the caregivers did not think those individuals understood the consequences for the families.

The authors of the study identified that the ethics of care (part of the narrative tradition in this text) can offer a broad approach, give new insight, and advance comprehensive understanding of the ethical dilemmas when individuals with cognitive impairment choose to live at home. Using an ethics of care to explore the dilemmas emphasizes the importance of relationship and communication within the context of the situation. It takes into account the uniqueness of individuals and the need for empathetic understanding. They also identified the ability of both family and professional caregivers to respond to the vulnerability of the person with dementia as a prerequisite for combining dependency and autonomy in dementia care. They stressed that professional knowledge is required in order to respond appropriately to the other person's needs, and that the virtues of sensitivity and empathy used in the ethics of care do not reduce ethics to an emotional response. They recognized that caring may be more than making the right decision at a certain moment. Rather, caring is a dynamic process that demands continuous involvement and decision making. Finally, they recognized that paternalism is an issue when autonomy conflicts with beneficence and non-maleficence. They acknowledged that paternalistic actions that prevent major harm or provide benefits while only trivially disrespecting autonomy have a plausible paternalistic rationale. However, they cautioned that acceptance of "soft" paternalism can prepare the way for using unnecessary "hard" paternalism and recommend starting with the least restrictive measures to avoid the probability of abuse (Smebye et al., 2016).

Discharge plans that involve placement in long-term care settings are often among the most difficult. The health delivery system may provide the older individual with little opportunity to choose either the site of care or its details. Discharge planners, including nurses, social workers, and others, often make the decisions with little opportunity to consult the patient or have a discussion with the family or caregiver. In some situations, the discharge plan is based primarily on the physician's judgment that the older patient "needs 24-hour care" and writes a subsequent discharge order. There are occasions when the patient is not informed that the discharge planner is following rules for referral to a post-acute care setting. Frequently, the older individual must make this critical life decision without adequate time, and may be advised by professionals who have not fully disclosed the constraints imposed on them by their organizations. If the physician and rehabilitation professionals believe that discharge to home is risky, they may give little consideration to the individual's right to make an informed, autonomous decision to return home (Wharton, 2014).

In spite of the factors that make discharge to long-term care complex, these decisions are becoming increasingly necessary as the availability of family caregivers diminishes and people reach extreme old age. These discharges have unique challenges for the older individual, the remaining family, and the rehabilitation team. The transition from independent living to long-term care is often characterized by distress, grief, feeling powerless, lack of control, time pressure, and crisis, and point to the need to plan for timely and collaborative transitions. The older individual in essence is put in a situation of sacrificing autonomy and other valued attributes of their life, including loss of their home, neighborhood, privacy, and independence in exchange for safety. Family members and rehabilitation professionals are in a position of exerting influence over the older person's decision but are conflicted by thoughts of violating that individual's personal goals and right to continue to live independently. There are common goals when faced with a decision to choose long-term care, including desire for the best outcome for the older person, but there are also differing values and conflicting ethical priorities, including different beliefs about what is a good discharge plan and how that plan should be decided. Studies of stakeholders' experiences in making decisions for discharge to long-term care have concluded that professionals express health related values, while relatives focused on care, and the older adults prioritize self-identity and autonomy. Other values considered included independence, security, privacy, quality of life, and trust. Denson, Winefield, and Beilby's (2013) qualitative study on discharge planning for long-term care needs noted a difference in the values of stakeholders. Younger family and professional respondents recognized the rights and autonomy of frail elders, but struggled with protecting them. While they emphasized safety, many also suggested discharge to home. They recognized that the capacity of the older person is a key factor. They believed that the older person should make the decision, provided they had the capacity to do so, and recognized that discharge planning became more ethically complex when issues of mental capacity and proxy decision making were involved. Older stakeholders recommended safe and restrictive options for a less able elder, but autonomy for themselves. The health professionals focused on safety, then autonomy, and personal care. All stakeholders acknowledged the importance of individual personality and preferences. The authors of the study recognized that the ethical theories and frameworks developed within the context of acute medical services have limited value in facilitating the decision. They suggest that analyzing personal values and narratives have more influence than principle-based ethics (Denson, Winefiled, & Beilby, 2012).

Brindle and Holmes (2005) identified that one variable in discharge planning may be that the healthcare providers' prescription for long-term care may not sufficiently respect individual autonomy. They recognized that the mental status exams typically used to determine an individual's ability to participate in decision-making process are of limited value in judging capacity to make complex decisions related to discharge. They note that such examinations fail to account for an elderly individual's ability to function in the community, based on social ability and the strength of support networks, in spite of the fact that both these factors are strong predictors of success in community living. They suggest that an ethical decision related to discharge that truly accounts for patient autonomy should include some prediction of the individual's ability to address the challenges of independent living. For individuals with dementia that wish to be discharged to their own home, that option should be considered in view of the individual's age, physical dependency, cognitive impairment, and competency to perform physical, mental, and functional tasks. An assessment should be performed to determine whether the individual has adequate insight into his or her level of dependency in order to address safety issues encountered when living at home. For successful discharge to home, an assessment must determine whether that individual's needs could be met through a holistic flexible care plan that utilizes community teams and ongoing assessment and observation (Brindle & Holmes, 2005).

A recurring theme seen when determining discharge from acute care to long-term care for older patients involves the situation in which discharge is planned for patients who are medically ready, but a discharge location that meets the patient's and family's need is not available. In these situations, the discharge order may be in conflict with the values and needs of both the patient and family. While it may be argued that hospitals are held to a higher standard than a patient's medical status alone, an ethical response would consider that discharge not be put into effect until there is adequate care and support in the home or in an appropriate healthcare facility. The institution might argue that the patient is entitled to be discharged to a facility as long as it meets minimally acceptable criteria, and the patient and family have no right to demand discharge to the best possible facility that meets their needs and values. Other factors that may preclude an ethical discharge plan are the reimbursement and length of stay constraints that are in effect in acute care settings. In response to these types of regulations, the hospital may assume that the patient has no right to prolong their stay simply because they are comfortable or the desired discharge destination is not available. They assert that patient autonomy is not absolute, that questions of distributive justice must be considered, and that a patient's rights must be balanced against legal, institutional, and reimbursement policies. In attempting to do the right thing in these cases, the rehabilitation professionals, including the discharge planner, are continually presented with a hopeless choice and an unfair set of circumstances. There are no easy answers at the individual case level. As a result, a rehabilitation professional may consider looking to preventive ethics, which focuses on the overall problem rather than the individual case. The right thing to do, then, becomes the mandate to advocate for a change in regulations in order to effect a more equitable, ethical solution for future cases (Wharton, 2014; Moody, 2004).

Ethics and Long-Term Care

Long-term care in current health services delivery, refers to a broad range of services that are available to assist an individual who has functional impairments. These services can include personal care, social support, and health-related services. Settings for the provision of long-term care include an individual's home as well as a variety of institutional settings.

Ethical issues that arise in the context of long-term care are different than those arising in acute care. In hospitals, the patient is a temporary resident. In long-term care, some older individuals may be a temporary patient that is admitted for rehabilitation care with a planned discharge to a less restrictive environment, including a return to home or to an assisted living or personal care facility. However, the majority of individuals admitted to long-term care institutions require nonskilled or custodial care and are residents of the institution. For these individuals, the facility is, in essence, their final home. This fact calls for a different ethical framework, in which the emphasis shifts from meeting individual rights of a "patient" to upholding the rights of a "resident" with shared responsibilities between that resident, the family, and the staff. The resulting ethical concerns are not focused on extraordinary situations, but arise in the context of daily life.

A major concern for both patients and residents in long-term care institutions is the lack of autonomy that is experienced in that environment. Welford, Murphy, Wallace and Casey (2010) conducted a concept analysis to identify residential autonomy and its attributes for older people in residential care. They recognized that autonomy is often eroded in a long-term care facility, especially for the individual who is a "resident" of that facility. Their concept analysis identified six attributes of autonomy for older people in residential care:

1. Residents are involved in decision making while their capacity is encouraged and maintained.
2. Residents delegate care needs based on self-determination.
3. Delegation of care needs can be achieved by negotiating care plans that are encouraged through open and respectful communication.
4. Delegation of care needs can be facilitated by involving families or significant others when the resident is cognitively impaired.
5. The resident unit operates on a culture and atmosphere of flexibility based on a philosophy of maintaining resident dignity.
6. The presence of regular, motivated staff enables meaningful relationships that enhance the resident's opportunities to be autonomous.

A key concept is that individuals in long-term care facilities must be perceived as "residents" versus "patients". The authors identified that a key difference between person-centered care and autonomy is the focus on residents having meaningful relationships with care staff who are recruited and retained based on their motivation to work with older people and encourage them to be involved in the decision-making process regardless of their level of cognition. They also acknowledged that autonomy is achieved through negotiated care planning which is encouraged through open and respectful communication, and that avoids using paternalistic models for decision making (Welford et al., 2010).

In addition to previously noted implications for patient autonomy for older adults, the lack of autonomy in long-term care institutions may also be the result of the caregivers' and administrators' roles, their job descriptions, the physical environment of the facility, and the regulations that govern these institutions. Administrators and staff are typically trained to be task oriented, which provides little opportunity to consider autonomy or even clients' involvement in daily decisions about their own care. The physical environment is often one of little space for storage of clothing and personal possessions, minimal security for personal items, and limited privacy. Daily life of residents and patients is subject to care plans and routines that dominate the timing and the content of daily activities. These regulations, although designed to protect the welfare and safety of residents, allow for limited freedom of choice and frequently discourage residents' participation in the decision-making process. Examples include restricting what residents can keep in their rooms, requirements about supervision and the charting of patient activity, and safety requirements. Conversely, some regulations may enhance patient autonomy, such as those that mandate the availability of consumer information, enforce privacy regulations, and place limits on using restraints (Wharton, 2014; Kane, 1994).

Privacy and dignity are also major ethical concerns in everyday life of a resident in a long-term care facility. In institutional settings, sensitivity to issues of privacy and dignity must be heightened, as the environment, by its nature, is not conducive to either. Examples of situations that may lead to violation of these rights include multiple occupancy rooms, responsiveness to call buttons, and using first names without permission from the patient. Providers of geriatric rehabilitation services must be cognizant of individual dignity when assisting with personal care services such as bathing and toileting. They must also consider resident preferences for other daily activities that enhance the individual's dignity, such as participation in social interactions and activities, choices related to daily routine, and the need for solitude (Wharton, 2014).

Long-term residents of nursing facilities report specific challenges that impact everyday living. Bollig, Gjengedal, and Rosland (2016) studied residents and relatives views of a "good life" and ethical challenges encountered by long-term residents. They identified major themes related to dignity and challenges encountered in everyday life. The main findings were that residents and relatives experienced challenges with acceptance and adaptation, well-being and a good life, autonomy and self-determination, and lack of resources. None of the residents interviewed mentioned complex ethical issues such as those encountered in end-of-life care. The everyday issues they noted that were important to quality of a good life included a lack of resources to meet basic communication and care needs, social contact, participation in daily life, and self-determination. The implications of this study suggest that daily routines in nursing homes should be adapted to these challenges, and that long-term care facility staff should strive to meet the residents' wishes as far as possible to strengthen their feelings of respect for autonomy and dignity. They further suggested that ethics education should focus more on everyday issues instead of focusing solely on end-of-life care (Bollig et al., 2016).

In 2004, the Center for Advocacy for the Rights and Interests of the Elderly (CARIE) developed a curriculum for guiding and improving ethical decision making in long-term care. The program was based on the premise that long-term care involves the overall well-being of the resident, including the emotional, spiritual, psychological, and social well-being, as well as the physical health of the resident. It also takes into account that a resident's care may be strengthened by including family members and friends, along with staff. Finally, the care model developed by the Center recognized that traditional bioethics is inadequate to address the ethical issues confronting staff and residents. The CARIE Program identified five themes: health, safety, pain and suffering, respect for personhood, and life story. These themes are coupled to commitments to preserve and promote the resident's health, protect the resident's safety, palliate the pain and suffering, practice respect and care for the attributes of personhood, and provide opportunity and support for the continuation and completion of the resident's life story. The attention shifted from focusing on illness to maximizing functional ability and addressing safety issues to facilitate the resident's interaction with their environment. The care model also acknowledged that spiritual and emotional pain can be as important as physical pain. Life story was viewed as a continuation of that person's being, so the model fostered honoring, encouraging, and supporting the qualities associated with personhood including self-awareness, intentionality, decision making, agency, emotions, relationships, and creativity. CARIE developed a five-step process to provide a framework for working through care dilemmas and reach ethical solutions. The five steps, called IDEAS, are:

1. identify the ultimate issues, stakeholders, and other decision points
2. develop a resident narrative
3. explore all conceivable responses to the issue
4. assess each response in light of the provider's commitments to the residents; and
5. select a course of action and create an implementation plan.

This program contributes to the care providers' ability to identify ethical dilemmas and provides a process for examining and sensitively resolving problems that are unique to long-term care (Mathes et al., 2004).

More recently, the Veterans Administration recognized that quality of life for older veterans in long-term care could be enhanced by a care model that reflects more freedom of choice, individuality, and dignity. They based their assumption on the premise that respecting patient autonomy for the patient with capacity to make choices would improve their experience within the long-term care facility. Subsequently, the Veteran's Administration central staff office asked nursing home administrators throughout their healthcare system to modify the institutional environment to one that reflects a homelike setting, and encourages, promotes, and sustains resident autonomy through a resident-centered model of care. To accomplish this objective, the Veteran's Administration recognized that a cultural transformation would require changes in both staff and resident thinking. They also recognized that the healthcare providers have an ethical obligation to safeguard and promote resident autonomy in long-term care. One facility reported on changes that were made. These changes were initiated in social interactions, meal choices, and medical care practices. An example given was the transformation enacted to address social interactions. The belief was that residents would be more likely to be involved in activities when they are able to make their own choice regarding social interactions. The solution enacted was for staff to make every effort to consider resident choice when developing social interaction activities. The ethical intervention to support this premise is that the center's Ethics Committee makes recommendations to support residents' autonomy by recognizing the residents' preference to participate in or refrain from engaging in a planned activity. The overall outcome of this experience at one Veteran's Administration center was that both residents and staff responded to the cultural transformation, and that residents' autonomy was enhanced by the experience (Dunbar, Sink, Bailey, & Starnes, 2011).

Learning Point 7.19   Can you think of any other ways to overcome ethical challenges in everyday living that are typically encountered in long-term care placement?

End-of-Life Concerns: Challenges for the Interprofessional Rehabilitation Team

Rehabilitation professionals who care for patients facing the end of life must be prepared to meet unique challenges, both clinically and ethically. These challenges can involve participating in important issues such as making recommendations for an appropriate locus of care, including hospice and palliative care settings; determining how to modify rehabilitation goals to incorporate pain management and measures to sustain quality of life; and responding to the patients and families about concerns for end-of-life choices, including whether to withhold or withdraw life support. Other challenges include recognizing the loss of capacity for patients to make their own decisions; working with surrogate decision makers; determining whether to provide hope to patients and families as end of life approaches; and dealing with cultural or religious differences that conflict with rehabilitation goals (Wharton, 2018).

Ethical concerns at end of life frequently arise when there are conflicts in values between the rehabilitation team, the patient and family, and even among members

1. Decision making
2. Patient's right to refuse or withdraw care
3. Pain management at end-of-life
4. Patient autonomy
5. Capacity and competency
6. Informed consent
7. Advance Directives
8. Surrogate decision making
9. Conflicts in moral and legal rights of patients and families/caregivers
10. Policy and legal barriers
11. Inadequate resources
12. Spiritual and religious beliefs that shape end-of-life decisions
13. Cultural influences

FIGURE 7.4 Commonly identified issues in end-of-life care.
Based on Wharton (2018).

of the team itself. In these situations, traditional bioethics theories may provide minimal guidance to address the specific concerns. Using the active engagement model, and reflecting on more contemporary theories, such as virtue ethics, the ethics of care, active engagement, and the Dialogic Engagement Model provide more guidance to facilitate an ethical response to challenging situations.

Even though members of the interprofessional rehabilitation team rarely have direct responsibility for many of the decisions that the patient and family have to make, they do have an obligation to support those individuals and to respect the ultimate decisions that are made. In all of these situations, it is imperative that members of the interprofessional team recognize their role as moral agents, create a space for dialogue to pursue shared goals through a moral commons, and engage in dialogue that facilitates an ethical response.

One important role for rehabilitation professionals dealing with a patient facing end of life is to serve as an advocate to facilitate enrollment in a hospice program. While it is not common for therapists to initiate a conversation about transitioning to hospice, they must be prepared to answer questions posed by the family or patient with sensitivity and compassion. They must also assure that their evaluation findings and recommendations are sensitive to the patient's declining status and that their documentation meets criteria that will support admission to hospice services once the patient and family make that decision (Wharton, 2018). **FIGURE 7.4** delineates commonly encountered ethical issues at end of life for elderly patients.

For patients already enrolled in hospice, when the focus of care shifts from rehabilitation to quality of life, the interprofessional rehabilitation team must be skilled at designing and documenting treatment plans and goals that are consistent with both reimbursement policies and the philosophy of hospice. Perhaps even more importantly, the professionals who work within hospice settings must have astute observation and listening skills to respond to both the physical and emotional needs of the patient as they experience declining cognitive and functional capacity. They must also be sensitive and perceive the needs of families and caregivers who may experience increased frustration and stress. In both of these situations, care and virtue can play an important role in facilitating an ethical response.

To be effective in hospice care, therapists must aspire to be altruistic and be willing to go above and beyond a therapeutic plan in order to respond to the psychological, emotional, and spiritual needs of all involved. They must recognize that individuals may have different perceptions, beliefs, and values about dying. By listening to the concerns and stories of the patient and caregivers, and facilitating dialogue among all those involved, rehabilitation professionals working in hospice can use insight to provide ethical and compassionate care to achieve the ultimate goal of supporting a good life to the very end (Wharton, 2018).

Learning Point 7.20   What strategies would you consider essential when providing services to patients in hospice or palliative care?

Ethical Considerations Related to Reimbursement

Concerns related to care of geriatric patients that arise from the myriad of regulations affecting reimbursement and resources, in the context of the current U.S. healthcare delivery system, focus largely on the principles of autonomy, beneficence, and non-maleficence as they impact the individual patient. For example, older patients may be coerced into going to rehabilitation in order to preserve Medicare payment benefits, which may be suspended if the patient fails to attend the regulated number of daily hours or treatment days per week, depending upon the treatment setting – rehabilitation unit or skilled nursing facility respectively (Wharton, 2014). However, there has been a dearth of discussion and debate in the literature focusing on the pressures placed on health care and professionals to provide cost-effective rehabilitation within a limited set of resources. These constraints are related to the principle of justice, which fosters fair treatment of all individuals. These current pressures put health professionals in a position of having to consider the values and preferences of the patient; their clinical judgment of how health outcomes could be maximized; the time and resources required to work toward an equitable discharge goal; and the likely consequences of that goal. The reality of clinical work is that health professionals must not only focus on the patient, but must also focus on providing services for whole communities. At the individual level, the professional needs to decide about such factors as allocating a limited number of patient contact hours; making recommendations to extend the duration of a rehabilitation program to effect a desired outcome; and determining and applying for funds for assistive technology and other costly interventions. In these complex situations, the principle of justice, which holds that there should be an equitable allocation and distribution of resources among all people within a given population, comes into play. The focus is generally on how to determine equitable allocation, but stops short on how resources influence the choice of goals negotiated between rehabilitation professionals, patients, and caregivers. One alternative suggested by Levack (2009) is to focus on utilitarianism, which judges the morality of an action on consequences, and considers the overall utility of an action based on the effect for all people. Utilitarianism has been applied to resource allocation and is often used in health economics, especially when related to health expenditures. In terms of setting rehabilitation goals, Levack (2009) proposes that utilitarianism would require that individual patient autonomy must be tempered with an overarching view regarding the best use of healthcare resources for the whole community. He further suggests that a utilitarian approach to goal planning might not change current practice, but it could provide a moral justification for refusing to pursue certain goals that are primarily patient-centered and determined solely by the patient. He notes that a concern with a utilitarian approach could be an unfair distribution of healthcare resources if people with severe disabilities are judged in terms of their utility to society and are devalued because they may not contribute to the good of society. In part, this concern may be based on the fact that society underestimates the quality of life of people with disabilities, even though those individuals generally report no less quality of life than individuals who are able-bodied. Employing a utilitarian approach, therefore, must account for the research that individuals with disabilities have quality of life, rather than on uninformed assumptions. Another factor to consider when applying utilitarianism is the total effect functional gains that can be achieved from small improvements in functional abilities. Studies have illustrated that even small gains can have a substantial impact on reducing the cost of ongoing care for individuals with complex disabilities. Another concern about applying a utilitarian approach to goal setting is the potential adverse effect on the role of the rehabilitation professional as a patient advocate. Levack (2009) proposes that taking ethical responsibility for the appropriate management of limited rehabilitation funds does not mean that the clinician ought to lack compassion when dealing with individual patients or exclude the opportunity to advocate for greater financial support for rehabilitation at the societal level. Rather, he argues that a utilitarian approach provides a moral argument for greater investment in rehabilitation that maximizes the ability of people, including older adults, to participate in meaningful life roles and activities (Levack, 2009).

Learning Point 7.21   What additional ways can members of the interprofessional team use to advocate for equitable and just reimbursement for rehabilitation services?

▶ Summary and Conclusion

Ethical care for geriatric patients involves both complex issues such as discharge planning and end-of-life decisions, as well as everyday ethical challenges that affect the quality of life. Older adults are particularly vulnerable because of frailty, chronic illnesses, and cognitive decline. These challenges pose ethical concerns that are further complicated by multiple factors, including the impact on families and caregivers, and society. Rehabilitation professionals must be prepared to recognize, reflect, and make decisions that are person-centered and that also take into account all of the complexities identified in a given situation. They need to rely on codes of ethics, traditional and contemporary bioethics theories, and on person-centered and compassionate care. This chapter discusses some of the major ethical issues that impact on older adults, their caregivers, and the rehabilitation professionals responsible for their care. It outlines strategies that may be employed to promote ethical decisions, enhance the quality of life for older adults and protect vulnerable older adults from abusive practices. The premise is that rehabilitation professionals who reflect on ethics concerns enhance the dignity for older adults and foster an approach to geriatric care that is recognized as best practice.

Closing Reflections

Learning Activities

Case of Isabella

Isabella C. is a 78 year old widow who lives alone in a one bedroom apartment in a senior high rise. She has a longstanding history of rheumatoid arthritis, and has undergone several joint replacements over the years, including both knees, and PIP and MCP joints in her right, dominant hand. In spite of this diagnosis, Isabella has managed to live alone in her senior apartment, and has enjoyed the company of her neighbors in the high rise. She gave up driving several years ago, but her daughter, Maria, has been very helpful taking her to the grocery store, church on Sundays, and doctor's appointments. Recently, however, Maria has also needed to help her mother with some of the heavier housework such as vacuuming and cleaning the bathroom and kitchen as her mother has experienced more frequent and severe flare-ups of her arthritis.

Isabella began having severe right hip pain approximately 6 months ago, which significantly restricted her activities. After several medication changes and home care physical therapy and occupational therapy didn't produce a significant improvement in pain or ability to perform activities of daily living, Isabella's rheumatologist sent her back to her orthopedic physician who performed Isabella's previous joint surgeries. They discussed multiple options, but finally, decided mutually that a Total Hip Arthroplasty would be the best solution to keep Isabella functioning as independently as possible. The surgery was scheduled for the beginning of October. Initially, Isabella's post-surgery recovery went smoothly. She started physical and occupational therapy the afternoon of the surgery, and began walking with a rolling walker. However, on the second post-operative day, Isabella had a spike in temperature and began to exhibit confusion and disorientation. Laboratory work revealed that she had developed pneumonia so she was immediately placed on antibiotics. She continued to receive bedside physical and occupational therapy, but her program was limited to dressing, bed mobility, active exercises, bed to chair transfers, and limited ambulation with the wheeled walker. She initially required minimal to moderate assistance from the therapists for safety factors, but after several days, only needed verbal cues as her confusion began to improve. Finally, after ten days, she was medically stable, so continued stay in the hospital could not be justified. The caseworker assigned to the Isabella's case came to her room and told Isabella that she would need to go to a nursing home to continue recovery. He said that he found a bed at Long Meadows, a facility in a neighboring town. He told Isabella that she would be transferred the next day.

When Sandy, Isabella's physical therapist, came to her room later that morning for her therapy session, she found Isabella in tears. Sandy sat down next to her patient, asked her what was wrong, and reached for her hand. Isabella told Sandy that she was being transferred to a nursing home that afternoon, and that no one cared about her own feelings. She said that she didn't want to go to the nursing home, she wanted to go back to her apartment with her friends and have home care, like she did after her other joint surgeries. Sandy was surprised about this discharge plan, as no one had informed her or Alicia, Isabella's occupational therapist. Based on the hospital intake information, the projected plan was discharge back to Isabella's senior high rise apartment. Sandy was particularly distressed because she wondered if anyone, the caseworker or physician, had talked to rehabilitation or had been reading their daily notes. She knew that if they had, they would see that Isabella made steady progress both physically and cognitively every day since her diagnosis of pneumonia. In fact, Sandy's most recent physical therapy progress note and Alicia's occupational therapy progress note indicated that Isabella was aware of safety factors and could dress and bathe independently, transfer safely from bed to chair and toilet, and walk independently with her rolling walker for short distances. Both Sandy and Alicia recommended discharge to Isabella's apartment with a home care referral for physical and occupational therapy. Sandy didn't say anything to Isabella about the documentation or recommendations. She simply consoled Isabella. She promised she would talk to the caseworker, and with Isabella's permission, would share Isabella's concerns. Isabella agreed to this plan and then worked with Sandy on her exercises. As Sandy left Isabella's room, she was more perplexed. Isabella did even better this session, and all indications were that she could return home safely with home care support.

As soon as Sandy finished her morning patients, she sought out Alicia and explained the situation. Then, both Sandy and Alicia went to talk to Isabella's caseworker. He confirmed that Isabella would be going to Long Meadows the next day. He said that Isabella's physician had already signed the discharge papers. Sandy asked why that decision had been made, and asked whether the recommendations from both physical and occupational therapy were considered. The caseworker said that they were aware of the therapy recommendations, but that Isabella's daughter, Maria, was adamant that her mother be transferred to a nursing home. Maria told the caseworker that she was extremely concerned about her mother living alone, especially since she had been so confused after the surgery and also needed more help than ever. Sandy asked the caseworker if he explained to Maria that the confusion was from the pneumonia and the medications, and that it had cleared now that the infection was under control and the medications were no longer necessary. The caseworker said he tried, but Maria was insistent. In fact, the caseworker said that Maria had already talked to the apartment management and terminated Isabella's lease, effective next month. Sandy and Alicia were aghast! They knew Isabella was competent to make her own decisions, even if living alone was slightly risky. When they said this to the caseworker, he told them that they needed to think of Maria's point of view. Maria is a single mother with three teenage sons. She is their sole support, and therefore, works two jobs, one as a maid at a local hotel and the other as the receptionist at a local restaurant. She works long hours, and also plans her schedule around her son's activities. That doesn't leave much time for her to assist her mother, especially as Isabella requires more and more help with housework and transportation. Sandy and Maria are still perplexed. They ask the caseworker if he considered alternatives and his response is that there are only so many hours in a workday. He says that in acute care, discharge is the focus of his interventions.

At lunch, Maria and Alicia talk to the nursing supervisor. They all agree that Isabella is being short-changed, however, the wheels are in motion for discharge to the nursing home the next morning. They brainstorm about how to ethically handle the situation and come up with a solution that would at least consider Isabella's point of view.

Guiding Thoughts and Questions to Create a Moral Commons and Facilitate an Ethical Response in the Case of Isabella:

Ethical analysis of the facts in the case that influence the ethical response of the various team members:

1. What are the issues in this case that are creating ethical concerns?
2. What is your preferred ethical theory to address the dilemma posed in this case?

3. What are the preferred theories of others interprofessional team members?
4. How do the various theories influence a course of action and an ethical response?
5. What are the identifiable constraints in this situation that preclude a unified ethical response? (Laws, policies, differing cultural values, etc.)
6. What guidance can be found in the codes of ethics for the various rehabilitation professionals?
7. How does Isabella's documented capacity and competency influence the case?
8. What influence does respecting Isabella's autonomy play in determining an ethical solution to this discharge plan?
9. How does the concept of relational autonomy and the impact on Isabella's daughter Maria influence an ethical decision regarding this discharge plan?
10. What are the issues of the team that potentially impede reaching an ethical solution? (Barriers to facilitating dialogue, issues of status and power, varying cultural beliefs, and values)

Establishing the Moral Commons

1. Determine whether the team is able to engage in critical dialogue in order to come to a consensus and facilitate an ethical solution for this situation.
2. Identify how differing perspectives and beliefs influence the decision of team members and all involved in this case.
3. Discuss how analysis from each of the ethical traditions suggests a course of action for the team.
4. Consider the team's value of Isabella's right of autonomy versus the influence of relational autonomy as it impacts on Maria influences the discharge decision. Also consider how Isabella's competency and capacity impact on the discharge plan.
5. Discuss potential courses of action that would allow Maria's concerns to be met and still allow a safe discharge home for Isabella.

Summative Reflection

1. What, if anything, could have been done differently to avoid this ethical dilemma?
2. Reflect on personal, professional, and interprofessional identities that impacted on this case.
3. Consider beliefs or biases that may have influenced how the team made decisions in this case.
4. Discuss aspects of the organizational structure that may have affected the response of team members in this case (for example, workload job responsibilities and expectations, reimbursement and other policies related to discharge criteria).
5. Consider what could have been done to support team decision making and facilitate moral agency.

Take Away Messages

- Ethical issues in rehabilitation of geriatric individuals may be complicated by chronic conditions, diminished functional ability, environmental issues, complexity of family systems, and cognitive issues.
- Autonomy in patient decision making is essential to self-determination, vital to maintaining self-identity, and linked to quality of life.
- Although autonomy in decision making is a primary ethical goal in rehabilitation with elderly patients, complex medical, cognitive, and systems issues present challenges for accomplishing the goal of patient autonomy. Some elderly patients would be considered vulnerable from a legal and ethical perspective.
- Rehabilitation goals are developed at the intersection between the child's interests, parent and family values, and the values of the members of the interprofessional team.
- Simply referring to traditional codes of ethics or applying bioethical principles may not be adequate to address the complexity of the geriatric population. Rehabilitation professionals are encouraged to use narrative approaches, active engagement, and reflexive listening to consider the patients' living situation, support network, cognitive status, quality of life, and vulnerable status.
- Paternalism substitutes the judgment of the rehabilitation professional for that of the patient, compromising patient autonomy. Some believe that paternalistic decisions may be justified to prevent harm (non-maleficence).
- Competence is a legal term indicating the legal authority to make decisions. Capacity refers to the ability of the patient to make decisions and requires information disclosure, decisional ability, and voluntariness.
- Some professionals respond to the altered reality of patients with cognitive deficits through therapeutic lying to validate the patient's reality. While validation conflicts with the obligation of veracity and truthfulness, it may be defensible in some circumstances to produce a positive outcome.
- Surrogate decision makers may either use the substituted judgment standard (what the patient would have wanted) or the best interest standard (what is in the best interest of the patient from the decision makers perspective). Ideally, surrogate decision makers should have extensive knowledge of the patient's values, wishes, and life choices. Family members and rehabilitation professionals may conflict regarding the appropriate balance between independence and safety.
- Refusing rehabilitation treatment is a common occurrence. Treatment pressures (such as persuasion and inducement) may be ethically permissible in such situations, but threats, coercion, and compulsion are generally considered unethical because they seriously undermine patient autonomy.
- Discharge planning may be ethically challenging as it requires balancing competing needs and values for the patient, family, and rehabilitation team. Many patients would prefer to return home (autonomy and self-identity), even if the team views this as unsafe (non-maleficence). Balancing these principles, goals, and values is further complicated by healthcare teams' concerns of legal liability, financial or reimbursement considerations, and limited discharge options. This points to the need for rehabilitation professionals to advocate for better resources for patients with cognitive and physical challenges.

- Maintaining individual autonomy is challenging for residents in the long-term care setting. An important strategy in this setting is to focus on rights as a resident versus a patient, facilitating relationships with staff, and policies and procedures to support dignity and privacy.

References

Administration on Aging, Administration for Community Living, & U.S. Department of Health and Human Services. (2016). *A profile of older Americans.* Retrieved from https://www.acl.gov/sites/default/files/Aging%20and%20Disability%20in%20America/2017OlderAmericansProfile.pdf

American Occupational Therapy Association. (2015). *Occupational Therapy Code of Ethics.* Retrieved from https://ajot.aota.org/article.aspx?articleid=2442685

American Physical Therapy Association. (2010a). *Code of Ethics for the Physical Therapist.* Retrieved from http://www.apta.org/uploadedFiles/APTAorg/About_Us/Policies/Ethics/CodeofEthics.pdf

American Physical Therapy Association. (2010b). *Standards of Conduct for the Physical Therapist Assistant.* Retrieved from http://www.apta.org/uploadedFiles/APTAorg/About_Us/Policies/Ethics/StandardsEthicalConductPTA.pdf

American Speech-Language-Hearing Association. (2015). *Code of Ethics.* Retrieved from https://www.asha.org/uploadedFiles/ET2016-00342.pdf

Anderson L., & Delany, C. (2016). From persuasion to coercion: Responding to the reluctant patient in rehabilitation. *Physical Therapy, 96*(8), 1234–1240.

Applebaum, P. S. (2007). Clinical practice: Assessment of patients' competence to consent to treatment. *New England Journal of Medicine, 357*, 1834–1840.

Baker, K., Campton, T., Gillis, M., Kristjansson, J., & Scott, C. (2007). Whose life is it, anyway? Supporting clients to live at risk. *Perspectives, 31*(4), 19–24.

Brindle N., & Holmes, J. (2005). Capacity and coercion: Dilemmas in the discharge of older people with dementia from general hospital settings. *Age and Ageing, 34*(1), 16–20. doi:10.1093/ageing/afh228

Brock, D. W., Park, J. K., & Wendler D. (2014). Making treatment decisions for oneself: Weighing the value. *Hastings Center Report*, March-April, 22–25.

Bollig, G., Gjengedal, E., & Rosland, J. (2016). Nothing to complain about? Residents' and relatives' views on a "good life" and ethical challenges in nursing homes. *Nursing Ethics, 23*(2), 142–153. doi:10.1177/0969733014557719

Brauner, D. J. (2016). The structure of autonomy-paternalism: An exercise in framing and reframing. *The American Journal of Bioethics, 16*(8), 15–17. doi:10.1080/152655161.2016.1187226

Carrese, J. A. (2006). Refusal of care: Patients' well-being and physicians' ethical obligations. "But doctor, I want to go home." *Journal of the American Medical Association, 296*(6) 291–295.

Cohen, A. B., Wright, M. S., Cooney, L., & Fried, T. (2015). Guardianship and end-of-life decision making. *Journal of the American Medical Association Internal Medicine, 175*(10), 1687–1691.

Criss, M., Heitzman, J., & Wharton, M. A. (2016). Legal and ethical reasoning to enhance compassionate care in patients experiencing cognitive decline. *GeriNotes, 23*(6), 18–23.

Daly, L., & Fahey-McCarthy, E. (2014). Re-examining the basis for ethical dementia care practice. *British Journal of Nursing, 23*(2), 81–85.

Delany, C. M., Edwards, I., Jensen, G. M., & Skinner, E. (2010). Closing the gap between ethics knowledge and practice through active engagement: An applied model of physical therapy ethics. *Physical Therapy, 90*(7), 1068–1078. doi:10.2522/ptj.20090379

Denson, L., Winefield, H. R., & Beilby. J. J. (2013). Discharge-planning for long-term care needs: The values and priorities of older people, their younger relatives and health professionals. *Scandinavian Journal of Caring Sciences, 27*, 3–12.

Doherty, R. F., & Purtilo, R.B. (2016). *Ethical dimensions in the health professions.* (6th ed). St. Louis, MO: Elsevier.

Dunbar, B., Sink, P., Bailey, B., & Starnes, R. (2011). Ethical perspectives of sustaining residents' autonomy. A cultural transformation best practice. *Nursing Administration Quaterly, 35*(2), 126–133. doi:10.1097/NAQ,0b013e31820fbd80

Epstein, R. M. (1991). Mindful practice. *Journal of the American Medical Association, 282*(9), 833–839.

Eves, M. M., & Esplin, B. S. (2015). She just doesn't know him like we do: Illuminating complexities in surrogate decision making. *Journal of Clinical Ethics, 26*(4), 350–354.

Fetherstonhauge, D., McAuliffe, L., Bauer, M., & Shanley, C. (2017), Decision-making on behalf of people living with dementia: How do surrogate decision-makers decide? *Journal of Medical Ethics, 43*, 35–40. doi:10.1136/medethics-2015-103301

Fetherstonhauge, D., Tarzia, L., & Nay, R. (2013). Being central to decision making means I am here! The essence of decision making for people with dementia. *Journal of Aging Studies, 27*, 143–150.

Greenfield, B. H., & Jensen, G. M. (2010). Understanding the lived experiences of patients. Application of a phenomenological approach to ethics. *Physical Therapy. 83*(8), 1185–1197.

Ho, A., Pinney, S. J., & Bozic, K. (2015). Ethical concerns in caring for elderly patients with cognitive limitations. A capacity-adjusted shared decision-making approach. *Journal of Bone and Joint Surgery, 97*(e16), e1–e6.

Hughes, J., & Common, J. (2015). Ethical issues in caring for patients with dementia. *Nursing Standard, 29*(49), 42–47.

Haddad, A. (2000). Acute care decisions. Ethics in action. *Rehabilitation Nursing 63*(21), 22, 24.

Hunt, M. R, & Ells, C. (2011). Partners towards autonomy: Risky choices and relational autonomy in rehabilitation care. *Disability and Rehabilitation. 33*(11), 961–967. doi:10.3109/09638288.2010.515703

Jensen, G. M., Randall, A. D., & Wharton, M. A. (2012). Cognitive impairment in older adults: The role of ethical mindfulness. *Topics in Geriatric Rehabilitation, 28*(3), 163–170. doi:10.1097/TGR.06013e31825932d0

Kane, R. A. (1994). Ethics and long-term care. Everyday considerations. *Clinics in Geriatric Medicine, 10*(3), 489–499.

Kaizer, F., Spiridigliozzi, A. M., & Hunt, M. R. (2012). Promoting shared decision-making in rehabilitation: Development of a framework for situations when patients with dysphagia refuse diet modification recommended by the treating team. *Dysphagia, 27*, 81–87. doi:10.1007/s00455-011-9341-5

Levack, W. M. M. (2009). Ethics in goal planning for rehabilitation: A utilitarian perspective. *Clinical Rehabilitation, 23*, 345–351. doi:10.1177/0269215509103286

Moody, H. R. (2004). Hospital discharge planning: Carrying out orders? *Journal of Gerontological Social Work, 43*, 107–118.

Nuffield Council on Bioethics. (2009). An ethical framework. In *Dementia ethical issues* (pp. 19–33). London, UK: Author. Retrieved from http://nuffieldbioethics.org/wp-content/uploads/2014/07/Dementia-report-Oct-09.pdf

Paola, F. A., Walker, R., & Nixon, L. L. C. (2010). *Medical ethics and humanities.* Sudbury, MA: Jones and Bartlett Publishers.

Philipsen, N., Murray, T., Wood, C., Bell-Hawkins, A., & Setlow P. (2013). Surrogate decision-making: How to promote best outcomes in difficult times. *Journal for Nurse Practitioners, 8*(9), 581–587.

Post, S. G., & Whitehouse, P. J. (1995). Fairhill guidelines on ethics of the care of people with Alzheimer's disease: A clinical summary. *Journal of the American Geriatric Society, 43*(12), 1423–1429.

Rid, A., & Wendler, D. (2010). Can we improve treatment decision-making for incapacitated patients? *The Hastings Center Report, 40*(5), 36–45.

Rosin, A. J., & VanDijk, Y. (2005). Subtle ethical dilemmas in geriatric management and clinical research. *Journal of Medical Ethics, 31*, 355–359. doi:10.1136/jme.2004.008532

Sher, Y., & Lolak, S. (2014). Ethical issues: The patient's capacity to make medical decisions. *Psychiatric Times*, 1–4.

Smebye, K. L., Kirkevold, M., & Engedal, K. (2016). Ethical dilemmas concerning autonomy when persons with dementia wish to live at home: a qualitative, hermeneutic study. *BMC Health Services Research, 16*(21). doi:10.1186/s12913-015-1217-1

Spielman, B. J. (1988). Financially motivated transfers and discharges: Administrators' ethics and public expectations. *Journal of Medical Humanities and Bioethics 9*, 32–43.

Tuckett, A. G. (2012). The experience of lying in dementia care: A qualitative study. *Nursing Ethics, 19*(1), 7–20.

Welford, C., Murphy, K., Wallace, M., & Casey, D. (2010). A concept analysis of autonomy for older people in residential care. *Journal of Clinical Nursing. 19.* 1226–1235. doi:10.1111/j.1365-2702.2009.03185

Wharton, M. A. (2014). Ethics. In T. L. Kauffman, R. W. Scott, J. O. Barr, M. L. Moran (Eds.), *A comprehensive guide to geriatric rehabilitation* (3rd ed., pp. 527–537). Oxford, UK: Churchill Livingstone.

Wharton, M. A. (2018). *Physical Therapy and the Aging Adult: End of Life Ethics. An Independent Home Study Course for Individual Continuing Education.* American Physical Therapy Association Learning Center. Retrieved from https://learningcenter.apta.org//Student/Catalogue/Browse Catalogue.aspx?query=End%20of%20life%20ethics

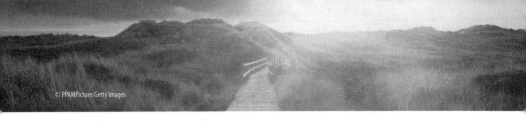

CHAPTER 8

Ethical Issues in Acute Care for Interprofessional Practice

Shirley A. Wells

CHAPTER OUTLINE

- Chapter Overview
- Guiding Principles
- Definition of Acute Care

- Ethical Challenges
- Navigating Ethical Challenges
- Summary and Conclusion

CHAPTER OBJECTIVES

At the conclusion of this chapter, the reader will be able to:

1. Define key terms used to discuss ethical challenges in acute care settings.
2. Identify potential areas of ethical challenges in the acute care settings.
3. Assess the ethical challenges of interprofessional collaborative practice in the acute care setting.
4. Discuss the impact of payment systems aimed at improving the quality, efficiency, and value of health care on ethical challenges for interprofessional decision making.
5. Analyze models that frame the patient-provider encounter in navigating ethical challenges.
6. Apply the Dialogic Engagement Model for Interprofessional Rehabilitation Ethics to acute care cases.

KEY TERMS

Reading these key terms before reading the chapter will introduce you to key concepts which will then be somewhat familiar to you as you read this chapter. This is an important learning technique that will enhance your learning as a multi-step process. You may even wish to make a flash card set of key terms and quiz yourself on them once or twice before reading the chapter. This will better prepare you to immerse in the language of ethics and better prepare you to integrate the content.

Accountable Care Organization (ACO): A shared savings arrangement in which groups of providers agree to coordinate care and to be held accountable for the quality and cost of their services.

Acute Care: The health system or delivery platform used to treat sudden, unexpected, urgent, or emergent episodes of injury and illness that can lead to death or disability without rapid intervention.

Bundled Payment: The reimbursement of healthcare providers, such as hospitals and physicians, by expected costs for clinically-defined episodes of care.

Fee-for-Service (FFS): A payment model where a doctor or other healthcare provider is paid a fee for each particular service rendered.

Hospital Value-Based Purchasing (HVP): A Centers for Medicare and Medicaid Services (CMS) initiative that rewards acute-care hospitals with incentive payments for the quality of care they provide to Medicare beneficiaries.

Macroallocation: The allocation of healthcare resources that involves distributing health-related materials and services among various uses and people through public health policies.

Microallocation: The allocation of healthcare resources concerned with selecting which individuals are to receive scarce or insufficient healthcare resources.

Pay-for-Performance: A payment model that rewards physicians, hospitals, medical groups, and other healthcare providers for meeting specific performance measures for quality and efficiency. It penalizes caregivers for poor outcomes, medical errors, or increased costs.

Rationing: Healthcare rationing is limiting healthcare goods and services to those who can afford to pay.

Resource Allocation: The distribution of resources, usually financial, among competing groups of people or programs.

▶ Chapter Overview

Healthcare providers in the acute care setting encounter difficult ethical decisions daily. They are asked to be the decision maker, to struggle with determining who benefits from interventions: you, your patient, the highest number of people or something else, and who pays for these for these services. In today's acute care environment conflict can arise among hospital policies, rules and cultures, fees and billing, limited resources, professional boundaries, informed consent, and quality of life. The ever-changing nature of healthcare delivery systems and increasing technologies are leading the way of ethical questions in the provision of care. Acute care practitioners have an obligation not only to their patients but also to the institution in which they work, their profession, and themselves. This clinical uncertainty affects their ethical decision-making skills. In this chapter, I will discuss the ethical principles inherent in clinical decision making in the acute care setting in order to promote understanding and interprofessional collaborative decision making, which in turn enhance patient care.

▶ Guiding Principles

In the acute care setting, there is the potential for misunderstanding and poor decision-making processes and poor outcomes (Bruce & Majumder, 2014; Smith-Gabai, 2011). It is important to have ethical guiding principles to serve as a framework for determining what particular action to take not only as an individual provider but also as an interprofessional collaborative team. Underlying justice and health care in the acute care setting, five principles might help healthcare professionals make well-reasoned and consistent decisions on a day-to-day basis. These principles will be applied across a range of issues in this chapter.

- Health equity is the commitment of providers, health systems, or payors to achieve the highest standard of healthcare quality for all people (National Academies of Sciences, Engineering, and Medicine, 2016). Healthcare providers should make efforts to ensure that all people have full and equal access to opportunities that enable them to lead healthy lives.
- Respect for autonomy recognizes an individual's right to hold views, make choices, and take actions based on their own set of personal views and beliefs (Purtilo & Doherty, 2011).
- Social Justice is the obligation to be fair in the distribution of benefits and risks (Slater, 2016). This includes fair opportunity, unfair discrimination, and a right to health care as well as rationing care. It involves how people are treated when their interest competes with the provider, institution, or payer.
- Situational ethics is a concern with those times when a person's belief and action change as their circumstances change. It is concerned with the outcome of an action as opposed to an action being intrinsically wrong (Pozgar, 2016).
- Beneficence is the obligation to promote the health and well-being of the patient and to prevent disease, injury, pain, and suffering (Slater, 2016).

▶ Definition of Acute Care

Acute care is the health system or delivery platform used to treat sudden, unexpected, urgent, or emergent episodes of injury and illness that can lead to death or disability without a rapid intervention (Dunn, 2013; Hirshon et al., 2013b; Masley, Havrilko, Mahnensmith et al., 2011). It encompasses clinical functions such as emergency medicine, trauma care, pre-hospital emergency care, acute care surgery, critical care, urgent care, and short-term inpatient stabilization. Simply put, acute care refers to inpatient or hospital-based care. A working definition of acute care would include the most time-sensitive, individually-oriented diagnostic and curative actions whose primary purpose is to improve health as well as the health system components or care delivery platform (Hirshon et al., 2013b).

Acute care is a level of health care in which a patient is treated for a brief but severe episode of illness for reasons such as illness, surgery, accident, or recovery from trauma. It is generally provided in a hospital by a variety of clinical personnel using technical equipment, pharmaceuticals, and medical supplies. Typical examples of acute care include receiving treatment for a cold, sprain or appendicitis, or recovering from the delivery of a baby. Acute care settings tend to be busy and open 24/7, and available for the sickest patients (Dunn, 2013). Acute services include promotive, preventive, curative, and rehabilitative or palliative actions whether oriented toward individuals or populations (Hirshon et al., 2013b).

Acute care plays a vital role in the prevention of disability. With the primary goal of stabilizing the patient's medical status and addressing threats to his or her life, the role of rehabilitation therapy services such as physical therapy, speech therapy, and occupational therapy in this setting tend to focus on restoring function, facilitating early mobilization, and preventing further decline (AOTA, 2012).

Learning Point 8.1   How do the unique goals of acute care influence the role of rehabilitation professionals?

Acute care functions as the triage for the rehabilitation process by coordinating care including transition and discharge planning. In this environment, there is a need for all healthcare members to provide safe, efficient, and effective care for their patients. The acute care decision-making process centers on the impact of the patient's current and evolving functional medical status. This includes the examination and interpretation of patients' health conditions, vital signs, lab values, co-morbid conditions, medications, possible adverse drug events, anticipated clinical course, and the possibility of multiple simultaneous precautions (Greenwood et al., 2015; Masley, Havrilko, Mahnensmith et al., 2011).

Understanding acute care as an integrated care platform allows effective and inexpensive intervention to be life-saving; it facilitates the coordination of acute care services; and it needs research methods to quantify the burden of diseases and injuries, including health economics and cost-effective components (Hirshon et al., 2013a; Horn & Kautz, 2007). Acute care practice encompasses the knowledge and skills suitable to thoroughly examine and appropriately intervene with patients in medically compromised situations encountered in any hospital environment across the lifespan, from children to adults. Helping individuals, families, and healthcare providers to manage the acute illness effectively can prove to be beneficial to everyone involved (Horn & Kautz, 2007).

▶ Ethical Challenges

Being a responsible professional necessitates an understanding of ethical challenges that may be encountered in professional practice. The complex and ever-changing acute care environment has led to an increase in the prevalence of ethical questions and dilemmas. In this era of healthcare reform, nearly every decision has ethical implications – for patients, for providers, and healthcare leaders. Some of the top ethical challenges facing today's healthcare providers revolve around balancing care quality and efficiency, improving access to care, building and sustaining the healthcare workforce of the future, addressing end-of-life issues, allocating limited medications and donor organs, and aggressive marketing practices (Larson, 2013; Singh, 2016). This section will focus on the impact of several specific changes: interprofessional collaborative practice, reimbursement changes, and allocation of resources, that have a direct bearing on acute care practice and the ethical challenges being faced.

Interprofessional Collaborative Practice

The ethical challenge for the acute care therapist is not looking beyond the specific medical condition but with the coordination of care within the hospital setting.

Learning Point 8.2   Why does the acute care setting pose challenges for communication, collaboration and coordination of care?

Creating and working collaboratively within the ambulatory setting challenges acute care providers to develop different types of structures to integrate and manage various healthcare services. Many assume that care within a hospital setting is inherently coordinated. However, coordinated care necessitates providers to all be in "sync." Coordinated care requires all healthcare providers to work together.

Interprofessional collaboration encourages various health and social care professions to work together to coordinate care, streamline services, and optimize treatment through mutual understanding of professional roles, team strategies, communication, and protocols (Fox & Reeves, 2015). However, because team members may have different care philosophies, specialized training and responsibilities, and business objectives, there are two possible ethical conflicts: within the team itself and between the team and patient (Blackmer, 2000; Dunn, 2013; Gucciardi et al., 2016). With each provider having their unique moral codes and standards, they bring individual and collective values into the team dynamics, fostering opportunities for disagreement and conflict in decision making regarding goal setting, treatment, and discharge planning (Engle & Prentice, 2013).

Conflict Between the Team and Patient

Patient care can be compromised when health practitioners lack access to the full range of skills or technology necessary to fully achieve their therapeutic goals. They must refer to other professions and practitioners to achieve their therapeutic objectives. The compromise can involve more expense, more time, and creation of vulnerabilities in care delivery (Nacarrow, 2015; Guicciardi, Espin, Morganti, & Dorado, 2016; Sharma, Ward, Burns, & Russell, 2012). From a patient perspective, accessible care requires the provision of appropriate health care in the right place at the right time. According to Gucciardi et al. (2016), in a study on integrating diabetes teams into primary care, interprofessional collaboration increased the interdependence between different types of services providers, effective communication among team members, and referrals and patient access to resources and services. The interprofessional collaboration led to a common understanding and holistic picture of the patient thereby enabling targeted patient care. They concluded that real-time interaction among team members facilitated the construction of solutions through group effort and reflected interdisciplinary expertise. Shared decision making between health practitioners and their patients is vital to providing collaborative care.

Learning Point 8.3   How do teams and patients engage in shared decision making?

This means both parties share information; the clinician offers options and describes their risks and benefits, and the patient expresses his or her preferences (Barry & Edgman-Levitan, 2012). Conflict can arise when the providers assume and expect that the patient will seek and generally follow their advice and they disagree with the patient's wishes or feel that the patient's goals are unachievable. This type of conflict raises questions as to whose interest is being served (Fox & Reeves, 2015). Is this client-centered or provider-centered care? This places the team in the position of conflict with the patient. Patients want to make their own goals and want to practice autonomy. Other team members want to do what they feel is best for the patient within the context of their professional training – and want to practice beneficence.

Conflict within the Team

With communication and relationship patterns deeply embedded in professional identities and organizational cultures, interprofessional and intraprofessional "turf wars" can impede the act of collaboration (Gittell, Godfrey, & Thistlethwaite, 2012).

Learning Point 8.4   How might turf wars undermine collaboration?

Poor collaboration can lead to inappropriate compromise. A team member may remain silent instead of objecting to decisions with which he or she may not agree. In order to maintain team harmony, he/she may be compromising patient care (Blackmer, 2000). As a means of promoting peace, this act may be at odds with the underlying concept of altruism which is a core attribute of a profession. Vulnerability is another feature of collaboration and source of conflict. Thistlethwaite, Jackson, and Moran (2013) expounded the need for members to make themselves vulnerable in order for the team to succeed.

Learning Point 8.5   Do you agree that effective teamwork requires that team members should become more open to each other?

Members need to trust each other as well as the process of collaboration. They ask, "Does this resonate with the ethos of the professional standing of self-regulation and professional autonomy (p. 52)?" Collaborative practice involves the relationship between various professions as they purposely interact to work and learn together to achieve a common goal. As custodians of professional knowledge, does the sharing and expanding of professional roles and skills serve to alter the power of difference among professions? Are they giving away professional secrets?

It is essential that the team provide consistent information to the patient and his or her family. Clinicians need to relinquish their role as the single paternalistic authority and train to become part of a team and to share the decision making (Blackmer, 2000; Barry & Edgman-Levitan, 2012). The conflict between members should be resolved and dealt with within the team context. This conflict can be a challenge if the issue being debated involves strongly held beliefs or is controversial. Because of overlapping of competencies, it would be useful to establish an ethical framework for the team to advance. Professional codes and standards of conduct can be used to find common grounds. The shared principles of respect for autonomy, beneficence, and situational ethics can establish a reasonable framework in providing services in an acute setting. It is also reasonable to consult the hospital's Ethics Committee when all efforts fail, and agreements on the ethical issue cannot be reached (Blackmer, 2000; Guicciardi, Espin, Morganti, & Dorado, 2016).

Driven by the "triple aim" of health care (better care, lower cost, and a healthier population), many providers and delivery systems are focusing on interprofessional collaborative care to improve patient care coordination and communication (Howlett, Rogo, & Shelton, 2014).

> **Learning Point 8.6** Some have identified a fourth aim—what are the goals? In your estimate how well is the U.S. healthcare system achieving each aim?

An ever-changing healthcare environment demands a degree of professional vigilance and critical reflection that encourage better coordination of care through the acute care process when patients are most vulnerable to least coordinated care.

Reimbursement Changes

As the landscape of acute care is transitioning, so is the model for reimbursement. High healthcare spending has been characterized as a barrier to affordable insurance and a long-term threat to the U.S. economy (Hussey, Eibner, Ridgely, & McGlynn, 2009; Mulvany, 2015). Pressure to reduce costs from employers to payors and on to providers has led to increased medical costs which are financially unstable. With healthcare reform, the burden of rising healthcare cost is shifting from payors to providers and driving the mandate to improve the overall quality, efficiency, and value of health care at a lower cost (Brown & Crapo, 2014; James, 2012). However, for providers and health systems who are not able to achieve this mandate, financial penalties and lower reimbursement can create ethical challenges.

For decades, the traditional or predominant fee-for-service (FFS) system of healthcare delivery has emphasized the processing of patients by rewarding providers for the volume and complexity of services they provide (Bolz & Iorio, 2016; Feder, 2013). Fee-for-service is a system of health insurance payment in which a doctor or other healthcare provider is paid a fee for each particular service rendered. Under this system, healthcare insurers pay physicians, hospitals, and other healthcare providers separately for each service furnished to a patient such as an office visit, test, procedure, or other healthcare service. Payments are issued retrospectively after the services are provided. This system gives an incentive for providers to deliver more treatments because payment is dependent on the quantity of care, rather than the quality of care (Bolz & Iorio, 2016; Brown & Crapo, 2014). Moreover, it does not align financial incentives between different providers. The FFS system does nothing to encourage low cost, high-value services such as preventive care or patient education (Calsyn & Lee, 2012). Does this type of system facilitate or deter ethical dilemmas for providers?

Efforts to control spiraling healthcare costs in the United States have resulted in dramatic changes in healthcare financial management. The transition from a FFS reimbursement system to a value-based system in which healthcare costs are compared with a goal and providers, and payors share in the saving and losses is driving the focus to how care is paid for. Value-based systems ask patients to trust that providers will spend money wisely on their behalf.

Learning Point 8.7 What are the differences between fee for service and value-based care?

The Patient Protection and Affordable Care Act includes a variety of payment provision and delivery system reforms designed to control cost and improve care, especially in the Medicare program. These alternative methods of payment including bundled payment, patient-centered medical homes, and accountable care organizations, create incentives to encourage preventive care and better coordination of care (Calsyn & Lee, 2012; James, 2012).

Pay-for-performance is an approach used to provide incentives to healthcare providers to achieve improved performance by increasing the quality of care or reducing costs (Trisolini, 2011). It encompasses a broad range of interventions and programs that pay for efficiency and value.

Under value-based programs, payments to providers are based on the quality of care they give patients. Several payment reform programs that will pay for performance in acute care are:

- Accountable Care Organizations (ACO) are shared savings arrangements in which groups of providers agree to coordinate care and to be held accountable for the quality and cost of the services they provide (James, 2012). Providers will share in savings if they collectively can provide high-quality care to their patients at lower costs.
- Hospital Value-Based Purchasing Program (VBP) is used by purchasers to promote the quality and value of healthcare services. Hospitals are paid for inpatient acute care services based on a set of quality measures as well as on how much they improve in performance relative to a baseline. The quality measures include process-of-care measures, patient experiences, mortality measures, hospital-acquired condition measures, and AHRQ patient safety indicators, inpatient quality indicators composite measures. Some say the program is built on penalties rather than incentives because the threshold for earning incentives points are set at the 50th percentile (Shoemaker, 2011).
- Bundled Payment creates financial incentives for providers to coordinate care over the full continuum of services and eliminate spending that doesn't benefit patients (Mechanic, 2015). The insurer will pay a fixed amount to all providers. Because the reimbursement amounts would depend in part on meeting quality and patient experience measures, the entire team of providers would be focused on improving quality. The potential saving from bundling includes reducing errors and complication during inpatient stays and managing post-acute care more efficiently. Bundled payment is designed to minimize inefficiencies, prevents duplication of effort, and encourage providers to keep better track of patients as they move through different care settings (Mechanic, 2015; Vertress, Averill, Eisenhandler, Quain, & Switalski, 2013; DeVore, 2016).

Learning Point 8.8 How do you think practice could change if there were team-based incentives for care?

These new valued-based models require providers to prove that they are meeting quality standards and benefitting patients while cutting costs. To successfully transition from FFS to value-based reimbursements, hospital and providers must effectively manage shared saving programs, streamline operations and eliminate waste, and understand their cost structure.

Managing financial decisions can be at odds with practice and professional codes of ethics. The principles of health equity, social justice, and beneficence often collide when a hospital's financial health influences its quality of care and patient outcomes. Minorities and more impoverished populations are more likely to be under or uninsured. If hospitals receive lower reimbursement for their service to these populations, it could exacerbate health disparities among patients at highest risk of receiving substandard care (Manary, Staelin, Boulding, & Glickman, 2015). This situation may require providers to cut services at the expense of quality. Healthcare professionals are obligated under professional ethical standards to act in patients' best interest, placing the patients' interest above all others including the financial interests of the provider. In a pay-for-performance approach, providers may avoid patients that are likely to lower their performance scores. The lack of trust in the healthcare provider, physician, hospital, and insurer have been pervasive throughout the healthcare system (Chien et al., 2012; Jha et al., 2011; Pozgar, 2016).

Allocation of Resources

When resources are limited, and demand exceeds supply, the ethical justifications for setting priorities in services are most acute. The purpose of allocating resources is to help people and act in the best interest of both the individual and the population (Hofman, 2011). However, because of the increasing demand for healthcare services, rising costs to provide these services and the introduction of new technology, Americans are being forced to choose how to allocate healthcare dollars. In the face of scarcity, resources are either explicitly or implicitly rationed (Brock & Wikler 2006; Kluge, 2007; Purtilo & Doherty, 2011). So, the ethical dilemma is how to balance the principles of autonomy, beneficence, health equality, and social justice.

Learning Point 8.9   What does "implicit rationing" mean? Have you seen examples of implicit rationing?

Resource allocation is the intentional decision of how to distribute resources among a competing group of people or programs (Teutsch & Rechel, 2012; Purtilo & Doherty, 2011). In acute care settings, hospitals do not have sufficient funds to meet the demands of expensive diagnostic equipment, a workforce who can deliver the care, or hospital beds-facilities. Therefore, the demand for healthcare resources will always be an allocation problem. The central question is not whether health care is rationed but how, by whom, and to what degree. Rationing means the distribution of any needed thing or procedure that is in short supply to those who need it in accord with a set of rules that assure fair distribution (Jones & Kelly, 2016). Autonomy suggests that individuals have a right to determine what is in their best interest while beneficence means that clinicians should act in the interest of their patient. Social justice implies fairness in that all groups have an equal right to clinical services regardless of race, gender, age, income, or other characteristics (Teutsch & Rechel, 2012).

Learning Point 8.10   Do you agree that all people should have an equal right to rehabilitation services? Does your profession have an official position on this?

The commitment of resources to one patient means that they cannot be used for others. Resources relate not only to financial factors but also to skills, time, and facilities. In the end, rationing has to be assessed against the broader societal and health system goals.

Acute care relies on a mix of public and private systems of financing and the decisions about rationing are made by both the public and private sector. Rationing, denying a potentially beneficial treatment to a patient on the grounds of scarcity, is unavoidable. Some degree of rationing of health care is necessary for the overall well-being of society (Scheunemann, Douglas, & White, 2011). Rationing decisions are reflected in coverage of health care. Unaffordable pricing, pre-existing conditions, eligibility exclusions or opting out of coverage, reduce the proportion of the population eligible for resources. Excluding services from the benefits packages reduces the quantity and quality of clinical care. Moreover, by rationing the extent or cost share to services covered (e.g., co-payments or value-based insurance) to specific groups of patients undermine access to care of lower income groups of the population (Teutsch & Rechel, 2012). Health insurers may ration care by limiting the doctors available to visit and through deductibles and caps.

Healthcare providers routinely ration their time, deciding which patients to see first and how much time to spend with each patient. How much time spent with each patient is not based on publicly disclosed reasons. This personal rationing is usually done by rules of common sense and professional obligations. Healthcare providers cannot provide every potential benefit to every critically ill patient, however small. Implicit rationing decisions are made at the bedside (Scheunemann & White, 2011).

Rationing can occur at multiple levels (Purtilo & Doherty, 2011). Allocating healthcare resources over other social needs such as defense, education, or infrastructure is called macroallocation. Decision making at this level occurs at the societal or community level and entails broad policies on how to distribute resources across populations. An example is organ donation policy which favors voluntary donation over routine salvaging or a commercial market in organs. The social "safety net" that acknowledges a moral duty to assure health care to those unable to pay is strengthened or weakened according to current societal commitments (Jonsen & Edwards, 2016). Microallocation decisions involve bedside decisions about whether an individual patient will or will not receive a scarce medical resource. Who gets the next available heart transplant? Alternatively, who sees the doctor first when many people are waiting in an emergency room? Most communities have policies and guidelines to ensure fairness in these situations. Explicit rationing (macroallocation) arises from stated principles and rules while implicit rationing (microallocation) occurs without formally stated rules or principles (Scheunemann & White, 2011).

Resources allocation in health should be cost-effective and equitable and follow a fair process. Daniels (2000) proposed four characteristics of a fair process: (a) oversight by a legal institution, (b) transparent decision making, (c) reasoning according to information and principles, and (d) procedures for appealing and revising individual decisions. Baum, Jacobson, and Goold (2009) added public engagement to a fair process as an essential step to identify unanticipated needs and values as well as to obtain public support for the allocation. The Oregon Health Plan (Oberlander, Marmor, & Jacobs, 2001) is an example of an allocation system that has many elements of procedural fairness. The plan serves to increase access to health care for more Oregon residents but cuts down on the range of services covered. A long list of medical procedures, ranked regarding their cost/benefit ratio, determines the reimbursement policy. Even with such a system, ethical criteria must be considered: How do we evaluate the quality of life? Is refusing medical care based on cost-effective ranking ethical? Does the method of ranking by the quality of life discriminate against people with disabilities? Rationing of health care is necessary, unavoidable, and ethically complicated. Some forms of allocations are unethical in any society that values justice (Jonsen & Edwards, 2016; Mitton & Donaldson, 2004). Thus, ethical rationing requires choices guided by applied principles and fair procedures (Hofman, 2011). How rationing occurs not only affects individual lives but also expresses what values are most important to society (Scheunemann & White, 2011).

Acute Care Environment

In the acute care environment, the concepts of autonomy and beneficence are at the forefront of healthcare services. Patients want to make their own decisions and practitioners want to assist their patients. For example, patients with diabetes are expected to take charge and manage their blood sugar level, diet, exercise, and pharmacological intervention to prevent long-term complications associated with the condition. When complications arise, the results are seen as patient negligence and failure to take responsibility for one's own health (Grog, 2013). Ethically, with increasingly complex technical health care, is it appropriate to delegate decision making to patients? Within the context of daily practice, whose interest is indeed being served?

Patient-centered interventions imply that the patient is actively engaged when the fateful healthcare decision must be made (Barry & Edgman-Levitan, 2012). It can transfer decision-making skills to healthcare providers via the institutional or professional environment. Hierarchical, restrictive policies and practices may complicate patient-centered practice. Most institutions are designed for the benefit of the organization first and professionals second.

Learning Point 8.11   What are the consequences of institutions putting the needs of the organization first?

Through active enforcement of institutional policies, processes, and practices, patients often see healthcare providers as willing collaborators in disabling and disempowering them (Hammell, 2007; Fox & Reeves, 2015). While healthcare providers might adopt patient-centered approaches in their practices, decisions are often made by professionals on behalf of the patients in a non-consultative manner (Fox & Reeves, 2015). Assessing a patient's decisional capacity is becoming one of the most common queries facing a hospital staff and team. Some providers suggest that severe illness robs patients of their right to autonomy because severely ill patients cannot make informed, reasoned decisions about their care. This is most often seen when the clinician feels strongly about the need to intervene in order to maximize outcomes, but the patient disagrees. This moral dilemma stems from the conflict between a patient's autonomy and the physician's paternalism (Bailey, 2006; McGrath, Henderson, & Holewa, 2006; Sher & Lolak, 2014).

Patients require information and resources to become active participants in health decisions. The information a health practitioner provides is an essential source of knowledge for the patient. Encouraging patients to become knowledgeable about their bodies and diseases, to monitor themselves and take appropriate action to become as healthy as possible is the role of the medical system (Fox & Reeves, 2015). Delany and Galvin (2014) expounded on the importance of healthcare providers to monitor their patients' readiness and capacity to receive information. Providers need to invest time and effort in order to build patients' understanding and to reach levels of equality sufficient for collaborative decision making. Patient-centered approaches arm individual patients with the right to advocate on their behalf as well as being responsible for maintaining their health. Clinicians need to relinquish their role as the single paternalistic authority and become active coaches or partners (Barry & Edgman-Levitan, 2012). Sharing information and fostering collaborative decision making is required in order to provide care that equitably addresses the needs of patients.

Learning Point 8.12   In what way does the acute care setting disempower patients?

▶ Navigating Ethical Challenges

Providing good patient care and avoiding harm are the cornerstones of ethical practice in acute care. Providers want to do the right thing, but it is not always clear how to proceed. Each situation is different and ethical dilemmas can arise even when hospitals have policies and procedures to address them. The potential for misunderstanding, poor decision-making processes and poor outcomes is always present. The Dialogic Engagement Model provides a framework for navigating the ethical challenges in acute care as an interprofessional team.

Dimension: Prepare

In the acute care setting, it is essential that the ethical principles inherent in clinical decision making be clearly defined. The foundation for dialogue and reflection starts with sorting out ethical perspective (ethical analysis) from both a personal and professional level. Creating the moral commons can be a challenge where models of reimbursement, relationships, resource allocations, and interprofessional collaborative practice can vary from hospital to hospital and service units. In acute care settings (a) healthcare providers' efforts should primarily be directed toward the best interest of the patient, (b) medical practice occurs in a social setting and societal considerations are relevant, and (c) providers are professionals and permitted to give weight to entrepreneurial concerns. Without clarity in the understanding of collaborative decision making, ethical challenges will remain unsolvable (Baily, 2013; Kluge, 2007; Blackmer, 2000).

Kluge (2007) described three models of relationship that frame the health provider-patient interaction: Hippocratic, social service, and business. Each model mandates a different method of resource allocation.

- In the Hippocratic model, the medical action revolves around the patient-provider encounter. Health providers are urged to serve the patients in the way they believe to be most suitable. The health of the patient should be the first consideration and driving force in ethical resolution. Providers should always act in the patient's best interest when providing medical care. This model establishes a fiduciary relationship between the health providers and the patient in that the providers should abstain from considerations such as the social cost of the treatment. Health providers are obligated to determine what is in the best interest of the patient and to acquire the resources that are necessary to meet those interests and to advance the good of the patient. Providers must be concerned with how to acquire the resources to fulfill their fiduciary duty of care. This is the traditional model of medical paternalism with little or no consideration of patient autonomy (Blackmer, 2000; Hammell, 2007; Kluge, 2007).

- In the Social Service model, healthcare providers are society's agents and as such have delegated authority in matters of healthcare delivery. This model approaches health care from a broader perspective. It sees medicine as a social enterprise with the purpose of advancing the health status of members of society. The provider-patient encounter is an expression of the profession's social role and as such society has accorded providers with certain privileges; for example, the ability to prescribe drugs, perform surgeries or engage in other health-oriented interventions that is prohibited to other individuals. The social service approach utilizes a utilitarian approach to resources allocation in which cost-benefit and cost-effectiveness are legitimate considerations in treatment choices (Kluge, 2007).

- The Business Model depicts health providers as entrepreneurs who have undergone a socially validated regimen of education and training that is necessary before receiving a license to practice just as accountants or airline pilots, who now have a socially approved service for sale. Professional medical ethics becomes a type of business ethics. The health provider-patient relationship is defined in purely contractual terms. Patients are provided with the right to make choices about the type and extent of care they receive, and providers are required to limit their treatment to those that are desired by the patients (Blackmer, 2000). Regarding resource allocation, the economics of the marketplace become the primary determinants, and allocation decisions become a financial matter. In other words, a patient's right to healthcare resources is defined by the patient's financial capacity. Fiduciary obligations become contract-driven.

> **Learning Point 8.13**   In considering the business model, do the terms patient or consumer evoke different ethical obligations or relationships?

In acute care, standards of care are established based on such factors as professional codes of ethics, case law, state and federals laws, professional standards, existing best practice, current professional guidelines, administrative rules and regulations, and licensing regulations. As a result, hospitals are looking inward at practices, policies, and even cultures and attitudes in their delivery settings to reduce ethical challenges. The rise in patients, medical interventions and technology, and therapies has significant implications for the quality and safety of patient care. The Institute for Family-Centered Care (2012) defined the core concepts of patient-centered care as:

- *Respect and dignity*. Healthcare practitioners listen to and honor patient and family perspectives and choices. Patient and family knowledge, values, beliefs, and cultural backgrounds are incorporated into the planning and delivery of care.
- *Information Sharing*. Healthcare practitioners communicate and share complete unbiased information with patients and families in ways that are affirming and useful. Patients and families receive timely, complete, and accurate information in order to participate in care and decision making effectively.
- *Participation*. Patients and families are encouraged and supported in participating in care and decision making at the level they choose.
- *Collaboration*. Healthcare leaders collaborate with patients and families in policy and program development, implementation, and evaluation; in healthcare facility design; and in professional education, as well as in the delivery of care.

When the patient knows what to expect, he or she is more aware of possible errors and choices thereby avoiding conflicts. Care must be customized to the personal expectations, cultural beliefs and traditions, and language needs of the patient. Providing patient-centered care means better meeting the needs of all patients including the underserved, the aged, and the chronically ill who will fill hospital beds in greater number (Fox & Reeves, 2015; Joint Commission, 2008).

In acute care, patient-centered ethical decisions can be dealt with by each interprofessional team member. Through their analysis, first, consider each factor that constitutes a minimal account of the quality of life and the extent to which each is affected, then weighing the significance of each factor affected, determine which factors should be considered relevant and which should be considered irrelevant to the process (Baily, 2013). This process allows the team member to prepare for understanding and collaborative decision making.

Dialogic Engagement Model

Ethically defensible decisions in interprofessional practice are those that are anchored by ethical principles or an ethical framework. To adequately address ethical challenges depends on engaging in collaborative teamwork and dialogue, sharing ownership of the patient-care experience, and creating a plan of action that supports learning and adapting to change. In hospitals and acute care settings, delivering safe, compassionate and ethical care is the primary mission. This critical collaboration includes responsibilities for the team members and implementation of the plan of action. Resource stewardship requires team ownership and accountability for decisions through an understanding of performance metrics such as financial indicators, patient results, and satisfaction which is critical to the overall sustainability of the clinical services. Health practitioners must strive toward a more collaborative and equal relationship in service of the patient (Al-Sawai, 2013; Browning, Torain, & Patterson, 2016).

Summative Reflection

Reflection is the deconstruction of events and interactions that allow practitioners to learn, grow and develop in and through practice (Harrison, 2012). Deliberate reflection provides the practitioners with a process to develop professional judgment and to choose a course of action. The capacity of the interprofessional team to reflect-on-action (looking backward) and reflect-for-action (looking forward) bridges learning and experiences (Wells, Black, & Gupta, 2016). Merging the reflections of interprofessional team members and sharing the decision making has the potential to generate new knowledge about the delivery of patient-centered care in modern healthcare systems.

Markey and Farvis (2014) found that reflective practice in an acute setting enabled nurses to examine their practice and challenged them to understand their patient's perspectives and experiences which in turn benefited their future work. When the staff was given time to reflect, they felt more valued by the organization. Kiron et al. (2017), also found reflective practice to be an essential part of career progression and could improve the skills of healthcare providers. It is widely accepted that the delivery of safe, high-quality, and sustainable health care depends upon increased levels of collaboration and reflection among healthcare professionals and the engagement of patients in their care (Dogba, Menear, Stacey, Briere, & Legare, 2016). Through the practice of critical reflection and role clarification, communication and collaboration are areas requiring continuing attention for the team to be successful.

▶ Summary and Conclusion

Advancing technologies and evolving financing models have intensified the ethical quandary in acute care. Many of the ethical actions taken today can have lasting effects on health care in the future. Acute care healthcare providers have unique challenges. Not only do they have obligations to the institution in which they work, their profession, and themselves, but also to do good and do no harm. Clinical uncertainty is further complicated by hospitals policies, and procedures. Poor interprofessional collaboration can adversely affect the delivery of health services and patient care. In critical care, team practices tend to occur in a parallel, multi-disciplinary manner instead of involving all team members in the decision-making process (Cappelle, Hui, & Yan, 2012). The conflict between, and within, team members can easily be detrimental and adversely affect patient care. Internal conflict, overlapping competencies, and job responsibilities can lead to confusion of the expected role within the team. Differences in professional identities and educational training and miscommunication can create a plan of action that fails to address the concerns of each profession and negatively affects the patient and family's hospital stay. Collaboration may not be prioritized due to the time needed for effective communication and coordination of heavy clinical workloads.

Interprofessional collaboration has the potential to improve professional practice and healthcare outcomes in acute care settings. Reeves, Pelone, Harrison, Goldman, and Zwarenstein's (2017) systematic review suggested that interprofessional collaboration may improve clinical process/efficiency and patient health outcomes compared with usual care or an alternative intervention. The use of interprofessional rounds, meetings, and checklists may improve the use of healthcare resources and adherence to recommended practices. Collaborative models enacted in the acute care settings continue to be the exception. In an acute care setting, hospitals must make interprofessional cooperation a priority and dedicate time to unifying perspectives and reflection.

As the interprofessional team attempts to reconcile competing obligations and identities, the principles of health equity, autonomy, social justice, and beneficence must be considered, and an attempt to strike a balance must be made. The combination of a professional code of ethics, the patient's capacity to be an autonomous individual, consensus of quality of life factors (i.e. pain and suffering, bodily integrity, and functioning), and regulations will increase the probability of a defensible plan of action (Bailey, 2006; Lachman, 2012; Hofmann, 2011). Applied, ethical principles help resolve ethical dilemmas, reduce burdensome and ineffective treatment, and reduce hospital stays. Creating an environment that encourages professional ethical analysis and critical dialogue will allow healthcare professionals, patients, and families to profit from the established benefit of interprofessional collaborative practice. With the goal of acute care being to give the best care possible while at the same time respecting the wishes and guidelines of the patient and society, promoting ethical reflection and creating a culture of moral commons may serve to prevent dilemmas or mitigate their effects.

Closing Reflections

Learning Activities

Analyze the following cases, using the Dialogic Engagement Model. Work with a team or group to determine a plan of action for the case. For moral deliberation for each case, consider the following questions:

- What ethical principle(s) appear(s) to conflict? Why? (Ethical Tradition)
- What additional information is needed by the team?
- What factors would contribute to or detract from the moral common?
- How should this conflict be resolved?
- How did the case make you feel?
- Were you satisfied with your ability to communicate with other team members?
- Did you work together as a team; why or why not?
- Is there anything else you would like to discuss?

Case of Mike

Mike, a 55-year-old long-haul truck driver who lives with his wife and one adult son, presents in the emergency room with excruciating shoulder pain after a weekend of playing touch football with his buddies. He is admitted to the orthopedic unit for an extensive assessment. An MRI and CT of the cervical and thoracic spines were ordered along with occupational and physical therapy evaluations. After the assessment, he was subsequently diagnosed with a right rotator cuff tear and scapular dyskinesis, Type III. Four treatment options were presented to Mike: surgery (aggressive), steroid injections (less aggressive), physical and occupational therapy (conservative), or no treatment (very conservative).

The orthopedic interprofessional team, which consisted of a physician, primary nurse, social worker, occupational therapist, physical therapist, and pharmacist, meet to discuss the treatment options. The physician preferred surgery, the other interprofessional team members opted for physical and occupational therapy, and Mike chose no treatment.

Case of Joan

Joan had been an avid hiker and bicycler, and passionate swimmer for most of her life. At the age of 40, she was involved in a major bike accident that changed her whole life. The accident resulted in a severe polytrauma including various fractures (ribs, breastbone, skull, bone spurs), internal bleeding, traumatic injury to the skull and brain, and complete paraplegia. After three months of rehabilitation, Joan begins to experience the neuropathic pain of constant burning and shooting. Over the subsequent months, Joan was treated for pain with medication and acupuncture. However, the pain management interventions offered little to no improvement, and the pain significantly lowered her quality of life. Pain prevented her from participating socially and negatively impacted her ability to complete her daily routine. She also experienced difficulties with sleeping and eating.

Joan was admitted to the hospital for pain management. An interprofessional team that consisted of a physician, nurse, social worker, occupational therapist, physical therapist, pharmacist, and psychologist collaborated to implement pain management. On the VAS scale, Jane rated the intensity of her pain as 8. The team classified the pain as neuropathic. Joan experienced poor sleep quality, i.e., she would sometimes wake up, due to pain. She presented with low motivation, emotional instability, and was afraid that the pain would get worse. This led to a diagnosis of minor clinical depression. Joan reported significant limitations in carrying out her daily routine. Her mobility-related issues included problems in transferring to and from the wheelchair and driving due to constant pain and the pain medications. This was supported by the team's assessment. These mobility problems severely limited her ability to meet friends and hindered her from working. As a result, Joan felt isolated.

Since previous efforts to manage Joan's chronic pain focused on pharmacological interventions and proved unsuccessful, a more comprehensive approach is needed. Under the fee-for-service system, Medicare would pay each provider along with the hospital for her care.

 # Take Away Messages

- Five ethical principles provide a foundation for analyzing ethical issues in the acute care setting: Health equity, respect for autonomy, social justice, situation ethics, and beneficence.
- Acute care is the health system that treats sudden, unexpected, urgent, or emergent injury and illness that may result in death or disability without rapid intervention. This treatment typically occurs in the inpatient hospital setting.
- The acute care setting plays an important role for rehabilitation in that triage, transition planning and preparation for discharge occur in this setting.
- Coordination of care presents a primary ethical challenge for rehabilitation professions in the acute care setting.

- Two primary types of ethical conflicts that arise in the acute care setting are conflict between the team and patient and conflict within the team. These conflicts typically arise in decision making about goal setting, treatment, and discharge planning

- Collaborative practice requires that various professions purposely interact to work and learn together to achieve a common goal. Communication and collaboration are essential. Lack of trust and poor collaboration can result in inappropriate compromises that undermine quality of care.

- Many healthcare system changes are being driven by the Triple Aim (better care, lower cost, healthier populations).

- Fee-for-Service health service delivery rewards providers for volume and complexity. Value-based systems provide incentives for quality of care. Bundling payment provides incentives for providers to decrease costs, eliminate duplication of care, increase efficiency, and track patients across the continuum of care.

- The principles of health equity, social justice, and beneficence may conflict when a hospital's financial health influences the quality of care and patient outcomes. For example, pay-for-performance systems may result in healthcare providers avoiding complex patients. Similarly, lower reimbursements may cause healthcare organizations to decrease services to underinsured or uninsured patients. Minority patients may be disproportionately affected by these types of actions.

- Explicit (macroallocation) or implicit (microallocation) rationing of resources, personnel, and time regularly occur in the acute care setting due to inadequate resources. Although rationing may be unavoidable for the welfare of society, it presents ethical challenges and some types of rationing are ethically unacceptable.

- The hierarchical structure and complexity of acute care settings may complicate patient-centered care and disempower patients.

- Kluge's (2007) three models of relationship (Hippocratic, Social Service, and Business) provide different models of relationships between rehabilitation professionals and patients and also of resource allocation.

- Rehabilitation team members must reflect-in-action (backward reflection) and reflect-for-action (looking forward) (Wells, Black, & Gupta, 2016). Merging the reflections of interprofessional team members and sharing the decision making has the potential to generate new knowledge about the delivery of patient-centered care in modern healthcare systems.

References

Al-Sawai, A. (2013). Leadership of healthcare professionals: Where do we stand? *Oman Medical Journal, 28*(4), 285–287. doi:10.5001/omj.2013.79

American Occupational Therapy Association. (2012). *Occupational therapy's role in acute care.* Bethesda, MD: Author.

Bailey, S. (2013). Decision making in acute care: A practical framework supporting the best interests principle, *Nursing Ethics, 13*(3), 284–290. doi:10.1191/0969733006ne864oa

Barry, M. J., & Edgman-Levitan, S. (2012). Shared decision making – The pinnacle of patient-centered care, *New England Journal of Medicine, 366*(9), 780–781. doi:10.1056/NEJMp1109283

Baum, N. M., Jacobson, P. D., & Goold, S. D. (2009). Listen to the people: Public deliberation about social distancing measures in a pandemic. *American Journal of Bioethics, 9*(11), 4–14. doi:10.1080/15265160903197531

Blackmer, J. (2000). Ethical issues in rehabilitation medicine, *Scandinavian Journal of Rehabilitative Medicine, 32*, 51–55. doi:10.1080/003655000750045541

Bolz, N. J., & Iorio, R. (2016). Bundled payments: Our experience at an academic medical center. *The Journal of Arthroplasty, 31*, 932–935. doi:10.1016/j.arth.2016.01.055

Brock, D. W., Wikler, D. (2006). Ethical issues in resource allocation, research, and new product development, In D. T. Jamison, J. G. Breman, A. R. Measham, G. Alleyne, M. Claeson, D. B Evans, . . . P. Musgrove. (Eds.), *Disease control priorities in developing countries* (2nd ed., pp. 259–270). Washington DC: World Bank.

Brown, B., & Crapo, J. (2014). *The key to transitioning from fee-for-service to value-based reimbursement.* Health Catalyst. Retrieved from https://www.healthcatalyst.com/hospital -transitioning-fee-for-service-value-based-reimbursements

Browning, H. W., Torain, D. J., & Patterson, T. E. (2016). *Collaborative health leadership: A six-part model of adapting and thriving during a time of transformative change.* Center for Creative Leadership. Retrieved from http://www.ccl.org/leadership/pdf/research /CollaborativeHealthcareLeadership.pdf

Bruce, C. R., & Majumder, M. A. (2014). The permanent patient problem. *Journal of Law, Medicine, & Ethics, 42*(1), 88- 8–92. doi:10.1111/jlme.12121

Calsyn, M., & Lee, E. O. (2012). *Alternatives to fee-for-services payments in health care: Moving from volume to value.* Center for American Progress. Retrieved from http://www.americanprogress .org/issues/healthcare/report/2012/

Chien, A. T., Eastman, D., Li, Z., & Rosenthal, M. B. (2012). Impact of a pay for performance program to improve diabetes care in the safety net. *Preventive Medicine,* (55 Suppl), S80–S85. doi:10.1016/j.ypmed.2012.05.004

Daniels, N. (2000). Accountability for reasonableness. *British Medical Journal, 321*(7272), 1300–1301. doi:10.1136/bmj.a1850

Delany, C., & Galvin, J. (2014). Ethics and shared decision-making in paediatric occupational therapy practice. *Developmental Neurorehabilitation, 17*(5), 347–354. doi:10.3109/17518423. 2013.784816

DeVore, S. (2016). Medicare "bundled payments" improve health, save money. Retrieved from http://www.statnews.com/2016/18/bundled-payments-medicare/

Dogba, M. J., Menear, M., Stacey, D., Briere, N., & Legare, F. (2016). The evolution of an interprofessional shared decision-making research program: Reflective case study of an emerging paradigm. *International Journal of Integrated Care, 16*(3), 4. doi:10.5334/ijic.2212

Dunn, L. (2013). *The Acute-Care Continuum: The future of Hospital-Based Care.* Retrieved from http://www.beckershospitalreview.com/white-papers/

Engle, J., & Prentice, D. (2013). The ethics of interprofessional collaboration. *Nursing Ethics, 20*(4), 426-435. doi:10.1177/0969733012468466

Feder, J. (2013). Bundle with care – Rethinking Medicare incentives for post-acute care services. *New England Journal of Medicine, 369*, 5, 400–401. doi:10.1377/hlthaff.17.6.69

Fox, A., & Reeves, S. (2015). Interprofessional collaborative patient-centered care: A critical exploration of two related discourses. *Journal of Interprofessional Care, 29*(2), 113–118. doi:10. 3109/13561820.2014.954284

Gittell, J. H., Godfrey, M., & Thistlethwaite, J. (2013). Interprofessional collaborative practice and relational coordination: Improving healthcare through relationships. *Journal of Interprofessional Care, 27*, 210-213. doi:10.3109/13561820.2012.730564

Greenwood, K, Stewart, E., Milton, E., Hake, M., Mitchell, L., & Sanders, B. (2015). *Core Competencies for Entry-Level Practice in Acute Care Physical Therapy.* Academy of Acute Care Physical Therapy. Retrieved from https://www.acutept.org/Resource/resmgr/Core_Competencies_of _Entry_Level_Practice.htm

Grog, R. (2013). The heart of patient-centred care. *Journal of Health Politics, Policy, and Law, 38*, 457–465. doi:10.1215/03616878-1966406

Gucciardi, E., Espin, S., Morganti, A. and Dorado, L. (2016). Exploring interprofessional collaboration during the integration of diabetes teams into primary care. *BMC Family Practice, 17*, 12. doi:10.1186/s12875-016-0407-1

Hammell, K. W. (2007). Client-centered practice: Ethical obligation or professional obfuscation? *British Journal of Occupational Therapy, 70*(6), 264–266. doi:10.1177/03080226070 7000607

Hirshon, J. M., Hansoti, B., Hauswald, M., Sethuraman, K., Kerr, N. L., Scordino, D., & Biros, M. H. (2013a). Ethics in acute care research: A global perspective and research agenda. *Academic Emergency Medicine, 20*, 1251–1258. doi:10.1111/acem.12271

Hirshon, J. M. Risko, N., Calvello, E. J. B., Stewart de Ramirez, S., Narayan, M., Theodosis, C., & O'Neill, J. (2013b). Health systems and services: The role of acute care. *Bulletin of the World Health Organization, 91*, 386–388. doi:10.2471/BLT.12.112664

Hofman, P. B. (2011). 7 factors complicate ethical resources allocation decisions. *Healthcare Executive,* May/June, 62–63. http://hdl.handle.net/10822/1017533

Horn, E., & Kautz, D. (2007). Promotion of family integrity in the acute care setting: A review of the literature. *Dimensions of Critical Care Nursing, 26*, 101–107. doi:10.1097/01. DCC.0000267803.64734.c1

Howlett, B. Rogo, E. J., & Shelton, T.G. (2014). *Evidence-based practice for Health Professionals: An Interprofessional Approach.* Burlington, MA: Jones & Bartlett Learning.

Hussey, P. S., Eibner, C., Ridgely, J. D., & McGlynn, E. A. (2009). Controlling U. E. care spending – Separating promising from unpromising approaches. *New England Journal of Medicine, 361*(22), 2109–2111. doi:10.1056/NEJMp0910315

Institute for Family-Centered Care (2012). *What are the core concepts of patient- and family-centered care?* Retrieved from http://www.ipfcc.org/faq.html

James, J. (2012). Health Policy Briefs: Pay for performance. *Health Affairs.* doi:10.1377/hblog20121011.024094.

Jha, A. K., Orav, E. J., & Epstein, A. M. (2011). Low-quality, high-cost hospitals, mainly in South, care for sharply higher shares of elderly black, Hispanic, and medicaid patients. *Health Affairs (Millwood), 30*(10), 1904–1911. doi:10.1377/hlthaff.2011.0027

Jonsen, A. R., & Edwards, K.A. (2016). Resource allocation, ethics in medicine. Retrieved from https://depts.washington.edu/bioethx/topics/

Kluge, E. H. W. (2007). Resource allocation in healthcare: Implications of models of medicine as a profession. *Medscape General Medicine, 9*(1), 57. PMC1925021.

Lachman, V. D. (2012). Ethical challenges in the era of health care reform. *MEDSURG Nursing, 21*(4), 248–245. PMID: 22966529.

Manary, M., Staelin, R., Boulding, W., & Glickman, S.W. (2015). Payer mix & financial health drive hospital quality: Implications for valued-based reimbursement policies. *Behavioral Science & Policy, 1*(1), 77–84.

Masley, P. M., Havrilko, C. L., Mahnensmith, M. R., Aubert, M., & Jette, D. U. (2011). Physical therapist practice in the acute care setting: a qualitative study. *Physical Therapy, 91*, 906–919. doi:10.2522/ptj.20100296

Mechanic, R. E. (2015). Mandatory Medicare bundled payment – Is it ready for prime time? *New England Journal of Medicine, 373*(14), 1291–1293. doi:10.1056/NEJMp1509155.

Mulvany, C. (2015). Are Medicare bundles in your future? *Healthcare Financial Management, 69*(8), 38–42. PMID: 26548136.

Mitton, C., & Donaldson, C. (2004). Health care priority setting: principles, practice and challenges, *Cost Effectiveness and Resource Allocation, 2*:3. https://doi.org/10.1186/1478-7547-2-3

Nancarrow, S. (2015). Six principles to enhance health workforce flexibility. *Human Resources Health, 13*, 1–12. doi:10.1186/1478-4491-13-9

National Academies of Sciences, Engineering, and Medicine (2016). *Accounting for social risk factors in Medicare payment: Criteria, factors, and methods.* Washington, DC: The National Academies Press. doi:10.17226/23513

Oberlander, J., Marmor, T., & Jacobs, L. (2001). Rationing medical care: Rhetoric and reality in the Oregon Health Plan. *Canadian Medical Association Journal, 164*(1), 1583–1587. PMCID: PMC81116.

Pozgar, G. D. (2016). *Legal and ethical issues for health professionals* (4th ed.). Burlington, MA: Jones & Bartlett Learning.

Purtilo, R. B., & Doherty, R. F. (2011). *Ethical dimensions in the health professions* (5th ed.). St. Louis, MO: Elsevier Saunders.

Reeves, S., Pelone, F., Harrison, R., Goldman, J., & Zwarenstein, M. (2017). Interprofessional collaboration to improve professional practice and healthcare outcomes. *Cochrane Database of Systematic Reviews, 2017*(6). doi:10.1002/14651858.CD000072.pub3

Scheunemann, L. P., & White, D. B. (2011). The ethics and reality of rationing in medicine. *CHEST,* *140*(6), 1625–1632. doi:10.1378/chest.11-0622

Sharma, S., Ward, E., Burns, T., & Russell, T. (2012). Training allied health assistants for telerehabilitation assessment of dysphagia, *TelemedTelecare, 18,* 287–291. doi:10.3109/175 49507.2012.689333

Sher, Y., & Lolak, S. (2014). Ethical issues: The patient's capacity to make medical decisions. *Psychiatric Times, 31*(11), Retrieved from http://www.psychiatrictimes.com/special-reports /ethical-issues-patients-capacity-make-medical-decisions

Shoemaker, P. (2011). What value-based purchasing means to your hospital. *Healthcare Financial Management Magazine, 65*(8), 61–68. PMID: 2186672.

Singh, R. (2016). *Impact and interpretation of regulatory, legal, and ethical issues.* Retrieved from http://complianceandethics.org/impact-interpretation-regulatory-legal-ethical-issues/

Slater, D. Y. (2016). *Reference guide to the Occupational Therapy Code of Ethics, 2015 Edition.* Bethesda, MD: AOTA Press.

Smith-Gabai, H. (2011). *Occupational therapy in acute care.* Bethesda, MD: AOTA Press.

Teutsch, S; Rechel, B. (2012). Ethics of resource allocation and rationing medical care in a time of fiscal restraint – US and Europe. *Public Health Reviews, 34*(1), 1–10. doi:10.1177/0969733018759831

The Joint Commission (2008). *Health care at the crossroads: Guiding principles for the development of the hospital of the future.* Retrieved from https://www.jointcommission.org/guiding _principles_for_the_development_of_the_hospital_of_the_future/

Thistlethwaite, J., Jackson, A., & Moran, M. (2013). Interprofessional collaborative practice: A deconstruction. *Journal of Interprofessional Care, 27,* 50–56. doi:10.3109 /13561820.2021.730075

Trisolini, M. G. (2011). Introduction to pay for performance. In J. Cromwell, M. G.Trisolini, G. C. Pope, J. B. Mitchell, & L. M. Greewald (Eds.), *Pay for performance in health care: Methods and approaches* (pp. 7–32). Research Triangle Park, NC: RTI Press. Retrieved from http://www.rti .org/rtipress

Vertrees, J. C., Averill, R. F., Eisenhandler, J., Quain, A., & Switalski, J. (2013). Bundling post-acute care services into MS-DRG payments, *Medicare & Medicaid Research Review, 3*(3). doi:10.5600/ mmrr.003.03a03

Wells, S. A., Black, R. M., & Gupta, J. (2016). Model for culture effectiveness. In S. A. Wells, R. M. Black, & J. Gupta (Eds.), *Culture and occupation: Effectiveness for occupational therapy practice, education, and research* (3rd ed., pp. 65–79). Bethesda, MD: AOTA Press.

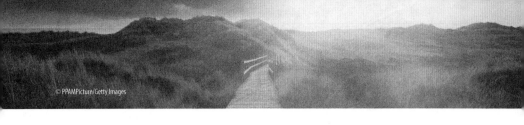

CHAPTER 9

Implications of Policy and Reimbursement for Interprofessional Rehabilitation Ethics

Penelope A. Moyers

CHAPTER OUTLINE

- Chapter Overview
- Distributive Justice and Freedom
- Values in Rehabilitation
- Business Model Related Conflicts of Interest in Rehabilitation
- Ethical Dilemmas Related to Reimbursement in Rehabilitation
- Moral Dialogue and Moral Agency
- Payment-Related Dilemmas Requiring Moral Agency
- Summary and Conclusion

CHAPTER OBJECTIVES

At the conclusion of this chapter, the reader will be able to:

1. Determine the underlying freedom and distributive justice values underlying alternative payment models for rehabilitation.
2. Examine the values inherent in team decision making in rehabilitation and how each of these values may be challenged when third-party payors make insurance coverage decisions.
3. Categorize the payment-related ethical dilemmas according to the ethical traditions.
4. Implement the moral agency required of rehabilitation teams in resolving payment-related ethical dilemmas.

KEY TERMS

Reading these key terms before reading the chapter will introduce you to key concepts which will then be somewhat familiar to you as you read this chapter. This is an important learning technique that will enhance your learning as a multi-step process. You may even wish to make a flash card set of key terms and quiz yourself on them once or twice before reading the chapter. This will better prepare you to immerse in the language of ethics and better prepare you to integrate the content.

Bundled Payment Methods: Flat-rate payment that includes all physician fees along with all costs of any related treatments, complications, or hospital readmissions within 90 days of the original operation (James & Poulsen, 2016).

Capitation: An insurance approach where "providers receive a fixed per person (or 'capitated') payment that covers all healthcare services over a defined time period, adjusted for each patient's expected needs, and are also held accountable for high-quality outcomes" (James & Poulsen, p. 104).

Co-payments: A small fixed fee to access the covered service, such as an office visit.

Co-insurance: What the patient pays as his or her portion of the healthcare insurance claim.

Conflict of Interest: Potentially occurs when the rehabilitation professional has competing allegiances among the interests of the patient and the family, the third-party payor, other rehabilitation team members, and the employing healthcare organization (Larkin & Lowenstein, 2017).

Distributive Justice: The fair allocation of goods in a society that represents a public policy focus on equality (Craig, 2010).

Fairness: The equity of health care.

Fee-for-Service or Volume-Based Reimbursement: Reimbursement that occurs when "...a provider supplies an approved billing code for (and may be required to justify) each unit of care consumed during a hospitalization, same-day procedure, or outpatient visit" (James & Poulsen, 2016, p. 105).

Freedom: Non-interference from the government to make life choices and to assume responsibility for the consequences of those choices (Gains, 2017).

Medical Necessity: An insurance term defining criteria for payment decisions based on the diagnosis, the evidence supporting the interventions, and the use of rehabilitation devices for non-medical purposes (Stinneford & Kirschner, 2004).

Pay for Performance or Value-Based Purchasing: Healthcare payment approach designed to increase value through rewarding the performance of the provider with contingent incentives that heighten motivation to improve quality and increase effort to reduce waste to cut costs (Siriwardena, 2014).

Per Case Method of Payment: Diagnostic categories based on the patient's primary disease, specific treatment, secondary chronic conditions, and care intensity to determine a flat rate for a single case (James & Poulsen, 2016).

Utilitarianism: "Maximizing the benefits of rehabilitation to the whole community served when negotiating goals with individual patients" (Levack, 2009, p. 345).

▶ Chapter Overview

Interprofessional rehabilitation ethics requires individual and team moral agency from rehabilitation professionals and are often preceded by discussion within the moral commons, or the "safe zone." Consequently, it is important to understand how views regarding the way in which health care should be paid may influence one's ethical stance and that of the other members of the rehabilitation team. The potentially contentious nature of discussions about access to insurance coverage versus the financing and cost of the Patient Protection and Affordable Care Act (PPACA), commonly called the Affordable Care Act (ACA) or Obamacare (Public Law 111 – 148, 2010), was clearly illustrated in the 2016 presidential election. The controversy has continued as Congress struggles to act regarding ways to fix the rising costs associated with the law's implementation. Some argue for the complete repeal and replacement of the ACA with strategies such as personal medical savings accounts for tax deferred deposits; others are proponents of incremental fixes of the current law, while still others call for a single payer approach to funding health care.

The debate represents the divide between proponents of distributive justice advocating for greater access to health insurance through redistribution of wealth and the proponents of free-market advocates arguing for reductions in government intervention to better respect the liberty of its citizens. There are gradations of beliefs along this continuum with distributive justice and less government intervention at the extremes. Public policy development in healthcare funding swings back and forth along this pendulum of equality (advocates of distributive justice) and freedom (free-market advocates). Because of the individual mandate for citizens to purchase insurance under threat of tax penalties (Starr, 2011) as the core funding approach for the ACA, the law represented a significant swing away from freedom to distributive justice.

Learning Point 9.1   How does the ACA pose a conflict between freedom and distributive justice?

This chapter contrasts the ethical reasoning for healthcare reform that was based on distributive justice due to the lack of access to care for the underinsured and uninsured (Lachman, 2009) with the potential changes in the law for which free-market advocates are supporting. Regardless of one's position along this continuum, healthcare professionals are concerned about how to provide high-quality care at the lowest cost. Understanding how these various funding proposals can modify or repeal the ACA, along with the current strategies within the law to control costs, all create ethical challenges for rehabilitation-team decision making.

This chapter examines the values inherent in team decision making in rehabilitation, and how each of these values may be challenged when third-party payors make insurance coverage decisions based on the concept of medical necessity. Other significant challenges to the values of rehabilitation providers arise from the evolving healthcare business models and payment methods to control costs, such as capitation and value based payment. It is therefore necessary for a rehabilitation team to use the Dialogic Engagement Model for ethical decision making when confronted with patient situations in rehabilitation that are contextualized within healthcare reimbursement policy.

▶ Distributive Justice and Freedom

The present healthcare system in the United States is not giving the benefit for the dollars spent. The infant mortality rate for the United States in 2014 was 5.8 deaths per 1,000 live births, ranking the United States as 30th in the Organization for Economic Co-operation and Development (OECD) countries. The rates were higher than most European countries, such as Finland, Sweden, and Denmark. These statistics are concerning, given that health spending is estimated to be 17.2% of GDP in the United States in 2016, which was the highest among OECD countries and was more than 8.2 percentage points above the OECD average of 9.0% (The Organization for Economic Co-operation and Development [OECD], 2017).

Learning Point 9.2   What other evidence supports the claim that the United States does not receive a good return on the amount of dollars dedicated to healthcare spending?

In fact, expenditure and infant mortality data supported the development of the ACA as a public policy method for driving down costs and increasing the numbers of insured in the United States. The ACA was a swing in political philosophy from freedom to purchase one's own insurance or to go without towards distributive justice where health care became a right offered through the government (see **TABLE 9.1**).

Learning Point 9.3   Does market freedom translate to freedom for individual patients?

Distributive justice involves the fair allocation of goods in a society and represents a public policy focus on equality (Craig, 2010). However, for some who advocated for a single payer system, the ACA did not go far enough to guarantee health care as a right.

TABLE 9.1 Equality Versus Freedom and Impact on Public Policy			
Basic Belief	**Values**	**Public Policy**	**Consequences**
Equality Health care is a right. Barriers to accessing health care must be removed.	Justice, equality, and community.	Single payer system	Finding balance between provision of adequate financial support for providers while assuring tax payors that the quality of care will be improved and spending will be lower.
Freedom Noninterference from government. Health care is a commodity.	Freedom and personal responsibility. Independence	Free market mechanisms	Preventing health insurance premiums from constantly rising and access to insurance coverage decreasing.

Learning Point 9.4   Do you believe that health care is a right?

Unfortunately, there has been a dramatic decrease in the affordability of healthcare premiums regardless of available subsidies for the insurance available on the ACA mandated insurance exchanges (Cox et al., 2016). These insurance programs are for those without employer-based insurance or for those who do not qualify for Medicaid. Consequently, it is equally unfair to mandate that all citizens have insurance if insurance is not affordable (Starr, 2011). Insurance mandates could cause significant harm to individuals and families already struggling financially, especially if they are not eligible for government subsidies.

Learning Point 9.5   In what ways is health care similar or different from other commodities in the marketplace?

▶ Values in Rehabilitation

As noted in Table 9.1, at either extreme of the pendulum between distributive justice and freedom, are a different set of values. Distributive justice proponents value community, social justice, and equality, which is contrasted to the free-market advocates who value freedom, independence, and personal responsibility. People holding a particularly strong opinion may not only have difficulty understanding or appreciating fully the values associated with their own view, but also may have difficulty respecting the values of those holding opposing beliefs. Without understanding these differences in values, it becomes tempting to vilify the positions of others on healthcare policy, especially when one's view in time is more popular than the other viewpoint. It is not uncommon for rehabilitation professionals to predominately advocate for distributive justice due to their many experiences with clients who cannot access appropriate and high-quality rehabilitation. A rehabilitation team member with a minority view may not share his or her beliefs with other team members who have the more dominantly held position. Having difficulty sharing values related to health policy is further complicated when rehabilitation professionals with the dominant set of values are also in positions with greater power.

These values associated with distributive justice and the free-market obviously lead to different policies, both of which have positive and negative consequences on the public. When government distributes wealth through the ACA, for example, tax payors must be assured the quality of care is appropriate for the cost. Free market policies, such as employer-based insurance coverage, must ensure rising costs of coverage do not result in reducing access to care. Rehabilitation professionals are also concerned with values as they play out in patient care, and the way in which payment policies may affect how these patient-care values are ultimately enacted (Dougherty, 1991). Values of happiness, freedom, and fairness operate daily in the provision of rehabilitation.

Value of Fairness

The fairness or equity of healthcare access is often expressed daily in terms of rehabilitation professionals advocating for the "medical necessity" of the rehabilitation intervention with third payors (Stinneford & Kirschner, 2004). The concept of medical necessity is replete with pitfalls, especially when it is not uncommon for insurance companies to deny payment for rehabilitation interventions they consider unnecessary due to being experimental, unproven, or medically futile. The availability of research, which is often a result of the illness or disease having a high public profile, is additionally dependent upon the rarity of the disorder, the lack of research funds examining rehabilitation interventions, and the rapidity of technological advances. Determinations of medical necessity is partly dependent upon the evidence from research and translational science.

Learning Point 9.6 In what way does the concept of medical necessity illustrate the policy values of fairness and free market?

In other instances, the payor may decide a service or item may be necessary, but it is not "medical" because it can be used for nonmedical purposes, such as bathroom home modifications (Stinneford & Kirschner, 2004). Granted there is potential for abuse when covering home modifications; however, such modifications may be critical for the person to remain in a noninstitutionalized setting and to prevent rehospitalizations due to falls. In many circumstances, the bathroom modification is clearly more cost effective when compared with hospitalizations and institutionalization. Now that hospitals are penalized for preventable rehospitalizations under the ACA of 2010, the concept of medical necessity as it has been applied in the past, may not make sense.

Learning Point 9.7 How has the ACA changed the understanding of medical necessity?

In other applications of medical necessity, the payor may determine that the patient is not responding quickly enough, the goals of treatment are not achievable, or the goals are not "necessary" in a medical sense (Stinneford & Kirschner, 2004, p. 70). It is frustrating to the rehabilitation team and to the patient and the family when the insurance carrier makes the decision of medical necessity without ever having met, talked with, or examined the patient, especially in the context of the person's environment and level of independence needed to remain in the home. The criteria for the patient to rapidly reach the rehabilitation goals is often based on little research. Medical necessity runs the risk of being heavily biased against elders in terms of their age as a proxy measure of rehabilitation potential, or in the case of the severely disabled, the disability becomes the proxy for determining potential to benefit.

Clinicians may thus be concerned with the utilitarian philosophy undergirding medical necessity of patient goals. According to Levack (2009), "A utilitarian approach to goal planning would necessitate a focus on maximizing the benefits of rehabilitation to the whole community served when negotiating goals with individual patients" (p. 345). Rehabilitation team members are typically concerned that the quality of life of people with a severe disability will be judged as being intrinsically low from a utilitarian perspective. However, the rehabilitation team is most likely equally conflicted when there is a large financial outlay expended to achieve small gains for persons with severe disability. Evidenced-based practice holds promise to help the rehabilitation team advocate for the appropriate interventions and the best dosage to produce specific outcomes within a reasonable time.

> **Learning Point 9.8**   Does a utilitarian view on goal planning in rehabilitation represent a fair balance between the needs of the individual and the community?

Value of Freedom

The value of freedom leads rehabilitation professionals to address the autonomy of the patient in terms of informed consent as a basis for shared decision making required of patient-centered care. The competition for providing rehabilitation that a third-party payor will cover places the rehabilitation professional often in tension with the healthcare organization, the insurer, and the patient as the central decision maker. For instance, the demands of the rehabilitation organization for high rates of provider productivity in order to maximize time spent in billable hours may inadvertently compete with the optimal needs of the patient that cannot be reduced to minutes of service. Previously, discussion about payor determinations of medical necessity indicate the way in which patient freedom in selecting interventions and treatment goals may be hindered. Freedom also is dependent upon price transparency so that the patient and family can select rehabilitation providers partially based on the cost of the service compared with other providers (Hilsenrath, Eakin, & Fischer, 2015).

> **Learning Point 9.9**   In what way does transparency about the price of rehabilitation promote patient autonomy?

Transparent price information is central in a consumer-driven marketplace because of high deductible insurance and other forms of cost sharing, such as co-payments (a small fixed fee to access the covered service, such as an office visit) and co-insurance (what the patient pays as his or her portion of the claim). Price transparency depends upon the organizational ability to measure costs across a cycle of care. Tracking costs is playing a greater role in the transition for which some advocate to value-based purchasing or pay for performance strategies similar to the ACA where quality of care is incentivized (Hilsenrath, Eakin, & Fischer, 2015). It is not clear, however, whether the new models of payment will alternatively favor capitation where an individual's risk-adjusted healthcare needs are covered for a defined time period regardless of actual service utilization as long as quality standards are achieved (James & Poulsen, 2016).

Value of Happiness

Happiness is associated with alleviating pain and suffering and is reflected in national quality measures to assure pain is adequately controlled while decreasing the potential harm. For instance, the ACA makes a portion of hospital reimbursement dependent on the hospital's performance as measured by 30-day readmission rates, clinical care metrics, and patient satisfaction (Wolosin, 2012).

The Hospital Consumer Assessment of Healthcare Providers and Systems (HCAHPS), which is required through the Centers of Medicare and Medicaid Services (2016), measures patient satisfaction within the following categories: communication, environment, responsiveness of staff, medication education, discharge instructions, pain management, and overall satisfaction. Based on a formula that incorporates patient satisfaction, CMS calculates provider payments leading to financial winners and losers in terms of hospital reimbursement (Fisher, 2016). Pain management scores are thus examined as a part of payment policy and are consequently a strong incentive for maximizing patient satisfaction related to happiness or the relieving of pain and suffering.

The unintended consequence of reimbursement policy focused on pain and suffering relates to the importance of prudent rehabilitation professionals who will not allow overmedication to satisfy the financial goals of the organization (Fisher, 2016). To achieve careful pain management and prevent the unintended consequence of opioid addiction, the rehabilitation team must assess the patient's pain carefully and regularly, while also instituting consistent, safe, and tailored pharmacologic and nonpharmacologic pain interventions that are ultimately self-managed by the patient and family.

▶ Business Model Related Conflicts of Interest in Rehabilitation

As has been the theme of this chapter, payment methodologies for rehabilitation services create ethical dilemmas in terms of conflict of interest where the rehabilitation professional is often torn among the interests of the patient and the family, the third-party payor, other rehabilitation team members, and the employing healthcare organization. Professional ethics requires a patient-centered focus. In contrast, the method or model for payment determines the "business model" of the practice in which a physician and the rehabilitation team operates thereby creating unavoidable conflicts of interest (Larkin & Lowenstein, 2017).

> **Learning Point 9.10**   In what ways do current payment models contribute to unavoidable conflicts of interest?

The rehabilitation services the physician selects under consultation with the patient and those the rehabilitation professionals subsequently selects and provides based on assessment and patient preference do directly affect a physician's income and the revenue of the rehabilitation service organization.

Regardless of these inherent conflicts of interest, it is clear that rising healthcare costs in conjunction with lower quality indicators in comparison to other countries (such as infant mortality rates) demand payment reform, which has been trialed under the ACA. Our learning thus far centers on the unrealistic expectation for physicians, hospitals, and rehabilitation providers to provide improved quality and reduced spending if there is not adequate financial support for the delivery of rehabilitation. On the other hand, it is also unrealistic to expect patients, employers, insurers, or the government to pay more without demanding that quality of care improve simultaneously with lowered spending. No one approach for payment will meet the needs of every community. More than likely, payment reform will involve a combination of strategies to realize cost reductions related to avoidable hospital admissions, reductions of unnecessary tests and treatments, selection of lower-cost tests and treatments, delivery of efficient services, use of lower-cost sites of service, reductions in preventable complications, and prevention of serious conditions (Miller, 2015).

Fee-for-Service or Volume-Based Reimbursement

Fee-for-service or volume-based reimbursement, provides incentives for physicians to order, and for the rehabilitation team to offer, more and different services than those that match patient need. The financial incentive of volume-based reimbursement influences the avoidance of less profitable treatments in favor of more expensive alternatives that may even be less effective. The primary method of controlling costs, other than co-payments and co-insurances, is for the third-party payor to set rates by procedure codes so that the amount paid may be less than the amount billed (James & Poulsen, 2016).

> **Learning Point 9.11** How might volume-based reimbursement undermine quality of care?

Regardless of attempts to control rates, there may, as a result, be incentives in the fee-for-service payment model for excessive use of expensive assessments and interventions that ultimately drives up the cost of health care. More importantly, fee-for-service does not lead to better control of the waste in the system related to cost of production (e.g., speed of lab test results), unnecessary or suboptimal use of services (e.g., inadequate pain control), and preventable illness or injury (e.g., falls or nosocomial infections), 5%, 50%, and 45% of the waste, respectively (James & Poulsen, 2016). Because there is no effort to reduce waste in the system, fee-for-service fails to allocate savings among providers, payors, and patients in a way that would fund continual improvements in rehabilitation and in health care. Unfortunately, this payment model remains as the dominant approach for paying for rehabilitation and other healthcare services.

Per Case Method

Diagnosis related groups (DRGs) common to Medicare payments to hospitals group patients into diagnostic categories based on the patient's primary disease, specific treatment, secondary chronic conditions, and care intensity in order to determine a flat rate for a single case (James & Poulsen, 2016). Physician payments associated with the case, however, have been reimbursed via fee-for-service models. Consequently, Medicare began experimenting with bundled payments for total hip- and total knee-joint-replacement surgery.

Bundled payment methods improve the DRG model by extending the single flat-rate DRG payment to include all physician fees along with all costs of any related treatments, complications, or hospital readmissions within 90 days of the original operation (James & Poulsen, 2016). The ethical dilemma obviously occurs when trying to provide fewer services than may be needed without inadvertently causing complications and hospital readmissions. In fact, hospitals and other providers may not be paid adequately for the actual costs of patient care. With safeguards to protect the healthcare organization from unrelated care or catastrophic cases along with risk adjustments, payments should be in line with costs (Porter & Kaplan, 2016). According to James and Poulsen (2016), case-based payment approaches may still fuel waste in the healthcare system since it is a volume-based approach where it is in the healthcare organization's financial interest to maximize the number of surgical cases. Increasing surgical cases may occur even if some patients would experience little improvement with joint replacements or would be harmed because of surgery not being the best option for care.

Pay for Performance

Payments in pay for performance (P4P) schemes are often linked to achievements against targets, such as with peers or similar organizations, or to improvements in the healthcare organization's own quality measures. The basic rationale for P4P is that rewarding performance with contingent incentives heightens motivation and increases effort, leading to better performance (Siriwardena, 2014). P4P requires answers to such questions as: a) what sort of performance should be reimbursed? b) how should performance be defined and measured? and c) how much should be paid for better performance and to whom should these payments be made? Many policymakers agree that health services should be paid for by a combination of capitation, work volume, and quality, with an increasing emphasis on quality as opposed to volume. Fortunately, quality of performance has converged to three main areas: effectiveness (and efficiency), safety, and patient experience related to timeliness, accessibility, and equity.

> **Learning Point 9.12**   Should organizations have performance incentives? What are the benefits and risks?

What is unclear is how payments should be determined in terms of the quality that should be incentivized. It has also been debated whether payment should be directed to individual providers or to a healthcare organization/system.

> **Learning Point 9.13**   How might individual versus team rewards impact team dynamics?

From an ethical perspective, P4P can be understood in terms of ethical systems of utilitarianism (utility for the greatest number), deontology (duty to others) or principlism (beneficence, non-maleficence, autonomy, and distributive justice) (Siriwardena, 2014). Increased quality under P4P might be a utilitarian payment approach until considering unintended consequences that arise from a focus on individual patient health indicators, such as in the control of hypertension or hyperlipidemia. By focusing on these individual indicators, there could be an unintended consequence of excessive drug treatment contraindicated in some patients. In terms of being a deontological approach to payment, providing incentives for quality seems to fundamentally conflict with the idea of doing something because of duty to others. Autonomy can be adversely affected if patients are unaware that their doctor and rehabilitation providers are incentivized to treat certain conditions, encourage specific interventions, or undertake tasks without first gaining trust from the patient and family. Despite evidence that P4P may have benefits, there is a need to build safeguards to reduce potential adverse consequences. Stakeholders should be involved in developing valid measures of quality while reducing the proportion of pay allocated to contingent rewards.

Capitation

Global payment schemes based on capitation involve a healthcare entity receiving a capped payment per patient based on the patient's conditions and health levels. The ethical dilemma created results from the incentives for physicians to choose too few services for patients. Each individual service directly reduces a patient's profitability given the contractually determined annual payment (Miller, 2015). A better capitation method involves a population-based payment system where care provider organizations would receive a risk-adjusted monthly payment that covers all necessary health services for each person.

> **Learning Point 9.14**   Why is population-based capitation superior to global capitation from an ethical perspective?

Responsibility for considering the cost of treatment options would be back in the control of physicians and rehabilitation providers as they consult with patients. Specific quality measures, patient satisfaction scores, and clinical standards are used to prevent underutilization of services. This population-based capitation approach rewards providers for improvements in quality and cost, while compensating for income lost if total care volumes decline because of waste elimination (James & Poulsen, 2016). The challenge remains with the difficulty in managing care of a population across multiple systems and the need to bring greater focus on prevention and lifestyle adjustments supportive of health.

▶ Ethical Dilemmas Related to Reimbursement in Rehabilitation

The values of rehabilitation professionals lead them to question reimbursement decisions that reduce patient involvement in decision making. There is a strong ethic to offer rehabilitation services such that there is respect for the patient's autonomy in selecting interventions and priorities for rehabilitation while balancing respect for the desires of the patient's family and the suggestions and guidance from other rehabilitation team members (Kassberg & Skar, 2008). Most healthcare teams, including those in rehabilitation, commonly express powerlessness stemming from ethical dilemmas involving the management of difficult interactions with patients and family, unease over unsafe and unequal care, and uncertainty over who should have power over care decisions (Rasoal, Kihlgren, James, & Svantesson, 2016). These situations can be exacerbated by reimbursement decisions of third-party payors since they enact alternative payment models (see **TABLE 9.2**).

TABLE 9.2 Alternative Payment Models & Payment of Uncovered Services

Opportunity to Improve Care and Reduce Total Spending	Barrier(s) in the Current Payment System	Potential Solutions Through Alternative Payment Models	Prevention of Ethical Dilemmas with Alternative Payment Models
Help patients better manage health problems and risk factors in ways that avoid the need for hospitalizations.	Lack of payment or inadequate payment for proactive outreach, care management, rapid response to problems, and non-hospital treatment options for rehabilitation issues.	Capitation Bundled Payments Pay for Performance	Ensure patients receive necessary services given tension to offer less care.
Reduce unnecessary testing and visits to specialists.	Insufficient payment to allow time for determining a good diagnosis. No payment to support phone or email contacts between physicians and rehabilitation providers to develop good diagnoses and treatment plans.	Capitation Bundled Payments	Ensure rehabilitation providers are not classified as unnecessary specialists. Protect assessment time of rehabilitation providers to select the most appropriate and effective interventions.
Use lower-cost procedures and services to treat patient conditions.	Loss of revenue when fewer services or less-expensive services are performed.	Capitation Bundled Payments	Position rehabilitation as a lower cost service compared with surgical interventions and other expensive procedures.
Reduce the total cost of delivering a specific procedure or treatment in a hospital or other facility.	Separate payments to the physician and hospital (or other rehabilitation services) prevent compensating physicians for additional time or costs needed to reduce costs for the hospital or rehabilitation facility.	Bundled Payments	Eliminate waste in rehabilitation service delivery that raises costs.

▶ Moral Dialogue and Moral Agency

Moral dialogue and moral agency assist the rehabilitation team in addressing payment related dilemmas often inherent in the funding of healthcare and rehabilitation services. Rehabilitation teams benefit from a guided process to address conflict in values related to the distributive justice and freedom principles on which public policy is often based. A rehabilitation team must understand the language associated with alternative payment models, thereby enhancing the ability to predict the unintended consequences of capitation, bundled payments, pay-for-performance, or a combination of these payment approaches.

Learning Point 9.15 Why is it important for rehabilitation professionals to understand the language of reimbursement?

Each of these payment methods entail a framework addressing the relative flexibility in care delivery, adequacy and predictability of payment, and accountability for costs and quality (Miller, 2015).

In terms of flexible care delivery, it is essential that rehabilitation services are delivered in the most efficient and effective way possible. Adequacy and predictability of payment requires the third-party payor to provide acceptable and predictable resources to cover the costs of delivering high-quality rehabilitation to patients. Achieving savings is only desirable if access or quality are not jeopardized (Miller, 2015). Making investments in facilities and equipment and in recruiting, training, and retaining high-quality personnel is impossible if the healthcare organization cannot predict how much it will be paid for the rehabilitation services.

Accountability for costs and quality means the rehabilitation services are designed to assure patients and payors that spending will be controlled or reduced and that quality will be maintained or improved. However, rehabilitation providers should only be held accountable for aspects of spending and quality they can control or influence (Miller, 2015). The rising cost of health care is not a problem of too few incentives for delivering care in a different way. In contrast, the current healthcare system provides inadequate support for more effective and efficient approaches to rehabilitation. Additionally, one of the largest barriers to value-based care inherent in these new payment models is staff knowledge. Value-based care demands coordinated, team-based care, which contrasts with the way in which physicians, care managers, and rehabilitation professionals have been trained in the past. Higher education curricula are dominated by teaching rehabilitation within the context of the fee-for-service model, thereby making it difficult for new rehabilitation professionals to be prepared for the payment models of the future.

Learning Point 9.16 How can educational programs prepare rehabilitation teams for the reimbursement models of the future rather than the old fee-for-service model?

▶ Payment-Related Dilemmas Requiring Moral Agency

It is not uncommon for rehabilitation professionals and their patients and families to be frustrated when third party payors refuse to cover needed rehabilitation services and equipment. The following are examples of reported coverage denials of rehabilitation patients (Stinneford & Kirschner, 2017, p. 70):

- Catheter kits categorized as hygiene items when the patient with paraplegia must follow an intermittent catheterization program
- Denial for payment of a brace to prevent pain due to a back injury when the previously issued brace was inappropriate for the patient's needs
- Denial of continued inpatient rehabilitation because the patient could walk a short distance, even though the patient's traumatic brain injury resulted in major deficits in judgment, orientation, memory, and depth perception creating serious safety issues for living alone
- Denial of a wheelchair for a patient because he could walk short distances, even though he was unable to ambulate in the community due to endurance and physical limitations

These payment-related ethical dilemmas and more like these can be classified as falling within the Rule-Based, Ends-Based, Virtue-Based, and Narrative-Based ethical traditions originally outlined in Table 9.2. Ways of determining whether the ethical dilemma fits with a tradition is described in **TABLE 9.3** as a way of fostering the agency of the rehabilitation team upon analysis of the payment issue. Often payment denials are Rule-Based because of statutes or corresponding regulations, such as is typical of Medicare and Medicaid. Other requests for payment coverage may be Ends-Based because of public policy, such as helping a patient in rehabilitation access smoking cessation programs and medications even though these services are not directly related to the rehabilitation needs of the person. However, the reduced lung capacity of a person with quadriplegia who also is struggling to quit smoking are serious factors in long-term mortality and morbidity and in the prevention of unnecessary costs. Narrative-Based payment-related dilemmas occur because of lack of access, such as difficulty affording the $50 co-payment for each outpatient rehabilitation visit along with the 20% co-insurance requirement for the total rehabilitation episode of care. Virtue-Based traditions are a result of values that guide payment-related dilemmas, such as including the patient in shared decision-making and trying to gain coverage for the patient's desires for intervention when the insurance payor pays for cheaper, but less effective alternatives. Use Table 9.3 to guide moral agency of the rehabilitation team once these payment-related dilemmas are understood within the ethical traditions. Go back to the examples of denied coverage and take them through the Dialogic Engagement Model to articulate opportunities for solutions in order to help the patient receive the necessary rehabilitation services and achieve the expected outcomes.

Learning Point 9.17   How can the rehabilitation team incorporate awareness of values undergirding payment related ethical situations?

TABLE 9.3 Dialogic Engagement Model to Guide Resolutions of Ethical Dilemmas Related to Payment Systems

Dimension	Goal or Process	Sample Questions
1. Moral Commons	Establish the climate of trust in preparation of politically charged dilemmas of distributive justice and freedom related to reimbursement policy.	• Is there a team culture that sanctions the legitimacy of some values over others as related to reimbursement policy? • What are the power differentials on the team that may influence the dominant view on the team regarding the policy aspects of payment?
2. Preparation	Determine the ethical values at stake within the payment decision for patient care and/or the process for obtaining payment.	• Do the payment decisions challenge values of patient freedom, happiness, or fairness? • How do perspectives from the ethical traditions, one's own identity in relationship to these values, one's clinical knowledge and experience in relationship to these values, and one's understanding of the context inform the understanding of payment issue?
3. Self-Reflection	Active listening from all stakeholders, eliciting opportunities to address the ethical dilemma related to the payment issue.	• Are there personal, team, organizational, or professional biases that reduce opportunities to address the payment issue? • What are the strengths and weaknesses of the team that affect opportunities to address the ethical dilemma related to the payment issue? • What is the level of the rehabilitation team's understanding of the processes for an appeal of the claims decisions? • Is the rehabilitation team addressing the autonomy of the patient in determining solutions to the payment issues?

(continues)

TABLE 9.3 Dialogic Engagement Model to Guide Resolutions of Ethical Dilemmas Related to Payment Systems *(continued)*

Dimension	Goal or Process	Sample Questions
4. Dialogic Process	The ability to engage in critical dialogue with the goal of reaching mutual consensus with the team and the patient regarding solutions to the payment related ethical dilemma.	• How do the ethical traditions suggest opportunities for solutions to the payment related ethical dilemma? • What course of action should be taken to solve the payment related ethical dilemma that also respects the autonomy of the patient? • How should any unintended consequences from the action of the rehabilitation team and the patient be addressed?
5. Summative Reflection	An iterative revisiting of thoughts and emotions by individuals and the group following reaching a decision or consensus regarding the payment- related ethical dilemma.	• What needs to be done to support future moral agency of the rehabilitation team related to payment-related dilemmas? • How will the rehabilitation team resolve any remaining disagreements related to the payment related ethical dilemma? • Are the team members fully aware of the values undergirding the solution to the payment-related dilemma?

▶ Summary and Conclusion

Due to rising costs of health care, payment approaches for covering rehabilitation are evolving away from fee-for-service or other types of volume-based payment models. Trying to address the question of how to control costs has led to approaches that create ethical dilemmas for the rehabilitation providers, such as cutting provider fees for services, shifting costs to patients, or delaying or denying care to patients. These strategies are perhaps a debatable win for the third-party payors, but are essentially lose-lose strategies. Patients do not get the care they need, which subsequently increases healthcare costs in the future. Small providers are forced out of business due to the inability to recover their costs. Additionally, health insurance premiums continue to rise while access to care decreases.

Consequently, alternative payment models are being developed that have the right focus on reducing spending that is unnecessary or avoidable, including the overuse of inpatient rehabilitation. These payment reforms rely on engaging and satisfying consumers, a value consistent with the ethical principle of autonomy.

Shifting toward population health through spreading risk and providing scale for implementing effective interventions is a utilitarian approach to decision-making characteristic of these alternative payment approaches. Continuing differentiation of rehabilitation services based on clinical quality and costs to produce value represents a growing focus on patient happiness or satisfaction, freedom to choose providers as the result of price transparency, and the fairness required to access effective care.

Closing Reflections

 ## Take Away Messages

- Different views regarding how health care should be financed may influence the ethical stance of members of the interprofessional team.
- Current health policy debates regarding the Affordable Care Act (ACA) illustrate the divide between proponents of distributing justice advocating for increased access to health insurance via wealth redistribution and free-market advocates who favor freedom from government control. The healthcare policy may be seen as a pendulum moving along a continuum between extremes of these two positions.
- Those who favor distributive justice embrace values of community, social justice, equality freedom, and independence while those who advocate for market freedom are committed to the values of freedom, independence, and personal responsibility.
- The return on investment for healthcare dollars spent is low in the United States, with significant funds invested in a health system that delivers outcomes inferior to those of other developed nations.
- The concept of medical necessity creates a number of ethical pitfalls in application as rehabilitation interventions may be denied due to lack of evidence, considered as non-medical or unnecessary. The ACA has changed our understanding of medical necessity because hospitals are now accountable for preventable rehospitalizations.
- Meeting third-party requirements for reimbursement places rehabilitation professionals in tension with the healthcare organization, the insurer, and the patient with regard to decision making.
- Payment methodologies create ethical dilemmas of conflict of interest whereby rehabilitation professionals are torn between the competing interests of the patient, family, third-party payer, other team members, and the healthcare organization.
- Fee-for-service or volume-based approaches to reimbursement attempt to control costs by setting rates for specific procedures. However, this creates incentives for providers to select more expensive interventions and there are inadequate controls for wasteful spending.
- There is some policy consensus that health services should be financed through capitation, work volume, and quality. Quality is considered to be effectiveness and efficiency, safety, and patient experience related to timeliness, accessibility,

and equity. It is not clear how and to whom quality payments should be disbursed. Ideally, relevant stakeholders (including patients) should be involved in developing standards of quality.

- Capitation by individual payment may create incentives for underutilization. Population-based capitation has the potential to reward organizations for cost and quality measures, while also compensating for lost income related to waste reduction.
- Rehabilitation teams must understand the language associated with alternative payment models, thereby enhancing the ability to predict the unintended consequences of capitation, bundled payments, pay-for-performance, or a combination of these payment approaches. "Payment literacy" is foundational for appreciating the ethical challenges of rehabilitation.
- Traditional curricula in the rehabilitation professions do not adequately prepare professionals to understand alternative payment models.

References

Centers for Medicare & Medicaid Services. (2016). *Hospital consumer assessment of healthcare providers and systems.* Retrieved from www.hcahpsonline.org

Cox, C., Long, M., Semanskee, A., Kamal, R., Claxton, G., & Levitt, L. (2016). *2017 premium changes and insurer participation in the Affordable Care Act's health insurance marketplaces.* The Henry J. Kaiser Family Foundation. Retrieved from http://www.kff.org/health-reform/issue-brief/2017-premium-changes-and-insurer-participation-in-the-affordable-care-acts-health-insurance-marketplaces/

Craig, H. D. (2010). Caring enough to provide healthcare: An organizational framework for the ethical delivery of healthcare among aging patients. *International Journal of Human Caring, 14*(4), 27–30.

Dougherty, C. J. (1991). Values in rehabilitation: Happiness, freedom, and fairness. *Journal of Rehabilitation, 57*(1), 7–12.

Fisher, S. K. (2016). Ethics, pain, and pay-for-performance. *Nursing, 46*(12), 55–58. doi:10.1097/01.NURSE.0000504679.57216.7c

Gains, K. (2017). Are we happy? Are we healthy? Is health care going 'Back to the Future'? *Urologic Nursing, 37*(4), 178–222. http://dx.doi.org.pearl.stkate.edu/10.7257/1053-816X.2017.37.4.178

Hilsenrath, P., Eakin, C., & Fischer, K. (2015). Price-transparency and cost accounting: Challenges for health care organizations in the consumer-driven era. *The Journal of Health Care Organization, Provision, and Financing, 52*, 1–5. doi:10.1177/0046958015574981

James, B. C., & Poulsen, G. P. (2016). The case for capitation. It's the only way to cut waste while improving quality. *Harvard Business Review, 94*, 103–111.

Kassberg, A., & Skar, L. (2008). Experiences of ethical dilemmas in rehabilitation: Swedish occupational therapists' perspectives. *Scandinavian Journal of Occupational Therapy, 15*, 204–211.

Lachman, V. D. (2009). *Ethical challenges in healthcare: Developing your moral compass.* New York, NY: Springer.

Larkin, I., & Lowenstein, G. (2017). Business model–related conflict of interests in medicine: Problems and potential solutions. *Journal of the American Medical Association, 317*(17), 1765–1768.

Levack, W. M. (2009). Ethics in goal planning for rehabilitation: A utilitarian perspective. *Clinical Rehabilitation, 23*, 345–351.

Miller, H. D. (2015). The building blocks of successful payment reform: Designing payment systems that support higher–value health care. *Payment Reform Series, 3*.

Porter, M. E., & Kaplan, R. S. (2016). How to pay for healthcare. Bundled payments will finally unleash the competition that patients want. *Harvard Business Review, 94*, 89–100.

Rasoal, D., Kihlgren, A., James, I., & Svantesson, M. (2016). What healthcare teams find ethically difficult: Captured in 70 moral case deliberations. *Nursing Ethics, 23*(8), 825–837. doi:10.1177/0969733015583928

Siriwardena, A. N. (2014). The ethics of pay-for-performance. *Quality in Primary Care, 22*, 53–55.

Starr, P. (2011). The mandate miscalculation Obama's health care blunder—and how to fix it. *The New Republic, 242*, 11–13.

Stinneford, M. K., & Kirschner, K. L. (2004). Concepts of medical necessity in rehabilitation. *Topics in Stroke Rehabilitation, 11*(2), 69–76. doi:10.1310/DE6C-WW93-DMR8P0W7

The Organization for Economic Co-operation and Development. (2017). *OECD health statistics 2017*. Retrieved from http://stats.oecd.org/Index.aspx?DataSetCode=SHA

Wolosin, R., Ayala, L., & Fulton, B. R. (2012). Nursing care, inpatient satisfaction, and value-based purchasing: Vital connections. *Journal of Nursing Administration, 42*(6), 321–325.

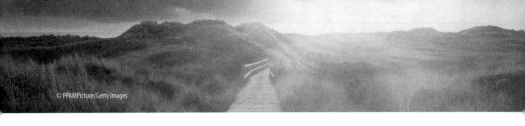

CHAPTER 10

Neuroethics: A Guide for the Perplexed[1] Rehabilitation Professional

Jeffrey Lee Crabtree and **Charlotte Brasic Royeen**

"Why are we so sensitive to ponder on neuroethics? Because it involves the brain, the organ responsible for our perceptions, our thoughts, and our conscience, and its knowledge and or manipulation entail the most genuine and nontransferable aspects of the human being."

Rabadan, 2015

CHAPTER OUTLINE

- Chapter Overview
- Interprofessional Habilitation and Rehabilitation
- How Neuroethics Applies to Interprofessional Rehabilitation and Habilitation

- Application
- Implications
- Summary and Conclusion

---

[1]Ode to M. J. Farah, who wrote the article *Neuroethics: A Guide for the perplexed*. The Dana Foundation, October 1, 2004. Retrieved from http://dana.org/Cerebrum/2004/Neuroethics_A_Guide_for_the_ Perplexed.

CHAPTER OBJECTIVES

At the conclusion of this chapter, the reader will be able to:

1. Appraise evolving information about neuroethics in the context of interprofessional habilitation and rehabilitation.
2. Understand how interfield theory helps to enlighten ethical issues in habilitation and rehabilitation.
3. Question standard approaches to ethical decision making that do not take neuroscience into consideration.
4. Determine the relevance of neuroscience in every day interprofessional practice.
5. Differentiate between habilitation and rehabilitation in practice and ethical decision making.
6. Value the moral insights found in the "long view" of rehabilitation and habilitation.

KEY TERMS

Reading these key terms before reading the chapter will introduce you to key concepts which will then be somewhat familiar to you as you read this chapter. This is an important learning technique that will enhance your learning as a multi-step process. You may even wish to make a flash card set of key terms and quiz yourself on them once or twice before reading the chapter. This will better prepare you to immerse in the language of ethics and better prepare you to integrate the content.

Interfield Theory: Theory that bridges two distinct fields or areas.
Neuroethics: The ethics of doing neuroscience pertaining to the ethical considerations of neuroscience research and related translational research (Roskies, 2002; Shrivastava & Behari, 2015). Alternatively, the neuroscience of ethics, pertaining to how we understand moral behavior related to our comprehension of the brain (Roskies, 2002; Shrivastava & Behari, 2015).

▶ Chapter Overview

This chapter explores neuroethics as applied to interprofessional rehabilitation and habilitation. To do this, we define rehabilitation and habilitation, interfield theory, and neuroethics itself. Additionally, we present a short history of neuroethics and we will apply neuroethics to interprofessional habilitation and rehabilitation using a multipart case study, reflecting upon the episodic nature of rehabilitation and habilitation and how neuroethics helps to explain and inform the ethical decision-making process. Finally, we delineate the interprofessional implications for neuroethics and habilitation and rehabilitation and provide a summary of the chapter.

Interprofessional collaborative practice is "…[when] multiple health workers from different professional backgrounds work together with patients, families, carers [sic], and communities to deliver the highest quality of care" (WHO, 2010, p. 7).

It could be said that the potential of interprofessional collaborative practice in rehabilitation and habilitation is the practical realization of interfield theory in that two or more professions, through collaboration, address and hopefully solve problems that no one profession, alone, is able to solve.

In many ways this chapter foreshadows more than it explains neuroethics applied to interprofessional rehabilitation and habilitation. Since "the Decade of the Brain" (President of the United States, 1990) researchers have generated an amazing amount of neuroscience research, data, models, ways of measuring activity and the nerve cells and pathways, and interventions. The momentum, therefore, of this dynamic, emerging field demands that we address it, but in no way will this be a definitive chapter regarding this robust and changing field. Rather, it will serve as an exploratory foray into neuroethics and its application to interprofessional habilitation and rehabilitation.

Neuroscience is growing explosively across the world and especially in China (Hu, Wang, Yin, & Wang, 2011) where speculations about how far neuroethics might go in the future, such as achievement of a human head transplant, challenge our current mores, culture, and philosophical views (Pascalev, Pascalev, & Giordfano, 2016). Neuroethics is even being pushed down into grade school education as evidenced by the website, Neuroscience for Kids: Neuroethics (Chudler, 2017). Other examples of the growth over the last two decades of relevant research in this field include corollaries to ethics such as:

- How the brain collects information required for decision making (Dimirov, Lazar, & Victor, 2011; Gold & Shadlen, 2007)
- The role working, episodic, and prospective memory has in shaping decision making (Berg, 2002; Berkman, Livingston, & Kahn, 2015; Umeda, Tochizawa, Shibata, & Terasawa, 2016)
- The role appraisal has in shaping decision making (Cowen, Davis, & Nitz, 2012; Hauser, Cushman, Young, Kang-Xing, & Mikhail, 2006; Schmitz & Johnson, 2007)
- The influence that emotional valence (Bechara, 2004; Berkman, Liningston, & Kahn, 2015; Greene, Nystrom, Engell, Darley, & Cohen, 2004) or anticipation of the action (Guitart-Masip, Duzel, Dolan, & Dayan, 2014) has on decision making
- How the brain engages in goal-directed and value-directed decision making (Solway & Botvinick, 2012).

And as interprofessional rehabilitation and habilitation grows, so too, we expect the neuroethics of interprofessional rehabilitation and habilitation to also grow.

Interfield Theory

Interfield theory brings together parts of different fields or disciplines in an attempt to answer questions that neither field nor discipline alone is able to answer. Interfield theories were well addressed initially by Darden and Mull (1977) who explained interfield theory as the theory that bridges two distinct fields or areas. In this chapter, the interfield theory of neuroethics bridges neuroscience (a biological science) with ethics (a philosophy).

Learning Point 10.1 Why might interfield theory be especially relevant to interprofessional education and practice?

Examples of additional interfield theories in which neuroscience is linked to another discipline are numerous and increasing. For example, neuroeconomics and neuromarketing seek to explain, and in some cases influence, decision making (Camerer, Loewenstein, & Prelec, 2005; Gordon & Ciorciari, 2017; Sanfrey, Loewenstein, McClure, & Cohen, 2006; Rangel, Camerer, & Mantague, 2008). Neuroesthetics studies the aesthetic perceptions of paintings, sculpture, music, or other expressions of art (Chatterjee, 2011; Conway & Rehding, 2013). Through neurocriminology, criminologists aim to better understand the causes of criminal behavior and thus help predict and prevent criminal behavior (Craver, 2005; Glenn & Raine, 2014). Neurooccupation "combines the idea that humans are occupational beings who both influence and are influenced by their nervous systems and the environment" (Crabtree, 2011, p. 880; Padilla & Peyton, 1997). For example, through neurooccupation occupational therapists attempt to better understand the relationship between the neuroscience related to posttraumatic stress and occupation (Lohman & Royeen, 2002), and neuroscience in general and occupation related to intention, meaning and perception (Lazzarini, 2004).

Neuroethics

Neuroethics seems to have first appeared in the literature in 1989 (Lombera & Illes, 2009). Neuroethics is a bourgeoning interfield theory that in many ways defies definition because neuroscience research continuously evolves and changes its application to health sciences, public policy, and law (Illes & Bird, 2006; Roskies, 2002; Shrivastava & Behari, 2015). Neuroethics, as Roskies (2002) describes it, became a headline in the popular press in 2002 and stimulated a number of high level conferences sponsored by well-known institutions from The Royal Institution in London to the Dana Foundation in collaboration with the University of San Francisco and Stanford University.

On the surface one might assume neuroethics is the application of ethical theories and principles to neurological cases such as identifying the moral implications of head transplants, then making ethical decisions and acting on those decisions. But that is only half of the story. To help situate neuroethics for this chapter, it is useful to understand two broad categories and characterizations of neuroethics. First, the ethics of neuroscience, or the ethics of doing neuroscience, pertains to the ethical considerations of neuroscience research and related translational research (Roskies, 2002; Shrivastava & Behari, 2015). Second, the neuroscience of ethics pertains to how we understand moral behavior related to our comprehension of the brain (Roskies, 2002; Shrivastava & Behari, 2015). Deceivingly simple while being contextually complex, **TABLE 10.1** presents these dual concepts side by side.

Learning Point 10.2 Consider the potential implications of each face of neuroethics for your profession and for interprofessional practice

TABLE 10.1 Juxtaposition of the Two Definitions of Neuroethics

Ethics of Neuroscience	Neuroscience of Ethics
Pertains to the ethical considerations of neuroscience research and related translational research (Shrivastava & Behari, 2015). For example, because of advances in neuroscience, scientists claim they can influence peoples' decision processes to modify their preference for food (Yoon et al., 2012). The ethics of neuroscience might address how this understanding of the nervous system could be used to help people gain control of their eating habits, on one hand, or to influence people to purchase certain brands of food on the other hand.	Pertains to how we understand moral behavior related to our comprehension of the brain (Shrivastava & Behari, 2015). For example, neuroscientists are beginning to explain how emotion influences why people make irrational or antisocial decisions (Naqvi, Shiv, & Bechara, 2006; Sobhani & Bechara, 2011). These decisions may result from dysfunction in certain parts of the brain and could help forensics distinguish between psychopathic behavior and the behavior of people with focal brain damage (Koenigs, Kruepke, & Newman, 2010).

Neuroethics, then, has two faces. One that looks inward to examine the ethics of neuroscience research and practice. The other face looks outward, using interfield theory to unite the results of neuroscience research and brain science and philosophy. Neuroethics helps us better understand behavior of any kind, and to the point of this chapter helps us better understand the challenges to what Purtilo (2000) has called "moral courage . . . . a readiness for voluntary, purposive action in situations that engender realistic fear and anxiety in order to uphold something of great moral value" (p. 4). Neuroethics is beginning to shed light on the nervous system's activity milliseconds before the action resulting from the ethical decision. That is, it is beginning to understand critical junctures and nervous system activity that occurs in the decision-making process that leads to action. These processes typically include:

- Receiving information required for decision making
- Appraising information; establishing emotional valence to the information; sorting information; and
- Storing information in working, episodic and prospective memory (Ballard, Murty, Carter, MacInnes, Huettel, & Adcock, 2011; Friston, 2012; Vossel, Weidner, Driver, Friston, & Fink, 2012)

Learning Point 10.3 How does emotion influence ethical decisions and behavior? Can you remember an ethical situation in which emotion was a critical factor?

Understanding any one, or all, of these processes can help us understand how ethical decisions are made. While the two faces of neuroethics are related, each is a distinct area of study. For example, the ethics of neuroscience pertains to the morality of basic and applied research involving the human brain, neuroimaging, pharmacology, cell transplantation, and any other neuroscientific interventions. In principle, the ethics of neuroscience is no different from the ethics of nursing or the ethics of occupational therapy in that they address moral implications of their services and research. Conversely, the neuroscience of ethics pertains to what we know about the brain, how brain function or dysfunction can and does shape moral decision making and action. A comprehensive review of neuroscience studies of morality and ethics can be found elsewhere (Darrah, Buniak, & Giordan, 2015) and for the most part is beyond the scope of this chapter.

Lombera & Illes (2009) suggests there are four broad ways of thinking about the impact or influence of neuroethics on society (see **TABLE 10.2**). The first impact is on science and the self and pertains to what we know about brain development-related cognitive functioning, and how we judge human behavior and make decisions. For example, earlier in this chapter reference was made to neuromarketing. In neuromarketing, techniques are employed to influence human decision making based upon what we know about the brain. Hence, in commercials you see correlation between strong visuals establishing a problem, or a cause of pain and then strong visuals of "relief" portrayed as a famous actor falling into a refreshing swimming pool. Such neuromarketing is pervasive in the United States, particularly among food vendors selling sugary and fat laden "treats" to children. This significant area of impact, and an impact that you also have seen in the 2016 Presidential contest, is based more upon emotions, values, and beliefs and less on discourse and dialogue.

The second impact area of neuroethics is on science and social policy. For example, check your current Code of Ethics. Is it currently influenced by neuroethics? Probably not yet, but within the next ten years it is likely to do so. As neuroscience develops, so will our understanding of how the nervous system influences professional behavior and decision making. And this understanding will likely influence and guide professional codes of ethics in the future. Currently, federal and state statutes limit the age of participation in various activities such as

TABLE 10.2 The Four Impact Areas of Neuroethics

Science and the Self	Science and Social Policy
Manifestation of moral responsibility, decision making, and free will related to neuroscience developments.	Development of organizational, legal, and codified initiatives, laws, and mandates related to health disparity, occupational justice, social justice, and societal determinants of health.
Ethics and the Practice of Brain Science	**Ethics and the Practice of Discourse**
Creation and validation of brain-based tests and interventions.	Lay understanding of neuroscience; how lay and science based folk interact and converse.
Use of neurotechnology to uncover "truths" such as lie detection.	
Determination of social and behavioral influences through data analytics of large data sets.	

Based on Lombera & Illes (2009).

voting, joining the military, and driving an automobile. While these limitations have always "made sense" to most people, with our evolving understanding of the nervous system, we understand that the frontal lobe does not fully develop until the early 20s, thus adding a neurological rationale and nuanced understanding of the role the nervous system places on making reasonable judgments and decisions-making. Additionally, strong drink affects brain function and is a social policy mandated to protect society from inebriated drivers. Thus, the act of drunk driving violates neuroethical standards in this category. The same could be said of any sort of occupational engagement while under the influence of any sort of mind altering medication or drugs such as marijuana, heroin, Adderall, etc. Many medical or health practitioners are negatively affected by various addictions and programs offering employee assistance are plentiful. The required drug testing that all students and health professionals must pass before clinical work is another example of the impact of neuroethics on science and society. Had you ever thought of your course of study or your work in the context of science and social policy ? You have likely been involved with the impact of neuroethics on society whether you had thought of it in this manner or not!

From a social policy perspective, there is yet another compelling reason to be conversant about neuroethics. According to Rabadan (2015) 30% of the U.S. population has some level of damage to their central nervous system; 35% of U.S. healthcare costs pertain to this population! Therefore, about one third of the U.S. population has challenges that may have behaviors and healthcare needs that are directly related to neuroethical considerations. Here is just one place where neuroethics and finance of modern health care intersect! For most of us, these figures are just too huge and daunting to really understand.

Ethics and the practice of brain science is the third area of impact for neuroethics. This area pertains to the development and standardization of brain related testing and brain-based interventions. To illustrate, the commonly used theoretical references of neurodevelopmental treatment and sensory integration both are brain-based interventions designed to enhance brain function through sensory manipulations. Current and ongoing research on parameters of safety testing for deep brain or neuronal stimulation fit this category, as do a myriad of other ways to view, look at, excite, or explore the brain. More recently in this impact area is the emergence of manipulation of large data sets to uncover behaviors or actions resulting from implicit or explicit messaging to orchestrate perceptions. For example, because of the ability to follow what you "click on" to explore in Google and other search engines, your record of online searches can be used to predict what you are or are not likely to buy and to make coupon offerings and "deals" to match those indicators. This emerging area of data analytics has the potential for huge impact upon manipulating peoples' decisions and thus their actions and the practice of brain science to manipulate or influence human behavior. We are just at the border of this frontier.

Fourth and finally, discourse is the last level of impact of neuroethics. Few of us "in the field" of habilitation or rehabilitation related to brain function have regular discourse with the lay public. Yet, the lay public is asked to make decisions about political leaders and legislative initiatives directly related to neuroethics. Legislation to legalize marijuana in various states or to restrict dispensation of opioid-based medications are just two examples. We speculate that effective dialogue and engagement in meaningful discourse between the scientific community, the rehabilitation community and the lay community could help to elucidate the issues, challenges, and dangers of neuroethics related to fragile and undeveloped brains growing up in poverty or the effect of extreme pollution on brain function, etc. To illustrate, the very nature of the conversation about alcoholism and drug addiction as a disease versus a behavioral choice – in fact, is a conversation related to neuroethics. These conversations could be the beginning of ongoing dialogue about the four impact areas of neuroethics on persons and society. What role will you play in facilitating discourse in these areas in both lay and professional groups?

Learning Point 10.4   How does a professional balance personal and religious values with professional values on controversial issues, such as, legalization of marijuana?

Given this overview of neuroethics and its impact on society, let us now turn to review interprofessional habilitation and rehabilitation.

Rehabilitation and Habilitation

Examining rehabilitation and habilitation from an interprofessional approach offers an opportunity to reexamine the meaning of rehabilitation and habilitation. If the structure of the term rehabilitation offers any clues to its meaning, re-habilitation might mean to habilitate again or to return to a habilitated state. Based on this structural analysis, if rehabilitation is a science, we take it to be the study of "how to return to a habilitated state." Put into the language of ethics:

> .... the essential meaning of rehabilitation, in the root sense of the term, cannot be defined solely in individualistic terms. To rehabilitate is to restore the power or capacity for living, where living does not signify merely biologic life and function but takes on a qualitative dimension. It is the restoration of the power of living well, living meaningfully, that rehabilitation essentially seeks. (Jennings, 1995, p. S26)

Breaking the word rehabilitation into its prefix and stem only helps a little, because we have yet to define habilitation. The etymology of the now nearly obsolete term habilitation[2] suggests the term came from Medieval Latin *habilitāre, habilitāt-*, to enable, and from an earlier Latin word *habilis*, or able (Oxford Dictionaries). So, we take habilitation to mean being able to function, or the initial learning of skills that allows an individual to function in society. Occupational scientists would say that habilitation is an issue of occupational justice, giving all the right to grow and develop to their potential regardless of socioeconomic status or environmental location.

Learning Point 10.5   Recall previous discussions of the UNCRPD and whether health care is a right. Do you agree that all people should have the right to develop their potential?

---

[2]It may be obsolete, but we believe it is the process by which the disenfranchised of America, during development, can and will learn to be contributory, productive members of society.

Over one hundred years ago, Jane Addams implemented a precursor to the occupational science movement known as the settlement house movement. At the settlement house known as the Hull House in "near west" of Chicago,[3] Jane Addams tried to implement an earlier form of social and economic habilitation with the immigrant populations in Chicago (Knight, 2010).

▶ Interprofessional Habilitation and Rehabilitation

Examining interprofessional rehabilitation and habilitation demands acknowledgement that adding to the number of people in a team, or the number of professional perspectives, does not necessarily change the dynamics of specific habilitation or rehabilitation interventions. Learning how to adapt to a limitation or how to use an adaptive device does not change when there are several professionals collaborating on the team. What changes in terms of interventions is the support and reinforcement that can occur in the collaborative environment. And from the perspective of ethical decision making, as we discuss later, adding to the number of people, or the number of professional ontologies, does not necessarily change the dynamics of the ethical dilemma. For example, from a deontological point of view, duty is duty whether it is applied by one person or by ten. What changes in terms of ethics is how the ethical dilemma is analyzed and whether all ten people can agree on the theory or ethical tradition to be used.

To help understand the expanded view of interprofessional rehabilitation and habilitation, it is useful to view them from two perspectives: from the insider view, the person, or the object of habilitation or rehabilitation, and from the outsider view, the interprofessional provider(s) of services. These perspectives are not meant to be mutually exclusive constructs, or views, but are hallmarks, or distinguishing characteristics, of the different views. For example, the person receiving the services reacts to the disease or injury and reacts to the interventions; the professionals react to the unfolding story of the client's habilitation. The insider, to paraphrase Adolf Meyer (1957), is the object of rehabilitation and habilitation— "...literally, an indivisible individual. To be more explicit, it is a unit of biology which functions always as a 'he' or 'she' or person, by itself and in groups. It is an experiential continuum in which the data are of a multi-relational character and appear in, and as, a state of flux. Constantly changing, it yet maintains a reasonably orderly internal and external structural and functional organization" (p. 6). To paraphrase Fischer and Sullivan (2002), recipients of these services are a "universe of one" and multiple "universes of one" do not make for good generalizations of people who need rehabilitation or habilitation services.

> **Learning Point 10.6**   Partner with one or more members of your interprofessional team, analyze the work of the team from both the insider and outsider perspective, and discuss your perspectives.

---

[3]The "near west" is in fact the area of Chicago where the second author currently lives.

Interprofessional rehabilitation and habilitation from the outsider view is one of a witness to the story or narrative and a change agent. As a witness each practitioner has her own personal and professional perspective but collaborates with other professionals who each have their own personal and professional perspectives. As a change agent each practitioner has a job to do, must gather information, and make sense of, and translate that information into interventions. With habilitation and rehabilitation, the information gathered tends to be of recurring episodes of a story or a narrative arc. To paraphrase Barwell (2009) each episode preceding the most recent one helps to explain or evaluate the previous one and contributes to an explanation or evaluation of the next episode. We submit that a uniqueness of rehabilitation and habilitation demands acknowledgment of the long story, the narrative arc that spans, in some cases, a lifetime. Thus, one cannot successfully evaluate the effectiveness of an intervention in isolation or evaluate the ethics of a given decision in isolation. One must situate the intervention and evaluations as episodes in the narrative, and their ethical importance is only fairly comprehended with reflection over time. The case of Henrietta, presented later in this chapter, will illustrate this concept of rehabilitation over time or the narrative arc of rehabilitation.

From the perspective of this chapter, we see habilitation and rehabilitation as a life process with recurring episodes of challenges to the recipient's sense of self and to the interprofessional team's sense of what is morally good. So, to understand interprofessional habilitation or rehabilitation is to understand the recipient's story and to become aware of related moral questions:

1. Is rehabilitation or habilitation a human right?
2. Is rehabilitation or habilitation a privilege afforded only to those who can afford it?
3. Why distinguish habilitation and rehabilitation from other human health services?
4. Does either habilitation or rehabilitation pose unique challenges to service providers?
5. What about interprofesisonal habilitation or rehabilitation makes it worthy of our efforts?

These questions are provided for you to ponder.

▶ How Neuroethics Applies to Interprofessional Rehabilitation and Habilitation

As stated earlier, since the 1990s there has been a veritable explosion of journals, books, and blogs on the topic of neuroethics. Many centers of ethics in various universities now have sub-specializations in neuroethics. In fact, every therapist who has ever worked with a patient who had a stroke (a very common event) has had to, in some manner, deal with neuroethics even if only peripherally or unknowingly or explicitly. The issues of who receives rehabilitation, for how long, where, and when are all neuroethical issues currently being driven by third party payors and those who can afford to pay out of pocket. Thus, the rehabilitation community has been deeply involved in neuroethical issues for a long time, even if not cognizant of it. One of the goals of this chapter is for sensitization of one and all to neuroethical issues that are at once commonplace and unrecognizable but are too often categorized under organizational policy or hidden in organizational procedures. But because of their significance for effective interprofessional interventions, these neuroethical issues need to be acknowledged and addressed throughout the full spectrum of rehabilitation science, our ideas about selfhood, our social policy, our ethics, practice, and discourse.

Please review **FIGURE 10.1** and revisit the four broad ways of thinking about the impact or influence of neuroethics on society, and apply them to interprofessional rehabilitation. How might these categories look if we applied them to our collective experiences in rehabilitation? This is speculated upon and presented in Figure 10.1.

Reviewing Figure 10.1 reveals a beginning level series of questions for self-analysis, group discussion, and teaching and learning activities to promote increased awareness of neuroethical impact on self, the professions, and society.

Science and the self	How does my profession view knowledge about science and the self? How does my profession view humans and decision-making abilities? Does my profession endorse free will? Does my profession recognize addiction as a disease? How is moral responsibility manifest?
Science and social policy	What is my profession's Code of Ethics? How does my profession and my organization view and work upon health disparity? How am I working on social determinants of health for myself and for those whom I serve?
Ethics and the Practice of Brain Science	What or how does my profession interact with brain based tests and/or interventions? How does informed consent operate at my institution? How should informed consent operate at my institution? How will I be influenced through data analytics in the future?
Discourse	With whom do I talk about the brain, behavior, society, habilitation and rehabilitation and neuroethics? With whom should I be talking about these things? Have I chatted with family members about these issues? Have I chatted with fellow students about these issues?

FIGURE 10.1 The four impact areas of neuroethics related to interprofessional rehabilitation and habilitation: Reflective questions for rehabilitation professionals to ponder.

▶ Application

Before reading the following case, think about what informed consent means in research and in clinical practice and what ethical principles might be at stake when informed consent is not upheld. Then, begin to read the case of Henrietta.

Case of Henrietta

Part One

Henrietta was a second-generation German-American from a small town in the rural Midwest where only German was spoken until World War II. She was one of four children wherein the two girls scored better in high school than the two boys, but the boys were sent to college and the girls were not, as was the custom in that region. She excelled at teaching and met her first husband in Chicago while teaching other young women how to use Burroughs's adding machines. She and her husband had three children. After the death of her first husband, Henrietta remarried and retired in a small southern town in the middle south. Taking care of the house and her husband was Henrietta's great joy, along with gardening and church activities. Surviving all three of her siblings, she eventually moved to a religiously affiliated retirement home near her youngest child, outside of a major metropolitan Midwestern city. She lived there for many years, but lamented the loss of friends and siblings, as she had outlived them all. Her children visited regularly, but the most locally located child became her medical guardian while her only son assumed management of her finances.

She retained a wicked wit and indomitable spirit as she aged. She suffered a series of small strokes (transient ischemic attacks) but was able to function well within the setting of a retirement home community. Her ongoing prescription of Coumadin® for prevention of additional strokes was discontinued since she vehemently disliked the medication. For some years she continued to function in her one-bedroom setting.

In her retirement home, she was able to continue "independent living" with the assistance of a caretaker who did not live in, but spent at least eight hours a day attending to Henrietta's activities of daily living and other needs. This arrangement was tacitly supported by the retirement home. There were ongoing signs of general deterioration of her cognitive functions (such as , smaller and smaller handwriting, inability to write checks, and inability to master the use of a mouse and computer), but nothing that signaled major intellectual decline until a primary care physician saw her for only a few minutes, and pronounced that she had Alzheimer's disease. He had administered typical diagnostic tests and prescribed an Alzheimer's related medication, which was not tolerated by Henrietta. She had a long history of not tolerating many medications and was extremely sensitive to anesthesia.

Henrietta continued what was considered a "good" quality of life, living on her couch and eating her main meal in the dining room of the retirement home. She began to complain, however, that no one liked her there and that she missed her friends from the south (who were all dead, but she had forgotten).

In hindsight, it was clear that Henrietta's general intellectual decline due to Alzheimer's prevented her from engaging in ongoing conversations in the dining room, and that she was likely truly excluded from conversations with others who were considered "typical" or "normal." Her nearby daughter feared that soon she would not be able to carry her food from the service area to a table for dining purposes. Henrietta's general love of reading *The Wall Street Journal* every day from cover to cover declined. *The Wall Street Journal* was cancelled at her request. Slowly, the only television she could focus upon was Fox News and that became her all day news show.

One day, when the caretaker arrived at about 5:00 a.m., she found Henrietta confused, cold, and delirious on the floor of her closet. The caretaker called Henrietta's daughter who arrived immediately and then called an ambulance. Henrietta was admitted with a diagnosis of hip fracture to the local hospital where she stayed for nearly one week. The time spent in the community hospital was disorienting for Henrietta and she had mild hallucinations as an in-patient.

Henrietta became bedridden. Hospital personnel asked her daughter, who had medical authority, to decide what were to be the next steps. Here are the options that were provided:

1.   Do nothing. Discharge her and admit her to the nursing home facility of the retirement community wherein she had resided. The personnel predicted that she would likely develop pneumonia and then pass away.
2.   Enroll her in rehabilitation. She could be physically rehabilitated. There was no discussion of what life would be like for Henrietta following rehabilitation.

Henrietta had always been very clear that she neither wanted nor desired any extraordinary measure to prolong life and that she disdained most medical intervention. These values were shared by her siblings in that her brother had experienced kidney failure, tried dialysis once, but ultimately elected to discontinue dialysis. The daughter felt that there was no option but to enroll Henrietta in rehabilitation.

Case of Henrietta

Part Two

Thus, Henrietta was enrolled in three months of inpatient rehabilitation at the retirement home. It was painful and confusing for Henrietta. She was feisty at times with others but committed to her rehabilitation. Once she was deemed "rehabilitated" with consistent use of a walker, the next issue arose.

Where would she go? She would not be allowed back into independent living since she was no longer considered independent. Previously, even with her Alzheimer's diagnosis, she could cope in independent living only with the assistance of a day time caretaker (who was not allowed by retirement home policy to stay overnight). But she could no longer go to her apartment in independent living. She would be permitted to return to the retirement home, but only if she lived in the Memory Care Unit (for those diagnosed with Alzheimer's disease). She moved to that unit. Henrietta hated it. She called all others there "crazy" and believed she was the only one with a "good" brain. The unit was always locked and the door would be opened when a staff member finally responded to the buzzer.

When her daughter visited, she noticed that the patients were typically involved in a large group activity with one staff member while 3–4 other staff members spent time away from the patients. Thus, Henrietta's life became a "herd like" existence of doing whatever the group was doing, with little to no individualization except when her daughter visited. Henrietta had always said she would never, ever, live with one of her children. It was clear to the daughter, however, that Henrietta was quite miserable in this setting and the daughter invited Henrietta to come live in her nearby home. Henrietta had lived in the Memory Care Unit for about nine months.

Case of Henrietta
Part Three

Henrietta moved into the daughter's home. There was no bedroom on the main floor, so the main floor "office" was transformed into a bedroom. There was not a full bathroom on the main floor, but there was a half bath and a laundry room that would allow Henrietta to perform what she had previously called "cat washing" or a sponge bath.

At this point Henrietta was about 93 years old. She had cancers removed from her face by a local dermatologist. Henrietta developed ulcers on various parts of her legs that required "wound care treatment." A local primary care physician who had been practicing for many years instructed the daughter in wound care so that she could care for her mother at home. Henrietta also had congestive heart failure at this point.

Henrietta lived comfortably in her daughter's house during the last six months of her life. On the advice of the primary care physician, the daughter eventually purchased a hospital bed, placing it in the middle of the living room. In this manner, Henrietta had center stage of all family activities and full view of the gorgeous park-like back yard and bird feeder. Over the course of three to four months, Henrietta lost her ability to talk. Her favorite activity was watching the birds and listening to Willie Nelson. Finally, the daughter decided to request hospice services. She returned to her original primary care provider, who refused to certify hospice because he did not think Henrietta was near death. It should be noted, however, that the primary care physician was associated with a different nursing home and historically only certified individuals for hospice who were residents of the nursing home with which he was affiliated.

Fortunately, hospice was able to accomplish the certification and initiated accessible pain medication and home-based visits for Henrietta two times a week. She died peacefully in her sleep on November 22, after having a gourmet meal of beef burgundy and an evening with her daughter and caretaker.

Learning Point 10.7   Which of the four ethical traditions is represented most prominently in this case?

Learning Point 10.8   Recall the discussion in Chapter 7 of challenges in decision-making for elderly patients. In your opinion, is the daughter a good choice to provide substituted judgment for her mother?

Learning Point 10.9   Do you agree with hospital personnel that these would be the only options for Henrietta? Do you believe that the daughter made the correct decision? Why or why not?

Learning Point 10.10   Is it ethically acceptable for the physician to have this relationship with a particular hospice? What recommendations do you have from a policy perspective about conflicts of interest that affect health care?

The Case of Henrietta: Discussion

From an ethical perspective, this case is replete with challenges to personal autonomy in the myriad opportunities for decisions about, with, for or despite Henrietta. From a neuroethical perspective, there were neurological processes going on with the caregivers and professionals that occurred as with any value-based decision-making processes which are, to varying degrees, without conscious awareness. In part one of the case, the daughter and family process information about Henrietta's changing health condition, especially her diagnoses of Alzheimer's disease. Again, without complete conscious awareness of their own neurological states, they are confronted with positive memories, negative possible actions that may be necessary, Henrietta's wants and desires, and the seemingly cold and abrupt diagnosis by the physician, all of which were taking place in various nerve cells and pathways of the brain. Their thoughts, conversations, and conclusions about what information to share with Henrietta are influenced by events and process at social and neurological levels.

Learning Point 10.11 Should rehabilitation professionals routinely incorporate their own emotional and other neurological responses into reflection on ethical situations?

Over time, Henrietta's condition changed, as did the roles of family members. New and often contradictory circumstances or options emerged that produced new information resulting in frustration and emotional distress. In part two, the family has enrolled Henrietta in inpatient rehabilitation at the retirement home. The daughter observes Henrietta , must make discharge planning choices, transitions to the Memory Care Unit, and is continuously taking in ever-changing information about her mother. How many of the decisions made along the way were a matter of convenience or expedience? These are legitimate ethical concerns and questions that inevitably arise from these situations. Again, these events all occurred without complete conscious awareness of the ever- changing information and emotions generated in the nervous system. This information and these experiences influence the nervous system at the cellular levels and pathways, ultimately influencing the decisions made and actions taken.

Once home (Part three) the daughter and caregiver take in additional intimate and pervasive information—sad and funny; frustrating and harmonious; enlightening and confusing—about Henrietta. The information has changed yet again; in some cases, contradicted by previous information; memories have faded, and new ones have emerged. While some emotions have been blunted, others are sharpened. We will leave to the reader ethical analysis regarding the decisions and actions taken in this case and whether Henrietta's autonomy was supported.

Learning Point 10.12 Was the daughter able to support "relational autonomy" (see chapter 7) for Henrietta throughout the multiple challenges?

Retrospectively, neuroethics contributes to this case through the potential for understanding what and how appraisal of information, emotional valence attached to information, anticipation of the consequences of action, prospective, episodic, and working memory affects decision making and thus potential insights into the ultimate action taken. Prospectively, one can use what has been learned through neuroethics to educate and even influence decision making and decision makers about neuroethical issue. For example, what was the effect of the potential conflict of interest on the decision making of the primary care physician who had refused to approve hospice care for Henrietta from a neuroethical perspective?

We often think of ethical cases as single events or phenomena, somewhat like a still photograph, which depicts a static, isolated situation such as whether a daughter has the right to place her mother in a nursing home without the mother's consent. The narrative of Henrietta, however, is more like a video which spanned the last two years of her life. Like many rehabilitation and habilitation cases, Henrietta's narrative was also a story of her family, of caregiver's stories, and therapists' stories. Her narrative was of multiple decisions, some ethically charged and others mundane, and services that ebbed and flowed throughout the narrative and that could never be fully understood as multiple still photographs. This case, therefore, presents the narrative arc of Henrietta's rehabilitation.

Learning Point 10.13   Consider the perspective that each of the ethical traditions provides on Henrietta's journey. How does this case illustrate the limitations of a singular focus on ethical principles and the Rule-Based tradition?

▶ Implications

Given this wide-ranging consideration of neuroethics, what are the additional implications that should be addressed? First, the active role of both perspectives of neuroethics in the Dialogic Engagement Model is acknowledged. The ethics of neuroscience related to neuroscience and translational research can be understood using the Dialogic Engagement Model (DEM). Also, the neurosciences of ethics, or how the brain works to process ethical decision making, underpins workings of the Dialogic Engagement Model. The DEM adopts not just a rationalistic process of thinking, but also incorporates intuitive and affective understandings of moral reasoning that have been highlighted by Felix (2014). Thus, the Dialogic Engagement Model takes us beyond limited rationalistic thinking and allows for incorporation of thinking, feeling and sensing in the neuroethical process of moral reasoning. The Dialogic Engagement Model includes dialogue and ethical deliberation toward resolution within the interprofesisonal moral commons. It is accessible and available for use by one and all as a process to address moral conundrums in their own right, but also moral conundrums that become difficult to address in interprofessional settings.

Second, neuroethics, as a way of enlightening the decision-making process, can be applied to any ethical tradition. It is not dependent upon a particular perspective, condition, or context of the moral conundrum. For our case example of Henrietta, a Narrative-Based tradition was used, but the same ethical elements can be found and addressed when using Rule-Based traditions, Ends-Based traditions, and Virtue-Based traditions. Neuroethics, therefore, accommodates the pluralism of multiple ethical traditions as manifest in decision making within the moral commons.

Third, the title of this chapter introduced the concept of neuroethics and the perplexed. That is, for some period of time we shall all struggle to define and refine our notions of the ethics of neuroscience and the neuroscience of ethics, particularly as applied using the Dialogic Engagement Model. As we grow within this process, uncertainty will reign, with perplexity being a constant companion. Just as wisdom incorporates tolerance for ambiguity, neuroethics with the moral commons using the Dialogic Engagement Model incorporates tolerance for iterations. That is, individuals and teams will work through, and repeatedly work through—again and again—moral deliberations where there is rarely a defined end point, but rather, a critical juncture in the narrative arc of an ethical story.

Fourth and finally, all in education are challenged to consider how best to incorporate neuroethics and the Dialogic Engagement Model into our educational milieu, regardless of profession or discipline or degree of interprofessional collaboration of the setting.

▶ Summary and Conclusion

This chapter on neuroethics has presented terms and concepts related to neuroethics applied to interprofessional rehabilitation and habilitation. Rehabilitation and habilitation, interfield theory, and neuroethics were defined and discussed. Additionally, neuroethics as applied to rehabilitation and habilitation in the context of interprofessional practice was considered. A short history of neuroethics was presented. How neuroethics applies to interprofessional habilitation and rehabilitation was discussed with a multipart case study of Henrietta reflecting upon the episodic nature of rehabilitation and habilitation over a narrative arc. How neuroethics helps to explain and inform the ethical decision-making process was explored. Finally, implications for neuroethics and habilitation and rehabilitation were delineated.

Closing Reflections

Learning Activities

10.1 Data analytics is mentioned in this chapter as related to neuroethics. Explore how data analytics is being used across disciplines and postulate how it may be used in interprofessional rehabilitation.

10.2 Explore parts of the central nervous system associated with problem solving and ethical reasoning, an aspect of neuroethics.

10.3 Why is rationality insufficient for solid ethical reasoning that should include feeling and intuition as well?

10.4 What do you see as the single largest impact of neuroethics on society? Why?

10.5 Review your professional Code of Ethics and confirm whether or not there are parts of it that may be related to neuroethics.

10.6 How is the concept of quality of life related to habilitation and rehabilitation?

10.7 Discuss how the narrative arc of a story of rehabilitation unfolds over time and identify why static points in time are chosen for ethical analysis.

10.8 How can you educate decision makers about neuroethics?

10.9 How does the Dialogic Engagement Model fit with neuroethics?

10.10 In the case of Henrietta, was there a conflict of interest for the primary care physician?

Take Away Messages

- Interprofessional collaborative practice is the heart of neuroethics.
- There has been an explosion of neuroethical scholarship since the 1990s.
- Interfield theory is an important dimension of integrating knowledge and understanding across two fields.
- The ethics of neuroscience relates to the doing of neuroscience in an ethical manner.
- The neuroscience of ethics relates to ongoing learning of how the brain functions to process moral deliberations.
- Neuroethics impacts society at the levels of science and the self, science and social policy, ethics and the practice of brain science, and discourse.
- It is important to talk about neuroethics with friends, family, leadership, and legislators.
- Discourse is an important part of neuroethics and the Dialogic Engagement Model.
- Occupational scientists would state that habilitation is an issue of occupational justice.
- The case of Henrietta illustrates an iterative process of ongoing ethical issues within a narrative arc.
- Neuroethics is a dynamic and evolving field that refers to the ethics of doing neuroscience or the neuroscience of ethics. The latter refers to how our understanding of the brain's function affects ethical decision making and moral behavior. The first sense of the term neuroethics might be viewed as its inward-looking face, while the second sense may be viewed as the outward-looking face that uses interfield theory to bridge neuroscience, brain research, and philosophy.
- Interfield theory brings different disciplines together to address questions that neither field alone is able to address. Neuroethics represents interfield theory that bridges neuroscience and ethics. Interfield theory is also relevant to interprofessional ethics.
- The four societal impact areas of neuroethics are science and the self, science and social policy, ethics and the practice of brain science, and discourse (Lombera, 2009).
- Habilitation and rehabilitation represent a life process with recurring episodes of challenges to the recipient's sense of self and to the interprofessional team's sense of what is morally good. So, to understand interprofessional habilitation or rehabilitation is to understand the recipient's story and to become aware of related moral questions.
- Neuroethics contributes retrospectively to ethical case analysis through the potential for understanding what and how appraisal of information; emotional valence attached to information; and anticipation of the consequences of action, prospective, episodic, and working memory affects decision making and thus potential insights into the ultimate action taken. Prospectively, one can use what has been learned through neuroethics to educate and even influence decision making and decision makers about neuroethical issues.
- Neuroethics, as a way of enlightening the decision-making process, can be applied to any ethical tradition. Neuroethics, therefore, accommodates the pluralism of multiple ethical traditions as manifested in decision making within the moral commons.

References

Arkowitz, H., & Lilienfeld, S. O. (2010). Do the "eyes" have it? *Scientific American Mind, 20*(7), 68–69.

Ballard, I. C., Murty, V. P., Carter, R. M., MacInnes, J. J., Huettel, S. A., & Adcock, R. A. (2011). Dorsolateral prefrontal cortex drives mesolimbic dopaminergic regions to initiate motivated behavior. *The Journal of Neuroscience, 31*(28), 10340–10346.

Barwell, I. (2009). Understanding narratives and narrative understanding. *The Journal of Aesthetics and Art Criticism, 67*(1), 49–59.

Bechara, A. (2004). The role of emotion in decision-making: Evidence from neurological patients with orbitofrontal damage. *Brain and Cognition, 55*, 30–40.

Berg, S. M. van den (2002). *Prospective memory: From intention to action.* Rotterdam, Netherlands: Universiteit Eindhoven.

Berkman, E., Livingson, J. L., & Kahn, L. E. (2015). Finding the 'self' in self-regulation: The Identity-Value Model. *Psychological Inquiry.* http://dx.doi.org/10.2139/ssrn.2621251

Camerer, C., Loewenstein, G., & Prelec, D. (2005). Neuroeconomics: How neuroscience can inform economics. *Journal of Economic Literature, 43*(1), 9–64.

Chatterjee, A. (2011). Neuroethics: A coming of age story. *Journal of Cognitive Neuroscience, 234*, 53–62.

Chudler, E. (2017, January 26). *Neuroscience for kids.* Retrieved from https://faculty.washington.edu/chudler/neuroe.html

Conway, B.R., & Rehding, A. (2013) Neuroaesthetics and the trouble with beauty. *PLOS Biology, 11*(3), e1001504.

Cowen, S. L., Davis, G. A., & Nitz, D. A. (2012). Anterior cingulate neurons in the rat map anticipated effort and reward to their associated action sequences. *Journal of Neurophysiology, 107*(9), 2393–2407. doi:10.1152/jn.01012.2011

Crabtree, J. L. (2011). Neuro-occupation: The confluence of neuroscience and occupational therapy. *Japanese Journal of Occupational Therapy, 45*(7), 879–886.

Craver, C. F. (2005). Beyond reduction: Mechanisms, multifield integration and the unity of neuroscience. *Studies in History and Philosophy of Biological and Biomedical Sciences, 36*(2), 373–395.

Darden, L., & Mull, N. (1977). Interfield theories. *Philosophy of Science, 44*(1), 43–64.

Darragh, M., Buniak, L., & Giordano, J. (2015). A four-part working bibliography of neuroethics: Part 2 – Neuroscientific studies of morality and ethics. *Philosophy, Ethics and Humanities in Medicine, 10*, 2. doi:10.1186/s13010-015-0022-0.

DeSanctis, C. H. (2012). Narrative reasoning and analogy: The untold story. *Legal Communication & Rhetoric: JALWD, 9*, 149–171.

Dimitrov, A. G., Lazar, A. A., & Victor, J. D. (2011). Information theory in neuroscience. *Journal of Computational Neuroscience, 30*(1), 1–5.

Farah, M. J. (2005). Neuroethics: The practical and the philosophical. *Trends in Cognitive Sciences, 9*(1), 34–40.

Farah, M. J. (2008). Neuroethics and the problem of other minds: Implications of neuroscience for the moral status of brain-damaged patients and nonhuman animals. *Neuroethics, 1*(1), 9–18.

Farrah, M. J. (2013). Neuroethics: A guide for the perplexed. *Cerebrum,* Retrieved from http://dana.org/Cerebrum/2004/neuroethics-A-Guide_for_the _perplexed

Felix, J. (2014). Education for ethical decision making: The contribution of neuroethics. In J. Reichel (Ed.), *CST trends: Beyond business as usual.* Todz, Poland: CSR Import.

Fischer, G., & Sullivan, J. P. J. (2002, June). *Human-centered public transportation systems for persons with cognitive disabilities.* Paper presented at the 7th Biennial Participatory Design Conference, Malmø, Sweden.

Friston, K. (2012). The history of the future of the Bayesian brain. *Neuroimage, 62*(2), 1230–1233.

Friston, K., FitzGerald, T., Rigoli, F., Schwartenbeck, P., & Pezzulo, G. (2016). Active inference: A process theory. *Neural Computation, 21*(8). doi:10.1162/NECO_a_00912

Glen, A. L., & Raine, M. A. (2014). Neurocriminology: Implications for the punishment, prediction, and prevention of criminal behavior. *Nature Reviews Neuroscience, 15*, 54–63. doi:10.1038/nrn3640.

Gold, J. I., & Shadlen, M. N. (2007). The neural basis of decision making. *Annual Reviews of Neuroscience, 30*, 535–574. doi:10.1146/annurev.neuro.29.051605.113038

Gordon, R., & Ciorciari, J. (2017). Social marketing research and cognitive neuroscience. In K. Kubacki & S. Rundle-Thiele (Eds.), *Formative research in social marketing: Innovative methods to gain consumer insights* (pp. 145–163). Singapore: Springer Singapore.

Greene, J. D., Nystrom, L. E., Engell, A. D., Darley, J. M., & Cohen, J. D. (2004). The neural bases of cognitive conflict and control in moral judgement. *Neuron, 44*, 389–400.

Guastello, S. J. (2015). The complexity of the psychological self and the principle of optimum variability. *Nonlinear Dynamics, Psychology, and Life Sciences, 19*(4), 511–527.

Guitart-Masip, M., Duzel, E., Dolan, R., & Dayan, P. (2014). Action versus valence in decision making. *Trends in Cognitive Sciences, 18*(4), 194–202.

Habilitate. (n.d.). English Oxford Living Dictionaries online. Retrieved from https://en.oxforddictionaries.com/definition/habilitate

Hauser, M., Cushman, F., Young, L., Kang-Xing, R., & Mikhail, J. (2006). A dissociation between moral judgments and justifications. *Mind & Language, 22*(1), 1–21.

Hu, J., Wang, T., Yin, J., & Wang, Y. (2011, October). Neuroethics: A research report from Chinese investigation. Presented at Internal Conference on Photonics, 3D – Imaging, and Visualization, Guangzhou, China. https://doi:10.1117/12.906102

Illes, J., & Bird, S. J. (2006). Neuroethics: a modern context for ethics in neuroscience. *Trends in Neurosciences, 29*(9), 511–517.

International Neuroethics Society. (2016). *Basics of neuroethics*. Retrieved from http://www.neuroethicssociety.org/

Jennings, B. (1995). Healing the self: The moral meaning of relationships in rehabilitation. *American Journal of Physical Medicine & Rehabilitation, 74*(1 Suppl), S25–S28.

Knight, L. (2010). *Spirit in action: Jane Addams.* New York, NY: WW Norton.

Koenigs, M., Kruepke, M., & Newman, J. P. (2010). Economic decision-making in psychopathy: A comparison with ventromedial prefrontal lesion patients. *Neuropsychologia, 48*(7), 2198–2204.

Lazzarini, I. (2004). Neuro-occupation: The nonlinear dynamics of intention, meaning and perception. *British Journal of Occupational Therapy, 67*(8), 342–352. doi:10.1177.030802260700803

Loftus, E. F. (1997). Creating false memories. *Scientific American, 277*(3), 70–75.

Lohman, H., & Royeen, C. (2002). Posttraumatic stress disorder and traumatic hand injuries: A neuro-occupational view. *American Journal of Occupational Therapy, 56*(5), 527–537.

Lombera, S., & Illes, J. (2009). The international dimensions of neuroethics. *Developing World Bioethics, 9*(2), 57–64. doi:10.1111/j.1471-8847.2008.00235.x

Mattingly, C. (1991). The narrative nature of clinical reasoning. *American Journal of Occupational Therapy, 45*(11), 998–1005.

Meyer, A. (1957). *Psychobiology: A science of man.* Springfield, IL: Charles C. Thomas, Publisher.

Naqvi, N., Shiv, B., & Bechara, A. (2006). The role of emotion in decision making: A cognitive neuroscience perspective. *Current Directions in Psychological Science, 15*(5), 260–264. doi:10.1111/j.1467-8721.2006.00448.x

Padilla, R., & Peyton, C. G. (1997). Neuro-occupation: Historical review and examples. In C. B. Royeen (Ed.), *Neuroscience & occupation: Links to practice.* Bethesda, MD: American Occupational Therapy Association.

Pascalev, A., Pascalev, M., & Giordano, J. (2016). Head transplants, personal identity and neuroethics. *Neuroethics, 9*(1), 15–22.

President of the United States (Bush). (1990). *The decade of the brain 1990–1999.* Washington, DC: Library of Congress.

Purtilo, R. B. (2000). Moral courage in times of change: Visions for the future. *Journal of Physical Therapy Education, 14*(3), 4–6.

Rabadan, A. T. (2015). Neuoethics scope at a glance. *Surgical Neurology International, 6*, 183.

Rangel, A., Camerer, C., & Montague, P. R. (2008). A framework for studying the neurobiology of value-based decision making. *Nature Reviews in Neuroscience, 9*, 1–13.

Roskies, Adina L. (2002). Neuroethics for the new millenium. *Neuron, 35*(1), 21–23. doi:10.1016/S0896-6273(02)00763-8

Sanfey, A. G., Loewenstein, G., McMclure, S. M., & Cohen, J. D. (2006). Neuroeconomics: Cross-currents in research on decision-making. *Trends in Cognitive Neuroscience, 10*(3). doi:10.1016/j.tics2006.01.009

Schmitz, T. W., & Johnson, S. C. (2007). Relevance to self: A brief review and framework of neural systems underlying appraisal. *Neuroscience & Biobehavioral Reviews, 31*(4), 585–596.

Shrivastava, M., & Behari, M. (2015). Neuroethics: A moral approach towards neuroscience research. *Archives of Neuroscience, 2*(1):e19224. doi:10.5812/archneurosci.19224

Sobhani, M., & Bechara, A. (2011). A somatic marker perspective of immoral and corrupt behavior. *Social Neuroscience, 6*(5–6), 640–652.

Solway, A., & Botvinick, M. M. (2012). Goal-directed decision making as probabilistic inference: a computational framework and potential neural correlates. *Psychological Review, 119*(1), 120.

Thomasma, D. C., & Pellegrino, E.D. (1981). Philosophy of medicine as the source for medical ethics. *Metamedicine, 2*(1), 5–11.

Umeda, S., Tochizawa, S., Shibata, M., & Terasawa, Y. (2016). Prospective memory mediated by interoceptive accuracy: a psychophysiological approach. *Philosophical Transactions of the Royal Society B: Biological Sciences, 371*(1708). doi:10.1098/rstb.2016.0005

Vossel, S., Weidner, R., Driver, J., Friston, K. J., & Fink, G. R. (2012). Deconstructing the architecture of dorsal and ventral attention systems with dynamic causal modeling. *The Journal of Neuroscience, 32*(31), 10637–10648.

World Health Organization. (2010). *Framework for action on interprofessional education & collaborative practice.* Geneva, Switzerland: Author.

Yoon, C., Gonzalez, R., Bechara, A., Berns, G. S., Dagher, A. A., Dubé, L., & Plassmann, H. (2012). Decision neuroscience and consumer decision making. *Marketing Letters, 23*(2), 473–485.

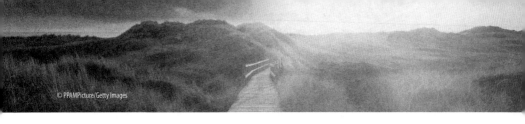

CHAPTER 11

The Future of Interprofessional Rehabilitation Ethics

Laura Lee Swisher and **Charlotte Brasic Royeen**

CHAPTER OBJECTIVES

At the conclusion of this chapter, the reader will be able to:

1. Discuss the future of rehabilitation ethics from a historical perspective.
2. Describe ethical issues that may be important for interprofessional rehabilitation practice in the future.
3. Discuss organizational ethics as the "elephant in the room" for interprofessional ethics.
4. Describe actions that rehabilitation professionals might take to break the moral silence and create the moral commons.

KEY TERMS

Reading these key terms before reading the chapter will introduce you to key concepts which will then be somewhat familiar to you as you read this chapter. This is an important learning technique that will enhance your learning as a multi-step process. You may even wish to make a flash card set of key terms and quiz yourself on them once or twice before reading the chapter. This will better prepare you to immerse in the language of ethics and better prepare you to integrate the content.

Everyday Ethics: The ethics of day to day practice which includes issues of relationships, organizational policies, team dynamics, turf wars, power, hierarchy, and other daily events. Everyday ethics stands in contrast to some preconceptions of ethics as classic ethical dilemmas addressing "life and death" situations.

Ethics Grand Rounds: An approach to ethical reflection whereby interprofessional or professional team members meet to discuss a patient case involving ethics, often a case involving an ethical dilemma. This process is often facilitated by an ethics expert.

Moral Case Deliberation (MCD): A structured model for ethical reflection developed in Europe that brings together members of the healthcare team to engage in a reflective and dialogic process with the goal of improving the quality of care (van der Dam et al., 2013, p. 126). Moral case deliberation differs from previous ethics approaches in its focus on the collective rather than the individual, everyday ethics versus topical cases, and on reflective dialogue versus decision making. MCD typically uses a facilitator to assist with the dialogic process. (See also "moral deliberation" in an earlier chapter.)

Organizational Ethics: Ethical issues that arise as a result of organizational structures, leadership, management, stakeholders and processes (Gibson, 2012). Also includes the goals, values, outcomes, and obligations. Gibson notes that an important consideration for organizational ethics in health care is balancing competing organizational goals of quality and financial well-being (Gibson, 2012, p. 37). An important characteristic of organizational ethics is its focus on collective entities and structures.

Paradigm: A systematic mental model that provides theoretical foundations for viewing a discipline. A paradigm suggests questions and issues to explore and resolve, and may become obsolete, necessitating a "paradigm shift" (Kuhn, 1970). The shift from Newtonian physics to the physics of relativity is an example of a paradigm shift.

Relational Ethics: Relational ethics grew out of the work of Carol Gilligan (1982) whose research indicated that women approached ethical decisions from the perspective of care and relationships versus abstract principles. The resulting "ethics of care" perspective has been associated with narrative and "voice." Ewashen et al. (2013, p. 327) describe four themes of relational ethics: relational engagement and connectedness, mutual respect, embodiment, and environment.

Topical Approach to Ethics: Approach to identification of ethical issues that categorizes issues based on topics (for example, end of life, confidentiality).

▶ Historical Context

In an article written in 1952, a leading rehabilitation physician, Arthur Watkins (1952), wrote a short article on the current trends in medicine and rehabilitation. Review of this article reveals that the current state of affairs today is much different than nearly 60 years ago. At that time, the physiatrist was the primary health professional responsible for rehabilitation and occupational therapy and physical therapy were considered "ancillary personnel" (1952). Speech language pathologists and others who may participate in rehabilitation teams of today were not even mentioned. At that time there were 31 educational programs in physical therapy and 24 programs in occupational therapy in the United States. Today, there are nearly 242 accredited professional level programs in physical therapy (Commission on Accreditation in Physical Therapy Education [CAPTE], n.d.) and 182 programs in occupational therapy (American Occupational Therapy Association, 2018). How things have changed!

Learning Point 11.1   How has your profession changed since its birth?

The dramatic increase in the number of educational programs in occupational and physical therapy (not without including speech language pathologists) correlates with the astounding statistic that one of every five U.S. citizens has a disability (U.S. Department of Health and Human Services, 2016). As the need for services has grown based upon the increased population, so has the number of educational programs in these areas. An additional variable that has affected personnel needs relates to the fact that most people with disabilities of today have comorbid conditions, which are existing health problems in addition to the disability. The presence of a disability plus comorbid conditions puts pressure on educational programs to educate professionals not only in rehabilitation but also in the myriad of co-morbid conditions that exist, including but not limited to diabetes, obesity, high blood pressure, and asthma.

Related to this, the future of rehabilitation is tied to the financial change occurring in health care. In 2001, individuals with disabilities constituted 50% of contact time with healthcare professionals, and 80% of healthcare costs overall (Greenwood, 2001). Accordingly, rehabilitation professionals will need to be conversant with health economics and that has further implications for our educational programming in these areas. Such financial literacy has not been a focus of our educational programs to date.

As stated, rehabilitation professions have evolved considerably since their birth during the 20th century. At the same time, healthcare delivery has undergone significant changes. Changes in professional identity and in healthcare delivery shape the ethical situations that occur, and our responsibility as professionals for those situations.

Learning Point 11.2   How has professional identity of your profession changed from its early days to current times?

In contrast to the picture provided by Watkins in 1952, many rehabilitations professions have secured some degree of professional autonomy in decision making. Although rehabilitation professionals may no longer be obligated to work directly under physician orders, all healthcare providers experience organizational and reimbursement constraints on their decisions. Organizational pressure for productivity and efficiency will undoubtedly continue to be a part of ethical issues in rehabilitation. Current reimbursement models in the United States demand that rehabilitation professionals have the economic, organizational, and policy skills to navigate a fragmented and complex healthcare system.

Learning Point 11.3   What are examples of fragmentation of the healthcare system?

At the same time, healthcare patients and clients are seeking a more active role in partnering with healthcare providers in determining their care.

▶ Chapter Overview

This text has described the historical evolution of interprofessional rehabilitation ethics, proposed the Dialogic Engagement Model for addressing interprofessional ethical issues, and applied the Dialogic Engagement Model to selected ethical issues based on setting or age. Of course, this discussion should not be considered exhaustive – as there are many settings and population groups that have not been addressed using the Dialogic Engagement Model. Our hope is that the reader will be able to apply the model to the patients and clients with whom they work. A major theme of this book is that the ethical approaches of the past may be inadequate to the current organizational and interprofessional environment. The list that follows indicates the ways in which the ethical models of the past may be inadequate for the current and future ethical issues confronting rehabilitation and healthcare professionals. The past has been focused upon:

1. Interpersonal ethical issues within the individual realm
2. Moral reasoning – deciding what the individual professional should do rather than moral deliberation by a group and subsequent team action
3. Uniprofessional perspectives about ethics rather than interprofessional team ethics
4. The topical content of ethical decisions rather than process thereof or relational issues
5. Ethics in isolation rather than the variation caused by organizational context in ethics
6. Ignoring issues of power differentials and top-down hierarchy that may undermine moral agency
7. Decontextualized "big ethical issues" rather than everyday ethics playing out pertaining to a particular individual at particular points in time within particular social or organizational contexts

Regarding the past focus upon the "individual realm," the Dialogic Engagement Model represents an "aspirational" model and a call to rehabilitation professionals to transform rehabilitation practice through team moral agency attending to multiple realms of ethics.

In his ground-breaking book, *The Structure of Scientific Revolutions*, Thomas Kuhn (1970) discussed the manner in which prevailing scientific models ("paradigms") work change. He argued that a prevailing "paradigm" provides a framework for agreements, discussion, and implicit questions to guide work. Every paradigm, however, has limitations and will inevitably fail in its assumptions and guidance, necessitating a new paradigm. The shift from Newtonian physics to theories of relativity is an example of this shift in paradigms.

Learning Point 11.4   Has health care previously undergone paradigm shifts with regard to its financing and delivery? Do you agree that the shift to value-based care would constitute a paradigm change?

The current shift in healthcare systems from fee-for-service to value-based care is another paradigm shift. In Kuhn's description, as a paradigm becomes more inadequate to emerging questions, other frameworks emerge and compete for commitment. One might argue that the emergence of principlism and the subsequent proliferation of competing theories (discussed in an earlier chapter), represents questioning of a dominant ethical paradigm and the foreshadowing of a paradigm revolution. The inadequacies of the traditional principle-based paradigm of ethics have undoubtedly been magnified by significant changes in the healthcare system over the last 50 years.

As previously discussed, the dominant paradigm or model of healthcare ethics that emerged in the 1970s may not be adequate to address the ethical situations that are emerging in interprofessional health care. This is especially true for the rehabilitation professions, many of whom were still in their infancy during the 1970s. The question as to whether interprofessional ethics is something entirely new (Schmitt & Stewart, 2011) or whether it is simply the same paradigm applied to a new area is important because the answer to this question has practical implications for approaching ethical situations. Whether or not healthcare ethics is undergoing a paradigm shift, we are undeniably in a time of significant challenges for interprofessional ethical dialogue.

Learning Point 11.5   Do the Code of Ethics and other ethical guidelines in your profession provide guidance for interprofessional ethical situations?

These challenges require changes in the process by which we address ethical issues. In this chapter, we provide suggestions for addressing interprofessional ethical situations in this new world.

Learning Point 11.6   What ethical obligations do members of the interprofessional tam owe to one another?

▶ "Topical Approach" to Interprofessional Rehabilitation Ethics

In thinking about the future of rehabilitation ethics, rehabilitation professionals often consider topical ethical issues that professionals will encounter. The topical approach to looking at the future of rehabilitation ethics attempts to determine the ethical concepts that professionals should have a thorough understanding and

TABLE 11.1 Potential Future Interprofessional Ethical Issues in Rehabilitation (Not Exhaustive)

Discharge Planning	Family Dynamics	Boundaries	Informed Consent
Scope of Practice & Turf Wars	Social Media	Patient Abuse	Shared Decision Making
Reimbursement Pressures	Research Ethics	Health Disparities	Confidentiality
Productivity	Leadership	Economic Disparities	Conflicts of Interest
Impact of Technology	Autonomy	Goal-setting	Healthcare Policy
Telehealth	Truth-telling	Team Dynamics	Big Data

ability to act upon. **TABLE 11.1** provides some examples of ethical topics that may be important in the future. Of course, this list is not exhaustive and there are many other ethical issues that may become important in the future. In the following paragraphs, we discuss several ethical issues that we believe will continue to be important for rehabilitation professionals.

Learning Point 11.7   What specific interprofessional ethical topics have been important in your profession? How do you think that these may change for the future?

▶ Future Ethical Issues in Rehabilitation Ethics

Goal-setting has historically been a central process for rehabilitation professionals because rehabilitation professionals typically establish goals for the plan of care treatment. Goals reflect desired outcomes from the perspective of the patient, the rehabilitation professional, and the rehabilitation team (in some settings). Reimbursement for treatment may also be tied to accomplishment of goals established for treatment. Given the central role that goal-setting has played in rehabilitation, it is surprising that there has been relatively little examination of the theoretical and ethical foundations for goal-setting. Establishing goals for rehabilitation have been assumed to have a variety of purposes. These include (Levack, Dean, Siegert, & McPherson, 2006; Levack & Dean, 2012, p. 94):

1. Involving the patient and the family
2. Facilitating patient autonomy and patient-centered care

3. Improving communication and relationships between patients, families, and professionals
4. Establishing outcomes
5. Improving teamwork
6. Supporting patient's adaptation, and:
7. Complying with legal, regulatory, or contractual requirements

As Levack et al. (2006) note, these multiple purposes of the goal-setting process may at times conflict.

Learning Point 11.8 Have you experienced conflict in an interprofessional team regarding goals? How did you resolve the conflict?

Notwithstanding the presumed value of goal-setting, a study of goal-setting by Levack et al. (2011) for patients after a stroke, revealed the existence of what he called "privileged goals." The term privileged goals refers to goals that were "prioritized or promoted" by the team because the goals had one of these three qualities: 1) focused on function, 2) had short timeframe for achievement, or 3) provided a conservative estimate of progress. The same study indicated that rather than promoting patient or family involvement, goal setting was often driven by professional or organizational priorities.

Learning Point 11.9 What is an example of professional or organizational priorities that might drive patient goals?

Additionally, goals that patients or families shared with the team were not integrated into the plan. For that reason, some organizations are now including the patient or family in team meetings. Early on in practice the second author experienced a case of privileged goals, or a goal set by the team and not the family. That is, in a public school setting a youth with paraplegia was expected to ambulate with canes. At home, the occupational therapist was surprised to discover that the family carried this youth around the house. In their culture, showing love and care by carrying the youth had greater importance than the therapist's goal of independent ambulation across school-based settings.

Levack (2009) examined goal setting using a utilitarian (Ends-Based) perspective. From an ethical perspective, goal-setting is often framed as facilitating patient autonomy. Levack argues that resource constraints justify selecting more limited goals based on the good of the entire community. At the same time, he acknowledges that this utilitarian perspective could result in discrimination or undermining the therapeutic relationship.

Goal setting will continue to play an important role in rehabilitation. As the previous discussion suggests, we are still in the early stages of understanding goal-setting. The fact that goal-setting is often performed by teams raises additional questions about team dynamics, involvement of the patient and family, purposes of goal-setting, conflicts that arise in the process, and a variety of other questions.

A second related ethical issue is balancing the competing demands of evidence-based practice (EBP) and patient centered care. Rehabilitation professionals have generally committed to the EBP model. However, there are aspects of the

EBP that present challenges for rehabilitation. For example, the focus of rehabilitation on function and disability presents challenges for conducting random studies. Additionally, one might argue that including "patient preferences" does not fully capture the collaborative process of goal negotiation necessary for rehabilitation professionals. Notwithstanding the fact that rehabilitation goals may, as Levack suggests, in reality be "privileged goals," consideration of patient preference or values represents a relatively weak commitment to patient centered care.

Learning Point 11.10   In your experience, to what extent are rehabilitation goals patient-centered?

Additionally, one might argue that the focus on evidence suggested by the term EBP represents a return to the ethics of paternalism where professionals are experts who are making decisions for their patients. This is further complicated by the fact that patients are in most cases not actively engaged in formulating research questions or interpreting research results that inform EBP (Brighton et al., 2018). Of course, others argue that "true EBP" includes a robust partnering and collaboration with the patient, especially as many patients are well-versed in the evidence. Nevertheless, there is a need for rehabilitation professionals to refine the EBP model to meet the needs of professional practice.

Learning Point 11.11   How did you personally incorporate the patient in making decisions?

A related area for future focus is rehabilitation research. The area of rehabilitation research is growing. Generally, rehabilitation research is seeking ways to regain function that has been lost (NIH, 2016). In this text, we have focused upon a tool (Dialogic Engagement Model) that can bring varied professionals and caretakers and others together in order to address the client and family needs to improve the life condition as they deem it necessary – not as we as professionals deem it necessary. Thus, rehabilitation research may address regaining lost function, but it may also include environmental and social redesign to allow for the person with the lost function to better operate in this world. We are not necessarily promoting the recapture of lost function…but are advocating for teams as well as research to work towards what the family and /or client need and want. Thus, we are, with this text, looking to expand the notion of rehabilitation to include not just restoration of function, but also effective and efficient ways to cope with lost function in order to achieve the quality of life (Schnall, 2016).

We hope that rehabilitation research will expand to include research into how the Dialogic Engagement Model can, and does promote a moral commons to allow for the team and the client and family to determine what needs should be addressed in rehabilitation. Such action would place ethics and the moral commons as front and center in any consideration of rehabilitation research. Additionally, this approach might expand the area considerably beyond a focus on outcomes to a focus on meeting client and family needs that may extend well beyond traditional notions of rehabilitation.

Why is this so important? In the United States in 2016 one in every five citizens had a disability (U.S. Department of Health and Human Services, 2016). This translates to 56.7 million individuals and 22.2% of the adult population. Traditional limitations to rehabilitation research including limitations in transportation, mobility, finances, and access to information that allows for participation in rehabilitation research studies (U.S. Department of Health and Human Services, 2016). With such an explosion of persons with disabilities, perhaps our past notions of rehabilitation research in laboratories and specialty clinics needs to be expanded to include living, working, and recreational environments, i.e., study of the individuals with disability in context. Further, the existing research methods of controlled clinical trials may not be consistent with the needs and situations of those with disabilities. At the policy level, rehabilitation research receives limited funding to address functional limitations and disability when compared with dollars dedicated to pharmacology, surgery, and medical interventions. Thus, new and innovative methodologies need to be developed to allow for authentic research in rehabilitation. Such change would result in another paradigm shift related to the field.

Another aspect of rehabilitation that will likely change in the future is the number of individuals undergoing rehabilitation due to cancer (Fu, 2017). The current rehabilitation focus on physical disabilities will expand to include psychical and psychosocial disabilities brought on by the presence of cancer.

Ongoing changes in how the federal government expects research data to be available and open to all for research speaks to the need for our educational programs to training future researchers in rehabilitation fields in the areas of data analytics and big data. For the open access and integration of research data sets, what Babbage (2014) calls "open and abundant data," will allow for new and innovative methods of statistical interpretation to guide practice.

The development of relevant models of informed consent and shared decision making represent another issue that rehabilitation professionals must address. The traditional medical model for informed consent presents challenges for rehabilitation professionals because it focuses on discrete encounters or procedures rather than a period of interaction with multiple processes, as occurs during rehabilitation. Further work is needed so that rehabilitation professionals are more effective in obtaining informed consent (Delany, 2007) and also in developing informed consent practices for team environments. In that regard, the idea of shared decision making represents a promising development of the idea of informed consent (Delany & Galvin, 2014; Kaizer, Spiridigliozzi, & Hunt, 2012; Korner, Ehrhardt, & Steger, 2013; Rose, Rosewilliam, & Soundy, 2017) Development of robust team processes for informed consent and shared decision making will be important for the future of interprofessional rehabilitation ethics.

Learning Point 11.12 Should shared decision making be implemented in rehabilitation? What does that mean?

Another rehabilitation ethical future issue is the role of technology. This includes using social media, electronic health record, telehealth, and big data. Advances in these areas have the potential to increase efficiency, extend the care of patients, provide insight into outcomes, and create new avenues for intervention. At the same time, technological advances have the potential to challenge traditional ethical obligations. For example, social media may pose challenges to confidentiality, privacy, and traditional boundaries if not implemented appropriately. Additionally, technological advances may exacerbate economic disparities and the ability to meet the rehabilitation needs of all patients in an equitable manner. For example, hearing equipment, wheelchairs, and software applications to support independent living may be available only to those with financial means.

A final consideration for rehabilitation is the separation of psychosocial rehabilitation of drug and alcohol addictions as distinct from traditional rehabilitation for those who have had a stroke, TBI, or other injury. Does it really make sense to have one aspect of rehabilitation focus upon the "physical" with traditional rehabilitation programs and drug and alcohol addictions placed in rehabilitation focused upon psychosocial issues when addiction is a function of the brain?

Learning Point 11.13   Recall the pervious discussion of neuroethics. How might neuroethics figure into decisions for a patient who is addicted to opioids?

It is not possible to anticipate the myriad of ethical issues confronting rehabilitation professionals in the future. The previous section has outlined a few of the major issues that we believe will continue to be relevant and it is not exhaustive. Consistent with the major themes of this text, discussion of topical areas for future ethics does not exhaust future concerns. In the next section, we discuss the importance of "everyday ethics."

Learning Point 11.14   What issues would you add to this list of future issues?

▶ Interprofessional Ethics as "Everyday Ethics"

Rasoal et al. (2016) use the moral case deliberation method to examine difficult situations encountered by healthcare teams. Based on 70 moral deliberations across 10 Swedish healthcare facilities, they found that the team members' concerns were best described as relational ethics rather than principle-based concerns. Three themes emerged from their analysis (Rasoal et al., 2016, p. 825):

- Powerlessness over the team regarding difficult interactions with patients and families.
- Concerns over unsafe or unequal treatment of patients.
- Uncertainty over who should have power to make decisions, the patient, the family, the provider or third-party payors (p. 825)?

Learning Point 11.15   Have you experienced situations that raised these team issues?

The authors described the difficult situations as "everyday ethics," more consistent with relational or virtue ethics rather than principle-based decisions. This illustrates the point that interprofessional teams must attend not only to being prepared for the content of ethically challenging situations (what to do) but the process by which teams address those issues (how to do it). Indeed, the ethical issues were not always clear to the participants in this study and emotion was one of the key issues that the team addressed. In their experience, it was important for team members to critically reflect on the emotions of patients and providers (Molewijk, Kleinlugtenbelt, Pugh, & Widdershoven, 2011). They note that emotions provide an important anchor for understanding context; additionally, it was important for the team to frame appropriate optimal responses in the face of strong emotions.

> **Learning Point 11.16** Can you think of an ethical situation where emotion was an important issue for you or others? How did you address emotion in that situation?

▶ Summary and Conclusion

The current emphasis on reimbursement and productivity in the healthcare system may overshadow ethical issues within healthcare organizations. Some providers fail to take note of ethical issues; others may be afraid to speak out regarding ethical concerns. Rehabilitation professionals and other healthcare providers must find ways to create "moral space" within the organization for moral dialogue; at the same time, we must find our moral voice. As previously discussed in an earlier chapter, literature about moral case deliberation and similar processes [e.g. ethics grand rounds (Schmitz et al., 2018) and ethics consultation] may provide support to the process of creating an interprofessional moral commons for addressing the moral dimensions of practice. Although the moral deliberation model has been used primarily in Europe, some have successfully adopted ethics grand rounds or similar models within the United States. Ideally, the process for moral deliberation should also involve organizational leadership. Gibson (2012) refers to organizational ethics as "the elephant in the room." Speaking about the Canadian healthcare system, she reminds us that ethics should be an important part of quality in health care:

> First, ethics needs to be acknowledged by health leaders as a constitutive component of good governance and effective leadership. Like quality and patient safety, ethics cannot be treated as an add-on or a "nice to have" investment. Rather, it must be treated as part of an uncompromising commitment to strategic and operational excellence. Second, there remain important knowledge gaps about how organizational ethics is experienced... (Gibson, 2012, p. 38)

Rehabilitation professionals and teams must play a role in the dialogue about ethics and values as a part of healthcare quality. This will require that rehabilitation professionals address the organizational "elephant in the room."

> **Learning Point 11.17** Why does Gibson refer to organizational ethics as the "elephant in the room"?

Writing about the potential consequences of healthcare reform in 1994, Ruth Purtilo (1994) addressed the role of the interdisciplinary team. Noting that the concept of the healthcare team was itself a relatively recent development, Purtilo distinguished two important functions of the interprofessional team: the instrumental and moral functions. The moral function of the team addresses the good of the "whole patient." This focus on respect for the whole person contrasts with the instrumental function of the team which focuses more on technical goals. As Purtilo indicates, most teams have elements of both instrumental and moral functions.

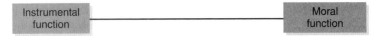

FIGURE 11.1 Instrumental and moral functions of the team.
Based on Purtilo (1994).

Learning Point 11.18   Think of teams that you have been a part of. Use **FIGURE 11.1** to indicate whether the team was more instrumental or moral in function.

For example, a team's goal may be, as Purtilo points out, cardiac catheterization. Purtilo mused that healthcare reform might advantage the instrumental aspects of team function at the expense of the moral functions of teams, especially as a result of evaluating cost and outcomes data. This will also have repercussions for who will remain on the interprofessional team, with the unfortunate result that the team may not be able to address the needs of the whole patient. Purtilo's forecast was amazingly prescient, as many of her concerns have been borne out in changes in the healthcare system and evidence-based practice, even without the implementation of proposed healthcare reforms of 1994. Purtilo's concerns point to the on-going need for rehabilitation professionals to focus on collective team moral agency, development of the moral commons, and attention to organizational and system forces that are shaping healthcare outcomes and the very nature of interprofessional teams. The goal of this text has been to provide tools for individual and collective moral agency for interprofessional rehabilitation practice. Our hope is that these tools will help the reader create a shared moral commons, engage in team moral agency, and maintain the moral functions of teams in the future.

Closing Reflections

Learning Activities

11.1   Think about what it would require for you to create a moral commons for discussion of difficult issues. Share this with your partner and learn what they would need. Determine if you are different and why.

11.2   Think back on examples of practice that you have observed or in which you have participated. Identify whose goal was being met – the client, the family, the therapist, or the payor.

11.3   Compare the moral function of a team versus the instrumental function of a team.

11.4   Consider a clinical context with which you are familiar. What opportunities exist in that setting to develop the moral commons? Could moral case deliberation or ethics ground rounds facilitate this process?

 ## Take Away Messages

- Rehabilitation is a relatively young field and has changed significantly since its birth.

- Some ethical issues in rehabilitation (such as goal-setting and shared decision making) will continue to be relevant in the future; however, many other ethical issues will depend on changes in the larger healthcare system.
- In additional to topical ethical issues, everyday ethics, relational ethics, and organizational ethics will continue to be a major focus for interprofessional rehabilitation teams.
- Development of the moral commons as part of the Dialogic Engagement Model of Ethical Decision Making can support the moral function of the team.
- Rehabilitation professions have undergone tremendous growth and change over the last 60 years. The number of rehabilitation professions, practitioners, and educational programs has grown enormously. Likewise, the work of rehabilitation professionals have gained more autonomy in scope of practice.
- The growth in rehabilitation is driven in part by the increasing number of people with disabilities and chronic conditions. Changes in professional identity and in healthcare delivery shape the ethical situations that occur and our responsibility as professionals for those situations.
- Rehabilitation professionals and all healthcare providers experience organizational and reimbursement constraints based on their decisions. Organizational pressure for productivity and efficiency will undoubtedly continue to be a part of ethical issues in rehabilitation. Rehabilitation professionals must have the economic, organizational, and policy skills to navigate a fragmented and complex healthcare system.
- A major theme of this text is that the ethical approaches of the past (such as principlism and rule-based approaches) may be inadequate against the current challenges of the organizational and interprofessional environment.
- Some ethical topics that may continue to be important to interprofessional rehabilitation ethics in the future are goal-setting, EBP, rehabilitation research, models of informed consent, and shared decision making relevant to rehabilitation, the role of technology, and integration of psychosocial aspects of addiction and substance abuse into rehabilitation.
- Rehabilitation professionals must be attentive to "everyday ethics" that involve relationships, difficult interactions with patients, uncertainty, team dynamics, and a sense of powerlessness. Emotion is a key anchor for navigating context in everyday ethics.

References

American Occupational Therapy Association. (2018). *Academic programs annual data report academic year 2017–2018.* Bethesda, MD: Author.

Babbage, D. R. (2014). Editorial: Open and abundant data is the future of rehabilitation and research. *Archives of Physical Medicine and Rehabilitation, 95,* 795–798.

Brighton, L. J., Pask, S., Benalia, H., Bailey, S., Sumerfield, M., Witt, J., & Evans, C. J. (2018). Taking patient and public involvement online: Qualitative evaluation of an online forum for palliative care and rehabilitation research. *Research Involvement and Engagement, 4,* 14. doi:10.1186/s40900-018-0097-z

Commission on Accreditation in Physical Therapy Education. (n.d.). *Welcome to CAPTE.* Retrieved from http://www.capteonline.org/home.aspx

Delany, C., & Galvin, J. (2014). Ethics and shared decision-making in paediatric occupational therapy practice. *Developmental Neurorehabilitation, 17*(5), 347–354. doi:10.3109/17518423.2013.784816

Delany, C. M. (2007). In private practice, informed consent is interpreted as providing explanations rather than offering choices: a qualitative study. *Australian Journal of Physiotherapy, 53*(3), 171–177. https://doi.org/10.1016/S0004-9514(07)70024-7

Ewashen, C., McInnis-Perry, G., & Murphy, N. (2013). Interprofessional collaboration-in-practice: the contested place of ethics. *Nursing Ethics, 20*(3), 325–335. doi:10.1177/0969733012462048

Fu, J. B., & Morishita, S. (2017). The future of rehabilitation in oncology. *Future Oncology.* https://doi.org/10.2217/fon-2016-0540

Gibson, J. L. (2012). Organizational ethics: No longer the elephant in the room. *Healthcare Management Forum, 25*(1), 37–39. doi:10.1016/j.hcmf.2012.01.003

Gilligan, C. (1982). *In a different voice: Psychological theory and women's development.* Cambridge, MA: Harvard University Press.

Greenwood, R. (2001). Editorial: The future of rehabilitation: Lies in retaining, replacement and regrowth. *British Journal of Medicine, 323*(7321), 1082–1083.

Kaizer, F., Spiridigliozzi, A. M., & Hunt, M. R. (2012). Promoting shared decision-making in rehabilitation: Development of a framework for situations when patients with dysphagia refuse diet modification recommended by the treating team. *Dysphagia, 27*(1), 81–87. doi:10.1007/s00455-011-9341-5

Korner, M., Ehrhardt, H., & Steger, A. K. (2013). Designing an interprofessional training program for shared decision making. *Journal of Interprofessional Care, 27*(2), 146–154. doi:10.3109/13561820.2012.711786

Kuhn, Thomas S. (1970). *The structure of scientific revolutions* (2nd ed., enlarged). Chicago, IL: University of Chicago Press.

Levack, W., & Dean, S. G. (2012). Processes in rehabilitation. In S. G. Dean, R. J. Siegert, W. J. Taylor (Eds.), *Interprofessional rehabilitation* (pp. 79–107). West Sussex, UK: John Wiley & Sons, Ltd.

Levack, W. M., Dean, S. G., Siegert, R. J., & McPherson, K. M. (2006). Purposes and mechanisms of goal planning in rehabilitation: The need for a critical distinction. *Disability and Rehabilitation, 28*(12), 741–749. https://doi/10.1080/09638280500265961

Levack, W. M. M. (2009). Ethics in goal planning for rehabilitation: A utilitarian perspective. *Clinical Rehabilitation, 23*(4), 345–351. doi:10.1177/0269215509103286

Levack, W. M. M., Dean, S. G., Siegert, R. J., & McPherson, K. M. (2011). Navigating patient-centered goal setting in inpatient stroke rehabilitation: How clinicians control the process to meet perceived professional responsibilities. *Patient Education and Counseling, 85*(2), 206–213. https://doi.org/10.1016/j.pec.2011.01.011

Molewijk, B., Kleinlugtenbelt, D., Pugh, S. M., & Widdershoven, G. (2011). Emotions and clinical ethics support. A moral inquiry into emotions in moral case deliberation. *HEC Forum, 23*(4), 257–268. doi:10.1007/s10730-011-9162-9

Purtilo, R. B. (1994). Interdisciplinary health care teams and health care reform. *Journal of Law and Medical Ethics, 22*(2), 121–126.

Rasoal, D., K., Annica, J., I., & Svantesson, M. (2016). What healthcare teams find ethically difficult: Captured in 70 moral case deliberations. *Nursing Ethics, 23*(8), 825–837. doi:10.1177/0969733015583928

Rose, A., Rosewilliam, S., & Soundy, A. (2017). Shared decision making within goal setting in rehabilitation settings: A systematic review. *Patient Education and Counseling, 100*(1), 65–75. https://doi.org/10.1016/j.pec.2016.07.030

Schmitt, M., & Stewart, A. (2011). Commentary on 'Interprofessional Ethics: A Developing Field?'—A response to Banks et al. (2010). *Ethics and Social Welfare, 5*(1), 72–78. doi:10.1080/17496535.2011.546181

Schmitz, D., Gross, D., Frierson, C., Schubert, G. A., Schulze-Steinen, H., & Kersten, A. (2018). Ethics rounds: Affecting ethics quality at all organisational levels. *Journal of Medical Ethics, 44*, 805–809. doi:10.1136/medethics-2018-104831

U.S. Department of Health and Human Services. (2016). National Institutes of Health research plan on rehabilitation: Moving the field forward. Retrieved from https://www.nichd.nih.gov/sites/default/files/publications/pubs/Documents/NIH_ResearchPlan_Rehabilitation.pdf

van der Dam, S., Schols, J. M., Kardol, T. J., Molewijk, B. C., Widdershoven, G. A., & Abma, T. A. (2013). The discovery of deliberation. From ambiguity to appreciation through the learning process of doing Moral Case Deliberation in Dutch elderly care. *Social Science Medicine, 83*, 125–132. doi:10.1016/j.socscimed.2013.01.024

Watkins, A. L. (1952). Current trends in physical medicine and rehabilitation. *The New England Journal of Medicine, 24*, 91–97.

Glossary

Accountable Care Organization (ACO): A shared savings arrangement where groups of providers agree to coordinate care and be held accountable for the quality and cost of their services.

Active Engagement Model: Model of applied ethics proposed by Delany, Edwards, Jensen, and Skinner (2010) that delineates three components or steps to active engagement: active listening, reflexive thinking, and critical reasoning. The active engagement model emphasizes connectedness and moral agency.

Acute Care: The health system or delivery platform used to treat sudden, unexpected, urgent, or emergent episodes of injury and illness that can lead to death or disability without rapid intervention.

Autonomy: The ethical principle obligating healthcare professionals to respect a patient's right to self-determination in health care. The ethical right to autonomy allows an individual to make choices and decisions about health care, and to have those choices honored and respected by others.

Axiology: Axiology is concerned with classifying what things are good, and what makes them good. For instance, a traditional question of axiology concerns whether subjective feelings have value.

Beneficence: The ethical principle obligating healthcare professionals to promote the good for the patient.

Best Interest Standard for Decision Making: A standard for decision making that may be used by surrogates when the preferences of that individual are unknown.

Blanket Consent: An all-encompassing consent that authorizes health care in a general way. For example: "I authorize so and so to carry out any test/procedure/surgery in the course of my treatment." This general consent may not be adequate to constitute full informed consent for specific interventions.

Bundled Payment Methods: Flat-rate payment that includes all physician fees along with all costs of any related treatments, complications, or hospital readmissions within 90 days of the original operation (James & Poulsen, 2016).

Bundled Payment: The reimbursement of healthcare providers, such as hospitals and physicians, by the aggregated expected costs for clinically defined episodes of care.

Capacity: The ability to make an informed decision. Capacity is linked to informed consent. According to Applebaum (2007), capacity includes the ability to communicate choices; the ability to understand information necessary for the specific decision at hand; the ability to appreciate the implications and significance of the information provided or the choice being made; and the ability to reason by weighing and comparing options and consequences of the potential decision.

Capitation: An insurance approach where "providers receive a fixed per person (or 'capitated') payment that covers all healthcare services over a defined time period, adjusted for each patient's expected needs, and where providers are also held accountable for high-quality outcomes" (James & Poulsen, p. 104).

Co-insurance: What the patient pays as his or her portion of the healthcare insurance claim.

Collectivism: Cultural term characteristic of cohesiveness among individuals and of placing the group over the individual. Members of collectivist cultures tend to value what supports the group over what supports the individual.

Community of Practice: In health care, this refers to a group of people who work alongside each other and share common professional interests and goals. For example, in pediatric rehabilitation practice, there may be many practitioners who bring different practice paradigms, but who share a common interest in order to provide a benefit to a child both within and, separate from, the family unit.

Competence: The ability of an individual to consent to or refuse treatment. Competence to make a medical decision must be legally determined. All adult persons are judged competent until legally judged otherwise. Patients who are deemed never competent include newborns, small children, and individuals who have been severely cognitively impaired since birth (Doherty & Purtilo, 2016, pps. 268, 269).

Conflict of Interest: Potentially occurs when the rehabilitation professional has competing allegiances among the interests of the patient and the family, the third-party payor, other rehabilitation team members, and the employing healthcare organization (Larkin & Lowenstein, 2017). A conflict of interest occurs in health care when a healthcare professional is unable to, or fails to, fulfill professional obligations due to competing interests. The highest ethical standard for professionals obligates them to avoid the appearance of any conflict of interest.

Co-payment: A small fixed fee to access the covered service, such as an office visit.

Culture: A socially constructed set of beliefs and values through which we view the world, ourselves, other professions, and our patients.

Decisional Capacity: Decision-making capacity includes the ability to make a choice, understand relevant information, appreciate the situation and its consequences, and process information (Menikoff 2001, p. 280).

Dialogic Ethics: Dialogic ethics emphasizes that ethics requires interactive dialogue or a "dialectical process" that resembles an interactive conversation (Abma, Molewijk, & Widdershoven, 2009). This dialogue takes place on multiple levels with regard to the self, other people, theory and practice, competing principles or values, and the perspectives of various stakeholders. It involves listening, reflexivity, and reciprocity.

Disability: An impairment, functional limitation, activity limitation, or participation restriction resulting from a negative interaction between the individual and context (environment and personal factors) (Based on the ICF). Note that older ideas about disability defined disability in terms of effects of disease on social role or task.

Distributive Justice: The fair allocation of goods in a society that represents a public policy focus on equality (Craig, 2010).

Documented Consent: Consent that is documented in the healthcare record either as recorded in the record as having occurred (example: "the patient agreed to these goals") or as a formal written consent document (Hall, Prochazka, & Fink, 2012).

Ends-Based Ethical Tradition: Ethical tradition that resolves ethical situations based on the ends, consequences, or outcomes. Utilitarianism is the classical historical example of ends-based thinking and it posits that we should seek the "greatest good for the greatest number of people."

Epistemology: Attempts to answer the question "what are the sources and necessary and sufficient conditions of knowing something?" These are possible justifications of our beliefs, and epistemology addresses issues such as whether these justifications must be internal or external to one's knowing.

Ethical or Moral Distress: An ethical situation where one knows the right thing to do but is unable to do it because of the lack of power or authority to do so.

Ethical or Moral Reasoning or Judgment: The dimension of moral agency that refers to making a decision about the "right" thing to do.

Ethical or Moral Sensitivity: The dimension of moral agency that involves recognition and interpretation of the situation.

Ethical or Moral Silence: Situation characterized by silence and lack of moral discourse when confronting an obvious ethical problem or issue.

Ethical or Moral Temptation: Situation where one is faced with a right versus wrong situation and is tempted to choose to do the wrong thing based on self-interest.

Ethical Pluralism: The idea that ethical truth is not a single unitary proposition, and that there are multiple perspectives on moral truth, all of which capture part of the truth, and none of which embrace the entire truth (Hinman, 2013, pp. 45, 364). Ethical pluralism is not synonymous with normative ethical relativism.

Ethical Principle: A normative concept that provides guidance for ethical conduct that is more general than a rule. Examples of ethical principles include the four-principles (autonomy, beneficence, non-maleficence, and justice), as well as informed consent, confidentiality, conflict of interest, and many others. The principles approach was popularized by Beauchamp and Childress (2009).

Ethical Reciprocity: Ethical reciprocity is the process of putting oneself in someone else's shoes. It extends the idea of treating others as one would like to be treated. Ethical reciprocity is one part of dialogic ethics.

Ethical Relativism: In contrast to absolutism, ethical relativism proposes that ethical values may vary across different cultures (descriptive relativism) and that these values are "right" within those cultures (normative relativism) (Hinman, 2013, p. 32).

Ethical Situation: A classification of different ethical contexts that may suggest a specific response. Situation types include ethical ambiguity/uncertainty, ethical issue or problem, ethical dilemma, moral distress, moral temptation, and ethical silence. Classifying an ethical issue into known types may provide insight into a correct response. For example, moral temptation should typically be resisted.

Ethical Theory: A comprehensive approach to ethics that provides a conceptual foundation delineating the fundamental nature of ethics and morality, how the component parts are inter-related, and how these relate to moral behavior. Examples of ethical theories include deontology, utilitarianism, virtue ethics, pragmatism, and cognitive moral development. While the majority of ethical theories are grounded in philosophy, the cognitive developmental theory is grounded in psychology. Most ethical decision making uses intermediate ethical concepts rather than fully developed ethical theory.

Ethical Tradition: An ethical perspective and related language that has developed over history with a specific focus on ethical analysis without consideration of its general theoretical adequacy. Kidder identified three major ethical traditions: rule-based, ends-based, and care-based. In this text, we refer to four ethical traditions: rule-based, ends-based, virtue-based, and narrative-based. Referring to "ethical traditions" creates common moral ground by grouping ethical theories and perspectives-based major emphases.

Ethics Grand Rounds: An approach to ethical reflection whereby interprofessional or professional team members meet to discuss a patient case involving ethics, often a case involving an ethical dilemma. This process may be facilitated by an ethics expert.

Ethics: Rational and systematic reflection on matters of morality, right, wrong, and the good.

Everyday Ethics: The ethics of day-to-day practice that includes issues of relationships, organizational policies, team dynamics, turf wars, power, hierarchy, and other daily events. Everyday ethics stands in contrast to some preconceptions of ethics as classic ethical dilemmas addressing "life and death" situations.

Evidence-Based Practice: In the simplest terms, evidence is something knowable like an outward sign that provides proof of something. Evidence-based practice in health care, then, entails making healthcare decisions based on intentional and judicious use of current evidence, individual clinical expertise, and patient values.

Explicit Consent: Consent process where the patient indicates definitive consent to a treatment either verbally or in writing (Satyanarayana Rao, 2008).

Fairness: The equity of health care.

Fee-for-Service or Volume-Based Reimbursement: Reimbursement that occurs when "…a provider supplies an approved billing code for (and may be required to justify) each unit of care consumed during a hospitalization, same-day procedure, or outpatient visit" (James & Poulsen, 2016, p. 105).

Fee-for-Service (FFS): A payment model where a doctor or other healthcare provider is paid a fee for each particular service rendered.

First Order Ethics: Ethical decisions based on the ethical values and principles learned through the primary cultural and social experiences of one's origin (See also morality) (Hinman, 2013).

Freedom: Non-interference from government to make life choices and to assume responsibility for the consequences of those choices (Gains, 2017).

Groupthink: Dysfunctional group dynamic identified by Janis (1972) where group members may ignore rational strategies in order to promote group harmony or avoid conflict.

Guardian: A person, generally appointed by a judge, who is responsible for making decisions for a person who is incapacitated.

Habilitation: The process of seeking maximal functional attainment.

Hospital Value Based Purchasing (HVP): A Centers for Medicare & Medicaid Services (CMS) initiative that rewards acute-care hospitals with incentive payments for the quality of care they provide to Medicare beneficiaries.

Implicit Consent: Process where consent is inferred or implied by the patient either through body language or silent assent (Carlisle, 2002).

Individualism: Cultural term characteristic of emphasizing competition and personal achievement. Members of individualist cultures tend to value what supports the individual over what supports the group.

Informed Consent: The right of the patient to make voluntary decisions about health care based on relevant information. The basic elements of informed consent include disclosure, delineation of the benefits and burdens of a proposed intervention, cognition (understanding), recommended alternative treatments, and questions and clarifications. In rehabilitation, informed consent is a process of interactive conversations and shared decision making between healthcare professionals and the patient and/or the patient's family (Caplan, Callahan, & Haas, 1987).

Interfield Theory: Theory that bridges two distinct fields or areas.

International Classification of Health, Disability, and Functioning (ICF): A conceptual model developed by the World Health Organization (WHO) that delineates how health, disability, environment, personal factors, and function are interrelated. The ICF also provides a taxonomy for standard evaluation and outcomes measures by developing shared language, terminology, and classification systems.

Interprofessional Collaborative Practice: "Collaborative practice occurs when multiple health workers from different professional backgrounds provide comprehensive services by working with patients, their families, care givers and communities to deliver the highest quality of care across settings" (WHO, 2010, p. 13).

Interprofessional Education: "When students from two or more professions learn about, from and with each other in order to enable effective collaboration and improve health outcomes" (WHO, 2010, p. 13.).

Interprofessional Ethics: Rational and systematic reflection on matters of morality, right, wrong, and the good encountered by healthcare professionals deliberatively working together in order to meet the goals of interprofessional collaborative practice. Interprofessional ethics should be patient/family centered, relationship focused, relevant across professions, and framed in language that is common to, and meaningful across professions (Interprofessional Education Collaboratve Expert Panel, 2011). Interprofessional ethics may refer to the process of ethical collaboration or to the emerging field of study that focuses on ethical issues in interprofessional collaborative practice.

Interprofessional Rehabilitation Ethics: Rational and systematic reflection on matters of morality, right, wrong, and the good encountered by the rehabilitation team with emphasis on interprofessional collaboration and the work of the interprofessional team.

Justice: The ethical principle obligating healthcare professionals to fairness in fulfilling their professional roles.

Macroallocation: The allocation of healthcare resources that involves distributing health-related materials and services among various uses and people through public health policies.

Medical Necessity: An insurance term defining criteria for payment decisions based on the diagnosis, the evidence supporting the interventions, and the use of rehabilitation devices for non-medical purposes (Stinneford & Kirschner, 2004).

Methodology: Is concerned with identifying the best approaches, such as systematic observation and experimentation, inductive and deductive reasoning, and the formation and testing of hypotheses and theories, to best gain knowledge or understanding.

Microallocation: The allocation of healthcare resources concerned with selecting which individuals are to receive scarce or insufficient healthcare resources.

Models of Disability: Conceptual model of the relationship between the individual person; illness, pathology, disease; impairment, functional limitation, activity limitation, or participation restriction and the environment.

Moral Agency: The capacity to act in an ethical manner. Individuals, teams, and organizations can exercise moral agency.

Moral Authority: Refers to the scope of authority a person has to make moral decisions on behalf of, and in the interests of, themselves or another. In the pediatric context, parents have moral authority to make decisions on behalf of their child. However, this authority does not extend to causing harm to their child.

Moral Case Deliberation: A structured model for ethical reflection developed in Europe that brings together members of the healthcare team in order to engage in a reflective and dialogic process with the goal of improving the quality of care (van der Dam et al., 2013, p. 126). Moral case deliberation (MCD) differs from previous ethics approaches in its focus on the collective rather than the individual, everyday ethics versus topical cases, and on reflective dialogue versus decision making. MCD typically uses a facilitator to assist with the dialogic process.

Moral Commons: A safe zone for ethical deliberation characterized by mutual respect for personal and professional identity, common language, inclusion of relevant stakeholders, and the dialogic process. The three key elements of the moral commons are identity (personal and professional), ethical traditions, and context.

Moral Deliberation: This refers to the dialogic process outlined, in part, in this text. It refers to deliberating about decisions of a moral nature through meaningful conversation, deliberation, and dialogue. In contrast to a traditional case discussion's focus on determining what to do, moral deliberation emphasizes facilitation of multiple perspectives. Moral deliberation views process and outcome as inseparably linked. Moral deliberation about patient care should include patient or family stakeholders (Abma et al., 2009, p. 223). In the pediatric rehabilitation context, it includes consideration of the interests of the child, the child's family, and the interprofessional team.

Moral Indeterminacy: Imprecise or uncertain outcome of moral discussion resulting from respect for diverse ethical, cultural, or personal values of perspectives of the participants. Given that there is no unitary or single ethical truth, analysis of ethical dilemmas or problems does not always produce a single best answer or course of action. Rather, moral indeterminacy refers to the multiple paths that may be a "right" course of action in response to an ethical situation. Moral indeterminacy may be a barrier for interprofessional ethics because the lack of one definitive "right" resolution may discourage professionals from persevering to determine the best course of action through moral dialogue.

Morality: Personal and social beliefs, customs, values, and behavioral conventions regarding right, wrong, and the good that are learned through enculturation and social institutions that are often taken for granted and not subjected to reflection or analysis. Some refer to morality as first order ethics because the beliefs about right and wrong are taken for granted and not subjected to critical analysis.

Narrative-Based Ethical Tradition: Ethical tradition that resolves ethical situations by listening to the experiences, voices, and perspectives of the participants and stakeholders. Responds to the criticism that healthcare ethics has been inattentive to patients' experiences.

Neuroethics: The ethics of doing neuroscience pertaining to the ethical considerations of neuroscience research and related translational research (Roskies, 2002; Shrivastava & Behari, 2015). Alternatively, the neuroscience of ethics, pertaining to how we understand moral behavior related to our comprehension of the brain (Roskies, 2002; Shrivastava & Behari, 2015).

Non-maleficence: The ethical principle obligating healthcare professionals to prevent harm to the patient.

Normative: Refers to considerations as to what one ought to do, typically grounded in consideration of duties and obligations. Normative ethics are a significant part of professional ethics. Normative ethics is often contrasted to descriptive ethics.

Ontology: Is on one hand, the study of what there is or what exists. On the other hand, it is the study of the general features and relations of those things that do exist.

Organizational Culture: The implicit and explicit values, culture, rituals, customs, or ways of behaving within an organization that are often "taken for granted."

Organizational Ethics: Ethical issues that arise as a result of organizational structures, leadership, management, stakeholders, and processes (Gibson, 2012). Also includes the goals, values, outcomes, and obligations of the organization. Gibson notes that an important consideration for organizational ethics in health care is balancing competing organizational goals of quality and financial well-being (Gibson, 2012, p. 37). An important characteristic of organizational ethics is its focus on collective entities, processes, and structures.

Paradigm: A systematic mental model that provides theoretical foundations for viewing a discipline or worldview. A paradigm suggests questions and issues to explore and resolve, and may become obsolete, necessitating a "paradigm shift" (Kuhn, 1970). The shift from Newtonian physics to the physics of relativity is an example of a paradigm shift.

Paternalism: Healthcare decision process that is driven or determined by the healthcare provider with minimal or no patient participation. It refers to a course of action (including decisions) for the assumed interest of the person, but without or against that person's informed consent (Sjostrand,

Eriksson, Juth, & Helgesson, 2013). Some contrast weak paternalism (healthcare provider making decisions to protect from harm) with strong paternalism (decisions made by the provider to promote the best interests of the patient as perceived by the provider).

Pay for Performance or Value-Based Purchasing: Healthcare payment approach designed to increase value through rewarding the performance of the provider with contingent incentives that heighten motivation to improve quality and increase the effort to reduce waste and to cut costs (Siriwardena, 2014).

Pay-for-Performance: A payment model that rewards physicians, hospitals, medical groups, and other healthcare providers for meeting specific performance measures for quality and efficiency. It penalizes caregivers for poor outcomes, medical errors, or increased costs.

Per Case Method of Payment: Diagnostic categories based on the patient's primary disease, specific treatment, secondary chronic conditions, and care intensity to determine a flat rate for a single case (James & Poulsen, 2016).

Polarized Discussion: Discussion characterized by participants asserting conflicting positions without willingness to listen or respond to the ideas or values of other participants and without the goal of reaching consensus.

Principle: Ethical principles are general normative standards or guidelines for ethical behavior. Beauchamp and Childress (2009) identified four major categories of ethical principles: respect for autonomy, beneficence, non-maleficence, and justice. Principles are less comprehensive than ethical theories and more specific than rules. Principles may conflict, requiring ethical analysis to resolve which principle may be more important in a situation.

Professional Ethics: Analysis of the ethical duties, obligations, virtues, and values for a specific profession.

Professional Identity: An internal sense of the professional self that evolves and matures over time and provides a basis for clinical and moral action.

Quadrant Approach: Ethical decision making approach developed first by Jonsen, Siegler, and Winslade (2006) and widely used in medicine. This approach analyzes ethical issues with four primary concerns: medical indications, patient preferences, quality of life, and contextual fairness.

Rationing: Healthcare rationing is limiting healthcare goods and services to those who can afford to pay.

Realms of Ethical Action: Distinguishes different ethical concerns based on whether the ethical situation is interpersonal (individual realm), within an organization or institution (organizational/institutional realm), or at the level of society as a whole (societal realm) (Glaser, 1994).

Reflexivity: A concept taken from qualitative research that involves self-reflection on one's beliefs, values, emotions, preconceptions, and social role assuming that cognitive reflection promotes the ability to "bracket" or set personal subjective experiences aside (Cutcliffe, 2003, p. 137). Reflexivity should examine hidden values, assumptions and aspects of everyday life that are so ingrained in life that they are "taken for granted."

Rehabilitation: The process of restoring function or seeking maximal functional ability (see habilitation) traditionally promoted by occupational therapists, physical therapists and speech & language pathologists. The contemporary rehabilitation team embraces members of any profession or discipline pursuing the goals of attaining functional ability.

Rehabilitation Ethics: Rational and systematic reflection on matters of morality, right, wrong, and the good encountered by the rehabilitation team or in the process of restoring function.

Relational Autonomy: The ability of healthcare professionals, family members, and friends to support an individual to make choices consistent with that person's sense of what is important to him or her and what makes sense for his or her life. Guided by the principle of beneficence, healthcare professionals and family should seek to promote the well-being of the individual, and endeavor to minimize the likelihood of harm (Kaizer, Spiridigliozzi, & Hunt, 2012).

Relational Ethics: Relational ethics grew out of the work of Carol Gilligan (1993) whose research indicated that women approached ethical decisions from the perspective of care and relationships versus abstract principles. The resulting "ethics of care" perspective has been associated with narrative and "voice." Ewashen et al. (2013, p. 327) describe four themes of relational ethics: relational engagement and connectedness, mutual respect, embodiment, and environment.

Resource Allocation: The distribution of resources, usually financial, among competing groups of people or programs.

Rights: An entitlement to possess something or behave in a particular manner. Duties are often viewed as corollaries of rights. If one has a fundamental human right to free speech, for example, society has an obligation to enable free speech.

Rule-Based Ethical Tradition: Ethical tradition that resolves ethical situations using duties, obligations, principles, and rules. Professional codes of ethics typically rely heavily on the rule-based tradition. Medical ethics has been criticized for its over-use of rule-based thinking grounded in ethical principles.

Shared Decision Making: Shared decision making involves an exchange of ideas between patient/family and the healthcare professional in the decision itself. Shared decision making occurs when real choice exists and the healthcare professional involves the patient in the decision (Whitney, McGuire, & McCullough, 2004).

Substituted Judgment Standard for Decision Making: Decision making that is based on what the person would have decided, if competent to do so.

Substituted Judgment: An appointed surrogate makes a statement that reflects what the surrogate believed the patient would have wanted when he or she was competent (Doherty & Purtilo, 2016, p. 269). In a case of substituted judgment the patient does not have an advanced directive or living will.

Surrogate Decision Maker: A person authorized to participate in or make decisions on behalf of an incapacitated individual.

Surrogate or Proxy: Consent provided when someone is appointed to consent on behalf of an individual who has been deemed legally incompetent (Doherty & Purtilo, 2016, p. 269).

Team Identity: The collective attitudes and beliefs held by a team regarding ethics, values, teamwork, relationships, power, hierarchy, and clinical roles.

Therapeutic Lying: A response to an individual with an altered sense of reality that involves validating that individual's own reality by acknowledging the truth of that person's experience, and is used with the intent to bring about good and minimize harm.

Topical Approach to Ethics: Approach to identification of ethical issues that categorizes issues based on topics (for example, end of life, confidentiality).

Utilitarianism: "[M]aximizing the benefits of rehabilitation to the whole community served when negotiating goals with individual patients" (Levack, 2009, p. 345).

Value: Values represent those commitments, qualities, and behaviors that are viewed as morally good and take priority over other commitments, qualities, or behaviors. Many professions have identified core values of professionalism.

Verbal Consent: A verbal consent occurs if and when a patient states his or her consent to a procedure verbally but does not sign any written form. Verbal consent may be adequate for routine treatment (Kakar, Gambhir, Singh, Kaur, & Nanda, 2014).

Virtue-Based Ethical Tradition: Ethical tradition that focuses on the cultivation of personal character, quality, or ethical virtues.

Virtue: A trait, characteristic, or quality that is desirable or good. Virtue ethics emphasizes the cultivation of virtues (for example, honesty, compassion, fairness).

Ways of Knowing: Acknowledges that there are many knowledge-based disciplines, such as mathematics, human science, history, and ethics, and within each one there are different "ways of knowing" which include, but are not limited to, emotion, faith, memory, reason, and what is perceived through our senses.

Index